Health Communication

Strategies and Skills for a New Era

Claudia F. Parvanta, PhD

Professor
Director, Florida Prevention Research Center
College of Public Health
University of South Florida
Tampa, Florida

Sarah Bauerle Bass, PhD, MPH

Associate Professor
Director, Risk Communication Laboratory
Department of Social and Behavioral Sciences
College of Public Health
Temple University
Philadelphia, Pennsylvania

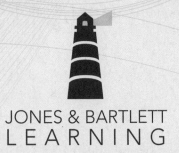

JONES & BARTLETT
LEARNING

World Headquarters
Jones & Bartlett Learning
5 Wall Street
Burlington, MA 01803
978-443-5000
info@jblearning.com
www.jblearning.com

Jones & Bartlett Learning books and products are available through most bookstores and online booksellers. To contact Jones & Bartlett Learning directly, call 800-832-0034, fax 978-443-8000, or visit our website, www.jblearning.com.

Substantial discounts on bulk quantities of Jones & Bartlett Learning publications are available to corporations, professional associations, and other qualified organizations. For details and specific discount information, contact the special sales department at Jones & Bartlett Learning via the above contact information or send an email to specialsales@jblearning.com.

Copyright © 2020 by Jones & Bartlett Learning, LLC, an Ascend Learning Company

All rights reserved. No part of the material protected by this copyright may be reproduced or utilized in any form, electronic or mechanical, including photocopying, recording, or by any information storage and retrieval system, without written permission from the copyright owner.

The content, statements, views, and opinions herein are the sole expression of the respective authors and not that of Jones & Bartlett Learning, LLC. Reference herein to any specific commercial product, process, or service by trade name, trademark, manufacturer, or otherwise does not constitute or imply its endorsement or recommendation by Jones & Bartlett Learning, LLC and such reference shall not be used for advertising or product endorsement purposes. All trademarks displayed are the trademarks of the parties noted herein. *Health Communication: Strategies and Skills for a New Era* is an independent publication and has not been authorized, sponsored, or otherwise approved by the owners of the trademarks or service marks referenced in this product.

There may be images in this book that feature models; these models do not necessarily endorse, represent, or participate in the activities represented in the images. Any screenshots in this product are for educational and instructive purposes only. Any individuals and scenarios featured in the case studies throughout this product may be real or fictitious, but are used for instructional purposes only.

13500-8

Production Credits
VP, Product Management: David D. Cella
Director of Product Management: Michael Brown
Product Specialist: Carter McAlister
Production Editor: Vanessa Richards
Senior Marketing Manager: Sophie Fleck Teague
Manufacturing and Inventory Control Supervisor: Amy Bacus
Composition: codeMantra U.S. LLC

Cover Design: Scott Moden
Rights & Media Specialist: Merideth Tumasz
Media Development Editor: Shannon Sheehan
Cover Image (Title Page, Chapter Opener):
  © Galkin Grigory/Shutterstock
Printing and Binding: LSC Communications
Cover Printing: LSC Communications

Library of Congress Cataloging-in-Publication Data
Names: Parvanta, Claudia F., author. | Bass, Sarah Bauerle, author.
Title: Health communication: strategies and skills for a new era / Claudia Parvanta, Sarah Bauerle Bass.
Description: Burlington, Massachusetts: Jones & Bartlett Learning, [2020] | Includes bibliographical references and index.
Identifiers: LCCN 2018009707 | ISBN 9781284065879 (pbk.)
Subjects: | MESH: Health Communication | Health Education
Classification: LCC RA423.2 | NLM WA 590 | DDC 362.101/4—dc23
LC record available at https://lccn.loc.gov/2018009707

6048

Printed in the United States of America
22 21 20 19 18   10 9 8 7 6 5 4 3 2 1

To our families, who love us unconditionally.

Contents

Contributors

The authors of chapters not written solely by the lead authors are listed below in alphabetical order.

Linda Fleisher, PhD, MPH, is a Senior Scientist at the Research Institute at the Children's Hospital of Philadelphia. She is also adjunct faculty at Fox Chase Cancer Center and Perelman School of Medicine at University of Pennsylvania in Philadelphia. Dr. Fleisher is co-author of Chapter 6.

Heather Gardiner, PhD, MPH, is Associate Professor and Director of the Health Disparities Laboratory in the Department of Social and Behavioral Sciences at Temple University, College of Public Health. Dr. Gardiner is author of Chapter 9.

Alesha Hruska, MPH, MS, MCHES, is Adjunct Instructor at the University of the Sciences, Department of Behavioral and Social Sciences. Ms. Hruska is co-author of Chapter 11.

Laurie Maurer, PhD, MA, recently completed her doctoral studies at Temple University in the Department of Social and Behavioral Sciences, College of Public Health and was a Research Assistant in the Risk Communication Laboratory. Dr. Maurer is co-author of Chapter 5.

Elisa Beth McNeill, PhD, MS, is Clinical Associate Professor and Coordinator of Health and Physical Education Teacher Certification in the Department of Health and Kinesiology at Texas A&M University. Dr. McNeill is author of Chapter 10.

Jeannine L. Stuart, PhD, is President of AREUFIT Health Services, Inc., in West Chester, Pennsylvania. Dr. Stuart is co-author of Chapter 11.

Case Study Contributors

Authors of case studies that appear in chapter boxes or appendices are listed below in the order in which their case material first appears in the book.

Appendix 3A: Use of Patient Activation Tool (PAT) for Shared Decision Making in Pediatric Appendicitis

Dani O. Gonzalez, MD
Center for Surgical Outcomes Research, The Research Institute, Nationwide Children's Hospital, Columbus, Ohio
Department of Surgery, Icahn School of Medicine at Mount Sinai, New York, New York

Katherine J. Deans, MD, MHSc
Center for Surgical Outcomes Research, The Research Institute, Nationwide Children's Hospital, Columbus, Ohio
Department of Pediatric Surgery, Nationwide Children's Hospital, Columbus, Ohio

Peter C. Minneci, MD, MHSc
Center for Surgical Outcomes, The Research Institute at Nationwide Children's Hospital, Columbus, Ohio

Appendix 5A: Demographic and Behavioral Targeting to Encourage Colonoscopy in Low-Literacy African Americans

Thomas F. Gordon, PhD
Professor, Department of Psychology, University of Massachusetts-Lowell, Lowell, Massachusetts

Box 6-3: Reaching Adolescents for HPV Immunization Using Facebook

Salini Mohanty, DrPH, MPH
University of Pennsylvania, Philadelphia, Pennsylvania

Emily Gibeau, MPH
Pennsylvania Department of Health, Harrisburg, Pennsylvania

Ayla Tolosa-Kline, MPH
Philadelphia Department of Public Health, Philadelphia, Pennsylvania

Caroline Johnson, MD
Philadelphia Department of Public Health, Philadelphia, Pennsylvania

Appendix 6A: Los Angeles County's Sugar Pack Health Marketing Campaign

Noel Barragan, MPH
Chronic Disease and Injury Program, Department of Public Health, Los Angeles County Health Agency, Los Angeles, California

Tony Kuo, MD, MSHS
Chronic Disease and Injury Program, Department of Public Health, Los Angeles County Health Agency, Los Angeles, California

Appendix 6B: Text4baby as a Surveillance/Information Dissemination Tool During Zika Outbreak

Jodie Fishman, MPH, MCHES
Zero to Three, Washington, DC

Appendix 6C: The Use of Virtual Worlds in Health Promotion

Joan E. Cowdery, PhD
Michigan University, Ypsilanti, Michigan

Sun Joo (Grace) Ahn, PhD
Grady College of Journalism & Mass Communication, University of Georgia, Athens, Georgia

Appendix 6D: Health Promotion and Social Change Through Storytelling Across Communication Platforms

Hua Wang, PhD, MA
University of Buffalo, Buffalo, New York

Arvind Singhal, PhD
The University of Texas at El Paso, El Paso, Texas

Appendix 7A: Using PhotoVoice in Formative Research

Rickie Brawer, PhD, MPH
Thomas Jefferson University, Philadelphia, Pennsylvania

Ellen J. Plumb, MD
Thomas Jefferson University, Philadelphia, Pennsylvania

Melissa Fogg, MSW
Mural Arts Philadelphia, Philadelphia, Pennsylvania

Brandon Knettel, PhD, MA
Duke University Global Health Institute, Durham, North Carolina

Margaret Fulda, MSW, LSW, MPH
JFK Behavioral Health Center, Philadelphia, Pennsylvania

Abbie Santana, MSPH
Thomas Jefferson University, Philadelphia, Pennsylvania

Melissa DiCarlo, MPH, MS
Thomas Jefferson University, Philadelphia, Pennsylvania

James Plumb, MD, MPH
Thomas Jefferson University, Philadelphia, Pennsylvania

Appendix 7B: Steps in Tailoring a Text Messaging–Based Smoking Cessation Program for Young Adults: Iterative Intervention Refinement

Michele L. Ybarra, PhD
Center for Innovative Public Health Research, San Clemente, California

Appendix 7C: Better Bites

Brian J. Biroscak, PhD, MPH
Yale University, New Haven, Connecticut

Ashton Potter Wright, DrPH, MPH
City of Lexington, Lexington, Kentucky

Anita Courtney, MS, RD
Lexington Tweens Nutrition and Fitness Coalition, Lexington, Kentucky

Carol A. Bryant, PhD, MS
University of South Florida, Tampa, Florida

Appendix 7D: Social Marketing to Increase Participation in WIC

Tiffany Neal, MPH, MCHES
Thomas Jefferson Health District, Virginia Department of Health, Richmond, Virginia

Appendix 7E: Asthma Self-Management Mobile Application for Adolescents: From Concept Through Product Development to Testing

Tali Schneider, MPH, CHES
Florida Prevention Research Center, University of South Florida, Tampa, Florida

Jim Lindenburger
Center for Social Marketing, University of South Florida, Tampa, Florida

Appendix 8A: The Challenges of Evaluating a Supplemental Nutrition Education Program for Low-Income Families

Kami J. Silk, PhD
Michigan State University, East Lansing, Michigan

Evan K. Perrault, PhD
University of Wisconsin-Eau Claire, Eau Claire, Wisconsin

Caroline J. Hagedorn, MA
Independent Researcher, Washington, DC

Samantha A. Nazione, PhD
Berry College, Mount Berry, Georgia

Lindsay Neuberger, PhD
University of Central Florida, Orlando, Florida

R. Paul McConaughy, MA
Michigan Fitness Foundation, Lansing, Michigan

Khadidiatou Ndiaye, PhD
George Washington University, Washington, DC

Box 9-4: Shared Decision Making: Decision Counseling Program at Thomas Jefferson University

Ronald E. Myers, DSW, PhD
Division of Population Science and Center for Health Decisions, Department of Medical Oncology, Sidney Kimmel Cancer Center, Thomas Jefferson University, Philadelphia, PA

Anett Petrich, RN, MSN
Division of Population Science and Center for Health Decisions, Department of Medical Oncology, Sidney Kimmel Cancer Center, Thomas Jefferson University, Philadelphia, PA

Acknowledgments

As with anything, it truly takes a village, and in this case, it took a village of dedicated and incredible people who helped us make this book happen. Many of the people who helped with ideas or materials for this book are credited where their contributions appear. We thank them for providing cutting-edge thinking as well as examples of health communication in action. Their work represents some of the best of the best, and we truly appreciate being able to showcase it in this textbook.

But we would be remiss to not shout out to those specific people who helped us every step of the way, without whose help this book would never have come to fruition. On the editorial side, Alesha Hruska, MPH, MS, at University of the Sciences and Laurie Maurer, PhD, MA, at Temple University contributed valuable critiques as well as editorial assistance in putting the book together. They also contributed to or co-wrote two chapters. Richard Harner, MD, provided his editorial touch everywhere. The book would simply not be here without their work. Thanks also to Virginia Liddell, BS, Shreya Kandra, MD, MPH, and Vijay Prajapati, BDM, at the University of South Florida, and Jessie Panick, BS, and Mohammed Al Hajji, MPH, at Temple University for their help with everything from editorial assistance to developing ancillary materials and helping us keep track of all the details.

The Jones & Bartlett Learning crew of Mike Brown, Carter McAlister, Vanessa Richards, Merideth Tumasz, Maria Leon Maimone, and Toni Ackley all provided great help and support. We thank Richard Riegleman, who originally came to us with the idea of having a book geared not only to public health students, but also to anyone who could incorporate health communication principles into their studies and work, for his insights and help with the process and conceptualization of the book.

Last but not least, we would like to acknowledge the support of our colleagues at Temple University, the University of the Sciences, and the University of South Florida for their support while we toiled away at getting this book done. And to our families, who endured us talking about, working on, and complaining fiercely about the book, we thank you for your patience and constant support.

—*Claudia F. Parvanta, PhD, and*
Sarah Bauerle Bass, PhD, MPH

About the Authors

Claudia Parvanta, PhD, is a Professor of Community and Family Health, College of Public Health, and Director of the Florida Prevention Research Center at the University of South Florida, Tampa. Her work in Florida focuses on reducing disparities in health through community-based prevention marketing. Between July 2005 and December 2016, she led the Department of Behavioral and Social Sciences at the University of the Sciences in Philadelphia where her research emphasized health literacy and culturally competent health communication. From 2000 to 2005, Dr. Parvanta headed the Division of Health Communication at the Centers for Disease Control and Prevention. She was central to the agency's communication response to the 9/11 attacks, anthrax, and severe acute respiratory syndrome. Before government and academia, Dr. Parvanta worked at Porter Novelli, a global social issues communication company. Dr. Parvanta has designed, managed, or evaluated health and nutrition social marketing programs in more than 20 countries. She is the 2016 recipient of the Public Health Education and Health Promotion Division of APHA's Distinguished Career Award.

Sarah Bauerle Bass, PhD, MPH, is an Associate Professor in the Social and Behavioral Sciences department in the College of Public Health at Temple University and Director of the Risk Communication Laboratory. With over 25 years of experience in health communication, her work focuses on development and testing of culturally and developmentally appropriate materials, specializing in use of commercial marketing techniques and new technologies to address health disparities. She teaches health communication at the undergraduate and graduate levels, as well as risk communication and community-based intervention development at Temple University. As Director of the Risk Communication Laboratory, her research has advanced the field of health communication by applying commercial marketing techniques to the development and testing of messages and interventions. Using perceptual mapping and vector modeling methods, Dr. Bass has shown how 3-D imaging can enhance message development and tailor it for specific behavior or attitude barriers. Dr. Bass is also utilizing psycho-marketing methods to assess emotional and physiological response to and processing of health messages through visual, graphic, web, or textual message elements using eye tracking, pupilometer, EKG, and skin conductance measures. She has a number of currently funded studies using these techniques to develop culturally and literacy appropriate health communication interventions to help audiences make better medical decisions. Prior to Temple, she was the Public Information Coordinator for the West Virginia Department of Public Health's HIV/AIDS program where she developed all communication materials and implemented statewide communication campaigns. She is the recipient of the Riegelman Award for Excellence in Undergraduate Public Health Education from the Association of Schools and Programs in Public Health, and the Great Teacher and Lindback Awards for distinguished teaching from Temple University.

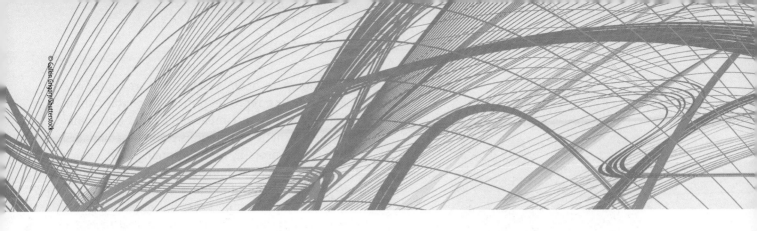

CHAPTER 1

Your World, Your Health

Claudia Parvanta

LEARNING OBJECTIVES

By the end of this chapter, the reader will be able to:

- Identify major factors affecting life expectancy and health outcomes.
- Define the approximate proportion of risk of premature death attributed to health care, genetics, social and environmental factors, and individual behavior.
- Explain how biological attributes of age, race, and sex are conditioned by social interpretations when it comes to health.
- Describe the leading causes of death for college-age individuals.
- Diagram an ecological model for a health issue.
- Explain how a communicator can use the people and places model to plan an intervention.

▶ Introduction

Mickey Mantle is known for saying, "If I knew I was going to live this long, I'd have taken better care of myself." There is a good chance that many readers will not know that Mickey Mantle was a center fielder and first baseman for the New York Yankees from 1951 through 1968, and is considered one of the greats in the game. After decades of alcohol abuse, Mantle died of liver disease and a heart attack in 1995 at the age of 63.

Jumping forward in time, an insurance company ran an ad in which it asked people to place a blue sticker on a wall to indicate the age of the *oldest* person they knew. The 400 participants created a histogram that peaked around the age of 95. The advertisers pointed out that the U.S. retirement age of 65 was developed around the time that Mickey Mantle was playing ball—and the average life expectancy was 61. By the year 2000, life expectancy had reached 74 for males and 79 for females,[1] and similar increases are projected through 2050. What does this increase in average life expectancy reflect?

▶ Major Factors Affecting Health Outcomes

Turning the question around, we can ask what factors are associated with dying "before your time," or as population scientists put it, **premature death**. FIGURE 1-1 illustrates the approximate contribution of major factors to premature death.

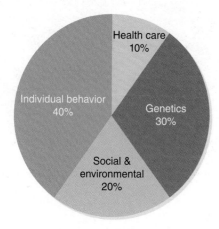

FIGURE 1-1   Risk of premature death attributed to different factors.

Data from Schroeder SA. We can do better—improving the health of the American people. *N Engl J Med.* 2007;357:1221-1228.

Are you surprised by this breakdown? Here is more about each major risk factor.

Health Care: The 10% Solution

Even though the United States spends more on health care than any other high-income country, Americans have the lowest life expectancy at birth and a greater prevalence of chronic diseases compared to the citizens of other high-income countries. Prior to the implementation of the **Affordable Care Act of 2010 (ACA)**, the United States spent 17.1% of its gross domestic product on health care. This was nearly twice what was spent in the United Kingdom (8.8%), for example. This spending was driven by greater use of expensive medical technologies (e.g., computed tomography scans) and higher healthcare and medication prices, but *not* more frequent doctor visits or hospital admissions.[2] So, Americans spend more money on drugs, tests, and fees but do not reap the benefit of healthier and longer lives. Why? Part of the reason is that so many individuals turn to health care only when something bad has already happened. In addition, many other factors contribute to our risk.

Genetics and Health: 30%[3]

The human genome contains about 20,500 genes. Of all these genes, we differ from every other human on earth by only about 1%. But it is this tiny percentage that determines our unique appearance, our potential for specific diseases, and our response to external factors, including therapeutic drugs.

As you learned in high school biology, in successful conception and pregnancy, the 23 chromosomes from your genetic father and 23 from your genetic mother develop into a 100-trillion-cell adult.

The 3 billion pairs of DNA letters that are copied and packaged during reproduction often contain slight variations that have no impact on health. But, sometimes these genetic instructions produce a damaged protein, extra protein, or no protein at all, which can result in a genetic mutation. Single gene mutations are responsible for more than 10,000 disorders. There are screening tests that parents can use prior to conception to identify autosomal recessive carrier status for more than 580 conditions. Autosomal recessive genes are not normally expressed in the heterozygous state, but if two carriers reproduce, they have a 25% chance that their offspring will be homozygous for the trait, and therefore have the condition. With appropriate genetic counseling, couples can avoid the heartache of giving birth to a child with a quickly fatal disease, such as Tay-Sachs, or a painful condition that shortens life, such as sickle cell anemia.

Women who carry a mutated form of either the BRCA1 or BRCA2 gene have an increased risk (i.e., greater than the 1 in 9 probability that all women carry) of developing breast or ovarian cancer at some point in their lives. Other adult onset diseases, such as colon cancer and heart disease, have genetic components. At this point in time, we have not discovered a genetic variation underlying most diseases.

The study of genetic variation, or genomics, is increasingly important in the development of treatments and drugs. These may be targeted to an individual's genome or the genome of the disease agent (e.g., a virus or a genetic form of cancer). As time goes on, we are discovering more genomic factors that may allow us to live more years free of disease. It is an exciting time for genomics, but for now, your best shot at being healthy is largely up to you—or is it?

Individual Behavior: 40%

Individual behaviors, which include what you eat, drink, or smoke; your sexual and reproductive activity; how fast you drive; how long you sit on the couch; and so on, play a significant role in determining your longevity. A study summarized the impact of six behaviors that the U.S. government has tracked in relation to changes in life expectancy and **quality-adjusted life expectancy** from 1960 to 2010.[4] Overall life expectancy increased by 6.9 years during this period. As shown in **FIGURE 1-2**, the authors of the study estimated that reductions in cigarette smoking and motor vehicle fatalities contribute nearly 2 of these years; however, the benefit of these gains is partially offset by the negative effect of rising obesity and accidental drug overdose.

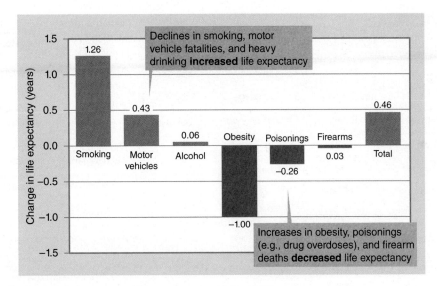

FIGURE 1-2 Impact of behavioral changes on life expectancy, 1960–2010.

Reproduced from National Bureau of Economic Research. How behavioral changes have affected U.S. population health since 1960. *Bull Aging Health.* 2015;1. http://www.nber.org/aginghealth/2015no1/w20631.html. Accessed July 2, 2015.

We still could add many years to our life span by adopting healthier behaviors; for example, fewer than 13% of Americans eat the recommended five to seven daily servings of vegetables and fruits. It takes more than just a friendly reminder to get most people to change from an unhealthy to a beneficial behavior. For many, the choice seems out of their hands, which brings us to a discussion of **social determinants of health (SDH)**.

Social and Environmental Factors: 20%

Although some social and environmental factors directly affect health (such as gang membership, air pollution, or toxic exposure to lead paint), others work indirectly by limiting or shaping access to resources or lifestyle options; for example, "…children born to parents who have not completed high school are more likely to live in [unsafe] neighborhoods… have exposed garbage or litter, and have poor or dilapidated housing and vandalism…."[5] A seminal meta-analysis concluded that social determinants are associated with a third of premature deaths in the United States.[6]

Because of the power of social determinants and the long history of disparities in the distribution of resources along societal lines, the World Health Organization (WHO)[7] and the U.S. government have adopted an SDH approach in setting priorities for action. For example, **Healthy People 2020**, launched in 2010 by the U.S. Department of Health and Human Services, organizes SDH around five key domains: (1) Economic Stability, (2) Neighborhood and Physical Environment, (3) Education, (4) Community and Social Context, and (5) the Health Care System. Other organizations include other factors, such as access to food, as shown in **FIGURE 1-3**.

Although problems with low literacy (listed under the Education domain) or playgrounds (listed under Neighborhoods) may seem outside the literal domain of health, not being able to read or understand English can have a tremendous impact on taking care of oneself or one's family. And access to safe playgrounds, sidewalks, and other green spaces is closely associated with risks of obesity. Your world is made up of social determinants, and because these determinants have a profound influence on your health, we will discuss them in greater depth in the sections that follow.

▶ Socially Defined You

For centuries, humans have been recording information about births, deaths, and significant illnesses and noting the individual's gender (male or female) and age, if known.

There were biological, social, and cultural forces that shaped these events. These forces still function today and determine, or at least provide a strong predictive contribution to, our own health outcomes.

There are protective factors, and similarly problems, associated with differences in:

- Sex and gender
- Race and ethnicity
- Age
- Environment
- Societal factors

Economic stability	Neighborhood and physical environment	Education	Food	Community and social context	Healthcare system
Employment	Housing	Literacy	Hunger	Social integration	Health coverage
Income	Transportation	Language	Access to healthy options	Support systems	Provider availability
Expenses	Safety	Early childhood education		Community engagement	Provider linguistic and cultural competency
Debt	Parks	Vocational training		Discrimination	
Medical bills	Playgrounds			Stress	
Support	Walkability	Higher education			Quality of care
	Zip code/geography				

Health outcomes
Mortality, morbidity, life expectancy, healthcare expenditures, health status, functional limitations

FIGURE 1-3 Social determinants of health.

Reproduced from Heiman HJ, Artiga S. Beyond health care: the role of social determinants in promoting health and health equity. KFF webpage. https://www.kff.org/disparities-policy/issue-brief/beyond-health-care-the-role-of-social-determinants-in-promoting-health-and-health-equity/. Published November 4, 2015. Accessed April 20, 2018.

These factors—added onto your genetic makeup—affect your personal health in ways that can be either beneficial or harmful.

Sex and Gender[8]

The term **sex** in biology refers to genetic expression of the genes inherited from one's parents. In most cases individuals are either XY or XX. Those with one X and one Y chromosome in every cell of the body are biologically male; biological females have two X chromosomes in every cell. Because these cells make up all the tissues and organs, there are sex-linked differences throughout our physiology, including but not limited to genitalia, hormones, and glandular development. In addition, biological males and females can express different symptoms when ill; may experience sensations such as pain differently; and respond differently to medications and substances, including addictive ones. Recognizing these biological differences, the U.S. government requires that clinical trials of new drugs or other medical interventions include both men and women, unless there is a clear rationale not to do so (e.g., a study of a prostate cancer drug or intrauterine device). For most of recorded history, individuals have been classified as "male" or "female" with little further thought. Medical science began documenting variations more effectively in the 20th century.[9]

Some individuals are born with undetermined genitalia at birth, which may also be true on a cellular level (i.e., some cells contain XX and others XY, or other variations). These conditions are referred to as *intersex*. It is possible for an individual to not be aware of subtle intersex variations, whereas others may be very aware of what they see and feel. Today's medical standards advise against surgical interventions until the affected individual can make that decision. The thought that a parent may wish to "fix" a child's body to look more like the sex they see most clearly expressed leads us to a discussion of gender.

Gender is a social or cultural concept that reflects how men and women, boys and girls, are meant to look and behave. By the age of 2 or 3, children will express strong identities as girls or boys, which are then reinforced or discouraged by their parents, teachers, or others in their social world. When children behave in ways that are discordant with their biological references (e.g., their genes, their genitalia), they may be labeled as *gender nonconforming*. This can be as casual as a girl playing with a truck and a boy playing with a doll. Some children eventually become comfortable adopting the societal roles assigned to their gender. Others may wish to change their outward appearance and fully behave in ways they feel are consistent with their internal concept of themselves. The term *transgender* refers to a range of behaviors associated with making this change. Some individuals go on to have *gender reassignment* surgery and take hormones to support this change.

As individuals mature to the point of seeking intimate partners, the term *sexual orientation* becomes meaningful. Sexual orientation refers to being sexually and romantically attracted to persons of the same or opposite sex. Kinsey and others have described a spectrum of attraction from consistently preferring the opposite sex (heterosexual), through preferring members of either sex (bisexual), to consistently preferring the same sex (homosexual).[10]

How Do Sex and Gender Affect Health Outcomes?

It is well known that, on average, women live longer than men, but they also experience more days of illness or disability. Setting aside the risks associated with childbearing, why should women experience more "sick time" and still outlive their male contemporaries?

Few researchers have separated the risks associated with the biological condition of being female or male from the lived experience of gendered identities. In other words, we have little data apart from birth outcomes that truly show the vulnerability associated with an XX or XY genotype versus the risks accumulated as a girl or a boy matures in a particular environment. Using the WHO's original *Global Burden of Disease*, published in 2002, Snow[11] noted that the XY genotype is a necessary (but not sufficient) condition for the risk of hemophilia, prostate cancer, and testicular cancer. Being born XX was associated with a greater risk of breast and ovarian cancer, and all maternal causes of death. **TABLE 1-1** shows conditions worldwide from which men and women lose more active years of life.

Most of the conditions in Table 1-1 are connected to social expectations for men and women. Virtually every human society expects boys and men to take risks and demonstrate courage or "manhood," often resulting in the higher rates of fatalities due to hunting accidents, local fights, warfare, or even car crashes. Women and girls too often fall victim to the ugly side of the same expectations, resulting in domestic violence, rape, conflict, and trafficking. Women also are more subject to culturally sanctioned traditions of bodily mutilation, limits on property ownership, or freedom of movement, which are upheld by both men and women in their societies.[12] Risks for girls can be even more extreme, as in the case of *femicide*.

Femicide. Along with other sex-linked traits, slightly more boys are born alive than girls, with a resulting 105 boys born for 100 girls. In most cultures, this imbalance evens out as slightly more girls survive infancy. However, there are many societies where the perceived need and desire for males leads to parents killing female infants at birth, through either neglect or force. When and where ultrasound technology became widely available, abortion replaced infanticide by allowing so-inclined parents to detect and abort a female fetus; for example, in China, the birth ratio is presently 120 boys for every 100 girls. In India, despite a 1994 law banning use of ultrasound for sex selection, for second-born children, there are only 76

TABLE 1-1 Conditions with Greatest Difference in Global Burden of Disease for Men and Women

Conditions for Men
War
Gout
Alcohol use disorders
Road and traffic accidents
Violence
Other intentional injuries
Drug use disorders
Lymphatic filariasis
Mouth and propharynx cancers
Lung cancer
Liver cancer
Drowning
Bladder cancer

Conditions for Women
Breast cancer
Gonorrhea
Chlamydia
Trachoma
Migraine
Posttraumatic stress disorder
Rheumatoid arthritis
Panic disorder

Data from Snow RC. *Sex, Gender and Vulnerability*. Population Studies Center Research Report 07-628. Ann Arbor, MI: Population Studies Center, University of Michigan; 2007.

females born for every 100 males.[13] In both countries, demographers warn of the stresses to society caused by these "missing" women. Numerous international agencies and voluntary organizations are working to reduce these gender inequalities. (A good place to start is with the United Nations Entity for Gender Equality and the Empowerment of Women at http://www.unwomen.org/en/.)

Sexual Orientation and Health

The National Health Interview Survey (NHIS) has been conducted annually in the United States for 57 years. **BOX 1-1** provides some information about the overall survey methods as well as questions pertaining to sexual orientation, used for the first time in 2013.

TABLE 1-2, reprinted from the National Health Statistics report, shows the sexual orientation among U.S. adults aged 18 and over, by sex and age group, based on data from the 2013 survey. Among all U.S. adults aged 18 and over, 96.6% identified as straight, 1.6% identified as gay or lesbian, and 0.7% identified as bisexual. Of the remaining 1.1% of adults, 0.2% identified as "something else," 0.4% selected "I don't know the answer," and 0.6% did not provide an answer.

The sexual orientation variables were analyzed against selected health behaviors, health status

---

BOX 1-1   National Health Interview Survey Methodology

Methods

NHIS is an annual multipurpose health survey conducted continuously throughout the year and serves as a primary source of health data on the civilian noninstitutionalized population of the United States.[a] Data are collected by trained interviewers with the U.S. Census Bureau using computer-assisted personal interviewing (CAPI), a data collection method in which an interviewer meets with respondents face-to-face to ask questions and enter the answers into a laptop computer. When necessary, interviewers may complete missing portions of the interview over the telephone.

Analyses in this report were based on data collected from 34,557 sample adults aged 18 and over. The conditional sample adult response rate (i.e., the number of completed sample adult interviews divided by the total number of eligible sample adults) was 81.7%. The final sample adult response rate, calculated by multiplying the conditional response rate by the final family response rate, was 61.2%.[b]

Sexual Orientation Questions

The first of the four cascading sexual orientation questions that were included in the 2013 NHIS, which is asked of all sample adults aged 18 and over, reads, "Which of the following best represents how you think of yourself?" It has five response options, which vary slightly by respondent sex.

For male respondents, they are:

- Gay,
- Straight, that is, not gay,
- Bisexual,
- Something else, and
- I don't know the answer.

For female respondents, the response options are:

- Lesbian or gay,
- Straight, that is, not lesbian or gay,
- Bisexual,
- Something else, and
- I don't know the answer.

Although not an explicit response option, respondents could refuse to provide an answer to any of these questions.

For the initial sexual orientation question (and the "something else" and "I don't know the answer" follow-up questions), flashcards listing the response options were handed to respondents in the face-to-face interview setting. Respondents were asked to report the number corresponding to their answer. When the questions were administered over the telephone, the interviewer read the response options. Complete text and details of the NHIS sexual orientation questions are provided in the 2013 Sample Adult survey questionnaire, which can be accessed on the NHIS website: http://www.cdc.gov/nchs/nhis.htm.

---

[a] National Center for Health Statistics. National Health Interview Survey, 2013. Public-use data file and documentation. Available from: http://www.cdc.gov/nchs/nhis/ quest_data _related_1997_forward.htm

[b] National Center for Health Statistics. 2013 National Health Interview Survey (NHIS) public use data release survey description. 2014. Available from: ftp://ftp.cdc.gov/pub/ Health_Statistics /NCHS/ Dataset_Documentation/NHIS/2013/ srvydesc.pdf

TABLE 1-2 National Health Statistics Report—Sexual Orientation

Sexual Orientation	Gay or Lesbian[a]		Straight[b]		Bisexual	
	Number in Thousands	Percent[c] (Standard Error)	Number in Thousands	Percent[c] (Standard Error)	Number in Thousands	Percent[c] (Standard Error)
Overall	3729	1.6 (0.09)	224,163	97.7 (0.11)	1514	0.7 (0.06)
Sex						
Men	2000	1.8 (0.14)	108,093	97.8 (0.15)	481	0.4 (0.06)
Women	1729	1.5 (0.12)	116,071	97.7 (0.15)	1033	0.9 (0.10)
Age Group (Years)						
18–44	2028	1.9 (0.15)	104,947	97.1 (0.18)	1153	1.1 (0.12)
45–64	1422	1.8 (0.16)	77,686	97.8 (0.17)	289	0.4 (0.07)
65 and over	278	0.7 (0.13)	41,531	99.2 (0.14)	73	0.2 (0.05)

Note: Estimate has a relative standard error greater than 30% and less than or equal to 50% and should be used with caution as it does not meet standards of reliability or precision.

[a] Response option provided on the National Health Interview Survey was "gay" for men, and "gay or lesbian" for women.

[b] Response option provided on the National Health Interview Survey was "straight, that is, not gay" for men, and "straight, that is, not gay or lesbian" for women.

[c] Percent distributions in this table may not equal exactly 100.0% due to rounding.

Reproduced from National Health Interview Survey. National Center for Health Statistics website. http://www.cdc.gov/nchs/nhis/index.htm. Accessed February 20, 2018.

indicators, and access to health care. **BOX 1-2** summarizes some of the results from this analysis.

This somewhat dry summary suggests that men and women who identified as lesbian, gay, or bisexual on this national survey were insured and participated in basic healthcare options in about the same proportion as their self-identified heterosexual counterparts. Those who self-identified as gay or lesbian were more likely to engage in smoking and drinking than their heterosexual counterparts. Although the NHIS asked about these health risks, it did not ask about unprotected sex or violence.

Other U.S. health data show that a higher percentage of lesbian or gay adults (56.4%) and bisexual adults (47.4%) report intimate partner violence compared to heterosexual adults (17.5%). In addition, although the Centers for Disease Control and Prevention (CDC) estimates that men who have sex with men (MSM) account for 4% of the U.S. male population aged 13 or older, the rate of new human immunodeficiency virus (HIV) diagnoses among MSM in the United States is 44 times that of other men.[14]

Another risk for individuals who identify as lesbian, gay, bisexual, or transgender (LGBT) that distinguishes them from their heterosexual counterparts is being the target of hate crimes. Even before the 2016 shooting rampage at a gay nightclub in Orlando, Florida, the Federal Bureau of Investigation (FBI) documented more hate crimes against LGBT people than any other collective group. Nearly 20% of the 5462 single-bias hate crimes reported to the FBI in 2014 were because of the target's sexual orientation, or how the perpetrator perceived their victim's orientation.[15]

So, your chromosomes, gender identification, sexual orientation, sexual behavior, and societal reactions to your gender identity and behavior all comprise how sex and gender influence your health risks.

BOX 1-2 Prevalence of Selected Health Indicators by Sexual Orientation for Adults Aged 18–64

Health-Related Behaviors

- Current cigarette smoking:
  - A higher percentage of adults aged 18–64 who identified as gay or lesbian (27.2%) or bisexual (29.5%) were current cigarette smokers compared with their counterparts who identified as straight (19.6%).
- Binge drinking:
  - A higher percentage of adults aged 18–64 who identified as gay or lesbian (35.1%) or bisexual (41.5%) reported having had five or more drinks in one day at least once in the past year compared with those who identified as straight (26.0%).
- Meet federal guidelines for aerobic physical activity:
  - There were no significant differences among adults aged 18–64 who identified as gay or lesbian (57.9%), bisexual (55.5%), or straight (52.3%).

Health Status Indicators

- Health status described as excellent or very good:
  - No significant differences were found by sexual orientation for the percentage of adults aged 18–64 with excellent or very good health, neither overall nor among men. Among women, however, a higher percentage of those who identified as straight (63.3%) were in excellent or very good health compared with women who identified as gay or lesbian (54.0%).
- Experienced serious psychological distress in the past 30 days:
  - A higher percentage of adults aged 18–64 who identified as bisexual (11.0%) experienced serious psychological distress in the past 30 days compared with their counterparts who identified as gay or lesbian (5.0%) or straight (3.9%).
- Considered "obese" based on calculated weight and height (i.e., not asked directly):
  - No significant differences were found overall in the percentage of adults aged 18–64 who were obese. A higher percentage of men aged 18–64 who identified as straight (30.7%) were obese than men who identified as gay (23.2%); among women aged 18–64, a higher percentage of those who identified as bisexual (40.4%) were obese than women who identified as straight (28.8%).

Healthcare Service Utilization and Access

- Received influenza vaccination in the past year:
  - A higher percentage of adults aged 18–64 who identified as gay or lesbian (42.9%) received an influenza vaccination in the past year compared with those adults aged 18–64 who identified as straight (35.0%).
- Ever been tested for HIV:
  - A higher percentage of men who identified as gay (79.5%) or bisexual (56.7%) compared to straight (33.0%) have ever been tested for HIV. Among women, the differences in testing were not statistically significant (51.6% identified gay or lesbian, 52.6% identified bisexual, and 40.2% identified straight).
- Has a usual place to go for medical care:
  - Among men aged 18–64, no significant differences in having a usual place to go for medical care were found (gay: 81.2%, bisexual: 74.5%, straight: 76.4%). Among women aged 18–64, by contrast, a higher percentage of those who identified as straight (85.5%) had a usual place to go for medical care than those who identified as gay or lesbian (75.6%) or bisexual (71.6%).
- Failed to obtain needed medical care in past year due to cost:
  - Among women aged 18–64, a higher percentage of those who identified as gay or lesbian (15.2%) failed to obtain needed medical care in the past year due to cost compared with those who identified as straight (9.6%). No significant differences by sexual orientation were found among men aged 18–64 for this indicator.
- Currently uninsured:
  - Among men aged 18–64, a higher percentage of those who identified as straight (21.9%) were uninsured compared with those who identified as gay (15.7%). Among women, 19.1% of those who identified as gay or lesbian, 24.9% who identified as bisexual, and 18.4% of those who identified as straight were currently uninsured, but the difference was not statistically significant.

Data from Ward BW, Dahlhamer JM, Galinsky AM, Joestl SS; Division of Health Interview Statistics, Centers for Disease Control and Prevention (CDC), U.S. Department of Health and Human Services. *Sexual Orientation and Health Among U.S. Adults: National Health Interview Survey, 2013.* Hyattsville, MD: National Center for Health Statistics. https://www.cdc.gov/nchs/data/nhsr077.pdf

Race and Ethnicity

FIGURE 1-4 shows the statistics from the 2010 U.S. census (reported in 2012) on how many people identified themselves by a specific **race** as well as Hispanic ethnicity. It also shows the projected population in 2060. The largest change predicted for the future will be the near doubling of the ethnically Hispanic population, with some small increases in Asian and "other" groups, which includes Native Americans as well as Native Alaskans, Hawaiians, and Pacific Islanders. What do these broad classifications mean in terms of health?

Changing Views of Race and Ethnicity

Have you sent a cheek swab to National Geographic to have your ancestry determined? Or maybe you have tried 23andMe.com? These fun activities compare your mitochondrial DNA (passed down from your mother) and some markers on your Y chromosomes (from your father) to detect your deep, deep roots. And by deep, we mean learning where your ancestors lived more than 500 years ago. From actual eons of migration, mixing, and mingling, humanity is incredibly diverse, with much more variation existing *within* a so-called "racial group" than *between* racial groups. Therefore, many social scientists assert that race is not based in biology but constructed by society.

For example, skin color, a 19th-century approach to defining race, is controlled by more than 378 genetic loci. These genes regulate melanin production and the skin's reaction to light of various wavelengths.[16] Anthropologist Nina Jablonski has pointed out that the geographical distribution of human skin color is related to distance from the equator. At more northern or southern latitudes, the level of ultraviolet B (UVB) rays hitting Earth's surface decreases due to the planet's tilt. The equator is bathed year-round in UVB rays, but seasonal variations mean that people in Northern Europe receive virtually no UVB exposure in winter. As a result, Jablonski said, humans living near the equator developed darker skin tones (to protect against the harmful effects of too much exposure), whereas those in northern climates developed lighter hues and are more efficient at synthesizing vitamin D from sunlight.[17]

Any population-level traits, including autosomal recessive conditions such as sickle cell disease (SCD) or Tay-Sachs, are carried down through generations due to social factors that have brought groups of people into gene pools (breeding populations) over time. (See **BOX 1-3** for more about these two conditions.) Sometimes populations had control over these groupings; at other times, they were against their wishes.

When many people share cultural traits, such as language, appearance, food, religion, dress, and meaningful symbols, and have a common ancestral homeland, they may be considered to have an **ethnic identity**. Does it match up with a set of physical or physiological traits? It can, if the population has lived and reproduced in the same place over a long period.

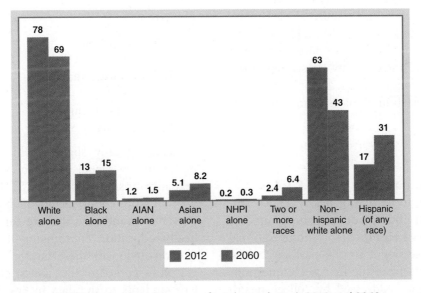

FIGURE 1-4 Population by race and Hispanic origin (percent of total population), 2012 and 2060.

Abbreviations: AIAN, American Indian and Alaska Native; NHPI, Native Hawaiian and Other Pacific Islander.

BOX 1-3 Diseases of Origin?

Sickle Cell Disease[a]

Red blood cells that contain normal hemoglobin are disc shaped, which allows the cells to move easily through large and small blood vessels to deliver oxygen. Sickle hemoglobin can form stiff rods within the red cell, changing it into a crescent or sickle shape. Sickle-shaped cells can stick to vessel walls, causing a blockage that slows or stops the flow of blood. When this happens, oxygen cannot reach nearby tissues.

People who have SCD inherit two abnormal hemoglobin genes, one from each parent. In all forms of SCD, at least one of the two abnormal genes causes a person's body to make hemoglobin S. When a person has two hemoglobin S genes, hemoglobin SS, the disease is called sickle cell anemia. This is the most common and often most severe kind of SCD. Hemoglobin SC disease and hemoglobin Sβ thalassemia are two other common forms of SCD.

A common myth about SCD is that it is an African disease affecting only people in Africa or their descendants. In fact, SCD occurs more often among people who come from areas where malaria was common, such as Africa, but also including the Middle East, India, some Mediterranean countries, and Latin America. Anthropologists theorize this is related to the protective effect that the sickle cell mutation provides against malaria infection in the heterozygous state.

Tay-Sachs: Not Only a "Jewish Disease"[b]

Tay-Sachs is a neurodegenerative disease that is fatal in the homozygous state. Babies born with Tay-Sachs disease appear normal at birth, but begin to show symptoms at 4 to 6 months of age. Children then gradually lose their sight, hearing, and swallowing abilities, and usually die by the age of 5 years.

Jewish individuals whose families originated in Eastern Europe, so-called Ashkenazi Jews, have long known to test for carrier status of Tay-Sachs before starting a family. Among the more orthodox populations that arrange marriages, rabbis often require blood tests before condoning a match. Of course, practicing Judaism as a religion had nothing to do with the disease directly, but because Jews in that part of the world limited their marriages to within their communities, and the carrier status was nonfatal, the gene was maintained at a higher rate within this ethnic group. Today, it is known that French Canadian, Cajun (Louisiana), and Irish populations also have higher than average rates of the disease. These days, due to more mixing of populations than was done in past centuries, all young adults are advised to get genetic screening before starting families.

[a] Data from Sickle cell disease. National Heart, Lung, and Blood Institute website. http://www.nhlbi.nih.gov/health/health-topics/topics/sca. Accessed February 13, 2018; Sickle cell disease (SCD). Centers for Disease Control and Prevention website. https://www.cdc.gov/ncbddd/sicklecell/data.html. Accessed February 13, 2018; About sickle cell: myths and misconceptions. The Sickle Cell Association of Ontario. https://sites.google.com/a/sicklecellontario.org/www/sickle-cell-101/myths-and-misconceptions. Accessed February 13, 2018.
[b] Data from Tay-Sachs disease. Einstein Healthcare Network website. http://www.einstein.edu/genetic/tay-sachs-disease/. Accessed February 13, 2018.

Therefore, although race may not be clearly defined biologically, it is very real socially, by which we mean that society may allocate valued resources based on this construct. Ethnicity tends to work through the transmission of cultural learning from one generation to another. As such, race and ethnicity can strongly affect health outcomes through the media of culture and society, including selection of mates from within only specific groups.

Age

Have you seen the questions in **TABLE 1-3** before? If so, you are likely to be one of nearly 23,000 students (graduate and undergraduate) who completed the American College Health Association's National College Health Assessment in the past few years. Table 1-3 shows data from the first set of questions that asks about topics addressed by college health information providers as well as student interest in these topics.

More than 50% of students wanted more information about the following topics, in descending order of interest:

- Stress reduction
- Nutrition
- Helping others in distress
- Sleep difficulties
- Depression and anxiety
- Physical activity

Lagging only slightly behind was information pertaining to sexual assault or violence prevention, sexually transmitted diseases (STDs), and suicide prevention. Runners-up included tobacco use, pregnancy prevention, and cold/flu/sore throats. If you were a health education coordinator at a university, what would you do with these data?

Now compare the issues of concern to college students to the data in **FIGURE 1-5** showing the CDC's depiction of the leading causes of death by age group in the United States. Examining the columns

TABLE 1-3 Items from the National College Health Assessment, 2015—Undergraduates

	Have You Ever Received Information on the Following Topics from Your College or University? (Percentage Saying Yes)	Are You Interested in Receiving Information on the Following Topics from Your College or University? (Percentage Saying Yes)
Alcohol and other drug use	80.5	28.0
Cold/flu/sore throat	45.4	38.8
Depression/anxiety	57.9	54.4
Eating disorders	31.2	33.2
Grief and loss	33.4	42.1
How to help others in distress	52.0	59.5
Injury prevention	38.3	41.6
Nutrition	54.2	60.0
Physical activity	59.6	56.1
Pregnancy prevention	44.0	35.1
Problem use of internet/computer games	20.3	24.6
Relationship difficulties	40.8	42.3
Sexual assault/relationship violence prevention	81.5	45.7
Sexually transmitted disease/infection prevention	57.9	42.0
Sleep difficulties	22.3	58.0
Stress reduction	58.4	68.4
Suicide prevention	52.5	46.1
Tobacco use	48.1	25.6
Violence prevention	56.4	43.0

Note: Data from 16,760 students at 40 schools across the United States.
Data from American College Health Association. *American College Health Association—National College Health Assessment II: Undergraduate Students Reference Group Data Report Fall 2015.* Hanover, MD: American College Health Association; 2016.

representing the ages when most individuals attend college (15–24 years and 25–34 years), the first thing to understand is that the total number of deaths in these columns is relatively low. For example, a total of 583 individuals died from HIV in 2014, and only in the older age group; however, there were more than 29,000 deaths from unintentional injury. The majority of these deaths were motor vehicle–related or caused by accidental poisoning, which chiefly refers to drug or alcohol overdose. More than 11,000 individuals took their own lives in 2014, and more than 8000 were killed by others.

Leaving homicide aside for the moment, the educational topics offered on most college campuses seem to correspond with the greater risks of self-harm experienced by this age group. Although students might not necessarily feel their schools need to share information with them about alcohol and drugs, studies make it clear that fatalities in this age group often involve substance abuse. Nearly one third of all traffic fatalities involve alcohol-impaired drivers, and drugs other than alcohol (legal and illegal) are involved in 16% of motor vehicle crashes.[18] According to the Substance Abuse and Mental Health Services Administration (SAMHSA), approximately 30% of 18- to 25-year-olds with mental health disorders had a co-occurring substance abuse disorder.[19]

Rank	\< 1	1–4	5–9	10–14	15–24	25–34	35–44	45–54	55–64	65+	Total
					Age Groups						
1	Congenital anomalies 4825	Unintentional injury 1235	Unintentional injury 755	Unintentional injury 763	Unintentional injury 12,514	Unintentional injury 19,795	Unintentional injury 17,818	Malignant neoplasms 43,054	Malignant neoplasms 116,122	Heart disease 507,138	Heart disease 633,842
2	Short gestation 4084	Congenital anomalies 435	Malignant neoplasms 437	Malignant neoplasms 428	Suicide 5491	Suicide 6947	Malignant neoplasms 10,909	Heart disease 34,248	Heart disease 76,872	Malignant neoplasms 419,389	Malignant neoplasms 595,930
3	SIDS 1568	Homicide 369	Congenital anomalies 181	Suicide 409	Homicide 4733	Homicide 4863	Heart disease 10,387	Unintentional injury 21,499	Unintentional injury 19,488	Chronic low. respiratory disease 131,804	Chronic low. respiratory disease 155,041
4	Maternal pregnancy comp. 1522	Malignant neoplasms 354	Homicide 140	Homicide 158	Malignant neoplasms 1469	Malignant neoplasms 3704	Suicide 6936	Liver disease 8874	Chronic low. respiratory disease 17,457	Cerebro-vascular 120,156	Unintentional injury 146,571
5	Unintentional injury 1291	Heart disease 147	Heart disease 85	Congenital anomalies 156	Heart disease 997	Heart disease 3522	Homicide 2895	Suicide 8751	Diabetes mellitus 14,166	Alzheimer's disease 109,495	Cerebro-vascular 140,323
6	Placenta cord. membranes 910	Influenza & pneumonia 88	Chronic low. respiratory disease 80	Heart disease 125	Congenital anomalies 386	Liver disease 844	Liver disease 2861	Diabetes mellitus 6212	Liver disease 13,278	Diabetes mellitus 56,142	Alzheimer's disease 110,561
7	Bacterial sepsis 599	Septicemia 54	Influenza & pneumonia 44	Chronic low. respiratory disease 93	Chronic low. respiratory disease 202	Diabetes mellitus 798	Diabetes mellitus 1986	Cerebro-vascular 5307	Cerebro-vascular 12,116	Unintentional injury 51,395	Diabetes mellitus 79,535
8	Respiratory distress 462	Perinatal period 50	Cerebro-vascular 42	Cerebro-vascular 42	Diabetes mellitus 196	Cerebro-vascular 567	Cerebro-vascular 1788	Chronic low. respiratory disease 4345	Suicide 7739	Influenza & pneumonia 48,774	Influenza & pneumonia 57,062
9	Circulatory system disease 428	Cerebro-vascular 42	Benign neoplasms 39	Influenza & pneumonia 39	Influenza & pneumonia 184	HIV 529	HIV 1055	Septicemia 2542	Septicemia 5774	Nephritis 41,258	Nephritis 49,959
10	Neonatal hemorrhage 406	Chronic low. respiratory disease 40	Septicemia 31	Two tied: benign neo./septicemia 33	Cerebro-vascular 166	Congenital anomalies 443	Septicemia 829	Nephritis 2124	Nephritis 5452	Septicemia 30,817	Suicide 44,193

FIGURE 1-5 The 10 leading causes of death by age group—United States, 2015.

Reproduced from 10 leading causes of death by age group, United States – 2015. Centers for Disease Prevention and Control website. https://www.cdc.gov/injury/wisqars/pdf/leading_causes_of_death_by_age_group_2015-a.pdf. Accessed June 15, 2018. Data source: National Vital Statistics System, National Center for Health Statistics, CDC. Produced by: National Center for Injury Prevention and Control, CDC using WISQARS™.

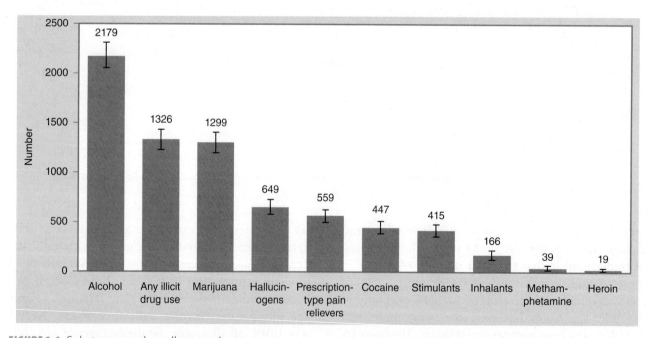

FIGURE 1-6 Substance use by college students.

Reproduced from Lipari RN, Jean-Francois B. A day in the life of college students aged 18 to 22: substance use facts. *The CBHSQ Report*. Center for Behavioral Health Statistics and Quality website. https://www.samhsa.gov/data/sites/default/files/report_2361 /ShortReport-2361.html. Published May 26, 2016. Accessed February 14, 2018.

Many college students will say they turn to alcohol, drugs, or tobacco (including e-cigarettes and vaping) to relieve the stress they feel from their academic or social environment. **FIGURE 1-6** shows the number of full-time college students who reported using an illegal substance for the first time. (Part-time student rates are much lower.) In addition, of the 9 million full-time college students in the United States, 1.2 million drank alcohol and 703,759 used marijuana on an almost daily or daily basis in 2015.[20]

So, it seems that in the United States, young adulthood is a fairly safe time of life from a disease perspective. The major health risks in this age group are behavior-related. Self-inflicted harm is the greatest cause of death, often in association with overdose or misuse of drugs and alcohol. Substance misuse and abuse can be triggered by elevated levels of stress or other emotional discomfort. Our environment plays a role in creating this stress.

The Environment

In the early part of the 20th century, the leading causes of disease and death in the United States were directly tied to environmental conditions such as close living quarters and poor sanitation, an unsafe and unhealthy food supply, and hazardous workplaces or occupations. In response to these health problems, the U.S. government at all levels created laws and regulations to clean up toxic waste, manage infectious disease outbreaks, ensure that food was safe to eat, and so on. These policies led to dramatic reductions in communicable diseases and maternal and infant mortality. In many low-income countries, however, much of the population continues to suffer from illnesses attributable to unsanitary and unsafe environmental and workplace conditions. According to the WHO, environmental factors account for 24% of the global disease burden and 23% of all deaths.

The environment is once again very much on our minds, whether because of mosquito-borne illness such as Zika virus, increases in childhood asthma, or populations affected by flooding, tornadoes, or other "natural" disasters. The environment affects all of us on a global level, such as through climate change, and on an individual level, such as how one reacts to heat, dust mites, cockroach droppings, pollen, and so on. The climatic trends associated with global warming indicate that we need to develop solutions to reduce environmental pollution and protect ourselves against environmental risks.

The CDC has published numerous infographics that depict different environmental health issues, some of which appear in **FIGURES 1-7** and **1-8**.

Although the environment affects everyone, the risk of exposure to poor quality environments or having access to safe and salubrious spaces is largely a matter of how society allocates resources. For example, **FIGURE 1-9** depicts the Washington, DC, subway (Metro) system showing life expectancy at various destinations.

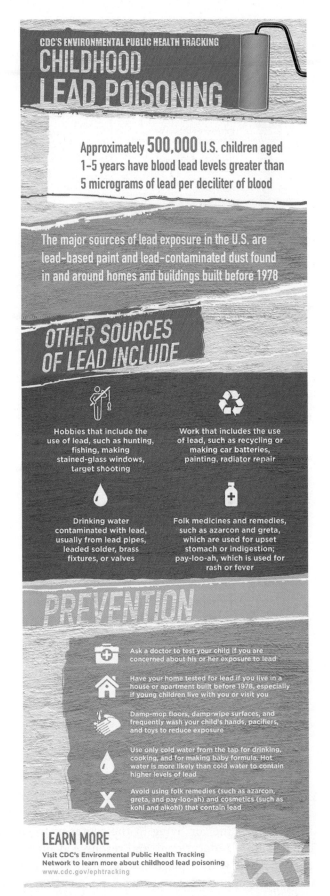

FIGURE 1-7 Childhood lead poisoning.

Reproduced from National environmental public health tracking: childhood lead poisoning communication tools. Centers for Disease Control and Prevention website. https://ephtracking.cdc.gov/showClpCommunicationTools.action. Updated October 26, 2016. Accessed February 21, 2018.

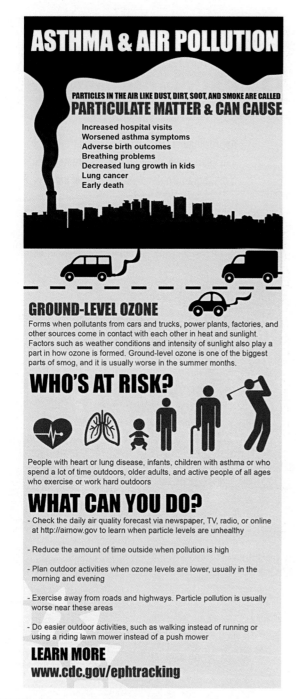

FIGURE 1-8 Asthma and air pollution.

Reproduced from National environmental public health tracking infographics. Centers for Disease Control and Prevention website. https://ephtracking.cdc.gov/showInfographics. Updated December 14, 2017. Accessed February 21, 2018.

People living at one end of the so called "Red Line" or "Yellow Line" have six to seven more years of life expectancy than those at the opposite end of the "Blue Line" or living in the center of town. The economic, educational, and resource availability associated with a place can be found in cities around the country.[21] So, growing up on the proverbial wrong side of the tracks not only is a matter of status, but it also is associated with health disparities.

► How to Change This Picture

The Ecological Model

Just as health problems arise from multiple sources (i.e., individual biology, family life, community resources), solutions can also be developed on multiple levels. Social scientists use an **ecological model**, such as that depicted in **FIGURE 1-10**, to begin identifying the roots of problems and potential points of intervention.

The basic idea in using an ecological model is to look at the outer layers of a problem and work on solutions to these. New policies and structural interventions will be more sustainable over time than individualized interventions. Take water contaminated by lead or other pollutants. Cleaning up the water supply will be more sustainable over time than handing out bottled water to individuals. Bottled drinking water should be viewed as a short-term, emergency intervention.

BOX 1-4 presents an ecological model for violence prevention, suggesting points of intervention at all levels of the model.

Sometimes a problem that appears to be individual has its roots in the outer layers of the model. **FIGURE 1-11** shows a simplified ecological model for childhood obesity, modeled after Davison and Birch.[22]

Points of Intervention

Health communicators work through a causal analysis to determine the modifiable factors existing at each level of an ecological model. With the example of students turning to drugs or alcohol to relieve stress, it would be important to go beyond simple interdiction of on-campus drug use or drinking and search for modifiable causes of the stress. A process to do this is root cause analysis.

Root Cause Analysis

Root cause analysis is a technique from engineering used to analyze what went wrong in a disaster. For example, if a building collapses, engineers look at what precipitated the event at a deeper level. The well-known parable attributed to Ben Franklin, "For the want of a nail, the shoe was lost; for the want of a shoe, the horse was lost . . .," ending up with the loss of a kingdom, is a kind of reverse root cause analysis. In relatively modern times, the Space Shuttle *Challenger*, with its crew of seven (including Christa McAuliffe, a science teacher), exploded a little more than a minute into its flight in 1986. Famed physicist Richard Feynman was among the group charged with the root cause analysis of this

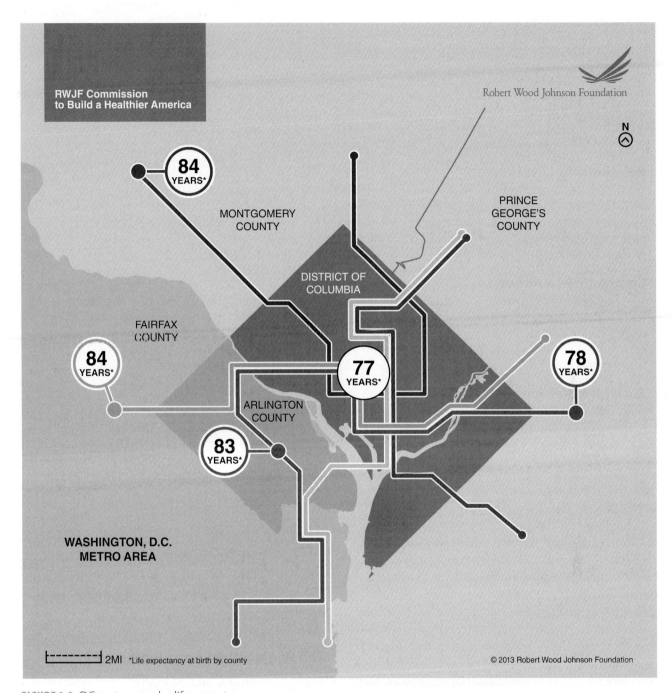

RWJF Commission to Build a Healthier America

Robert Wood Johnson Foundation

N

84 YEARS*

MONTGOMERY COUNTY

PRINCE GEORGE'S COUNTY

DISTRICT OF COLUMBIA

FAIRFAX COUNTY

84 YEARS*

77 YEARS*

78 YEARS*

ARLINGTON COUNTY

83 YEARS*

WASHINGTON, D.C. METRO AREA

2MI *Life expectancy at birth by county

© 2013 Robert Wood Johnson Foundation

FIGURE 1-9 DC metro map by life expectancy.

© 2013 Robert Wood Johnson Foundation. Reprinted with permission from the VCU Center on Society and Health.

Societal   Community   Relationship   Individual

FIGURE 1-10 Social-ecological model.

Reproduced from Krug E, Dahlberg LL, Mercy JA, Zwi AB, Lozano R, eds. *World Report on Violence and Health.* Geneva, Switzerland: World Health Organization; 2002.

disaster. In speaking to the National Aeronautics and Space Administration (NASA) engineers, the group discovered that the "O rings" seal of the solid rocket was sheared off by strong wind and cold temperatures. It was a shocking moment to the world watching the launch and set the space program back by several years. But the underlying cause, according to Feynman and the scientific commission, was the prevailing culture of "all systems go" that discouraged NASA scientists from raising issues that might impede a launch. A cultural and political change was necessary to prevent disasters like what occurred with the *Challenger* from occurring again.

BOX 1-4 CDC Ecological Model for Violence Prevention

Individual-Level Forces

The first level identifies biological and personal history factors that increase the likelihood of becoming a victim or perpetrator of violence. Some of these factors are age, education, income, substance use, and history of abuse. Prevention strategies at this level are often designed to promote attitudes, beliefs, and behaviors that ultimately prevent violence. Specific approaches may include education and life skills training.

Relationship-Level Forces

The second level examines close relationships that may increase the risk of experiencing violence as a victim or perpetrator. A person's closest social circle—peers, partners, and family members—influences their behavior and contributes to their range of experience. Prevention strategies at this level may include parenting or family-focused prevention programs, and mentoring and peer programs designed to reduce conflict, foster problem-solving skills, and promote healthy relationships.

Community-Level Forces

The third level explores the settings, such as schools, workplaces, and neighborhoods, in which social relationships occur and seeks to identify the characteristics of these settings that are associated with becoming victims or perpetrators of violence. Prevention strategies at this level are typically designed to impact the social and physical environment—for example, by reducing social isolation, improving economic and housing opportunities in neighborhoods, and improving the climate, processes, and policies within schools and workplaces.

Societal-Level Forces

The fourth level looks at the broad societal factors that help create a climate in which violence is encouraged or inhibited. These factors include social and cultural norms that support violence as an acceptable way to resolve conflicts. Other large societal factors include the health, economic, educational, and social policies that help to maintain economic or social inequalities between groups in society.

Reproduced from The social-ecological model: a framework for prevention. Centers for Disease Control and Prevention website. http://www.cdc.gov/violenceprevention/overview/social
-ecologicalmodel.html. Updated March 25, 2015. Accessed February 19, 2018.

Root cause analysis has found its way into health-care settings, particularly in eliminating intravenous line infections, mistakes in drug delivery, and similar human errors. It can also be used to prevent disasters, such as young adult suicide or drug overdose. For example, if a college student is feeling so stressed that they take drugs, what is causing the stress? It could be difficult coursework and tests, relationships not working out as hoped, financial difficulties, lack of sleep, and even poor nutrition. Why are students losing sleep and not eating well? How would you get to the root causes of any of these conditions?

Counseling might be an effective strategy for helping students cope with personal relationships, difficulties with coursework, or possibly addiction. However, communication to address parental pressure, clubs or fraternities, or how professors interact with students or set up testing might also be likely candidates for intervention.

Health communication strategies can be organized in terms of their relative utility within each level of the ecological model. Some approaches are more effective at influencing the outer layers, including the policymakers who develop regulations or implement programs that provide resources to communities and individuals. Other processes are more effective midway by influencing community dynamics, and others work by facilitating individual behavior change.

The People and Places Framework

Maibach, Abrams, and Marosits[23] have developed a framework to diagram the processes of communication in terms of its potential impact within an ecological model. They call this the *people and places model of social change* (**FIGURE 1-12**).

The people and places framework (PPF) asks, "What about the people, and what about the places, needs to be happening for all to be healthy?" Forces that affect people at the individual, social network, or community/population level are referred to as "people fields of influence." Forces that are linked to a higher administrative level (state, nation, world) are referred to as "place fields of influence." PPF suggests that business-to-business approaches and policy (legislative, corporate) advocacy mainly affect place fields of influence. Social marketing and health

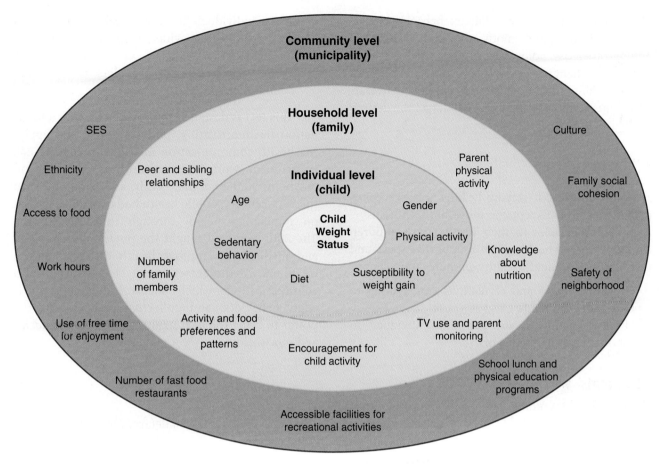

FIGURE 1-11 Ecological model for childhood obesity.

Modified from Gonzalez-Casanova I, Lucia Sarmiento O, Pratt M, et al. Individual, family, and community predictors of overweight and obesity among Colombian children and adolescents. *Prev Chronic Dis 2014*;11:140065. http://dx.doi.org/10.5888/pcd11.140065

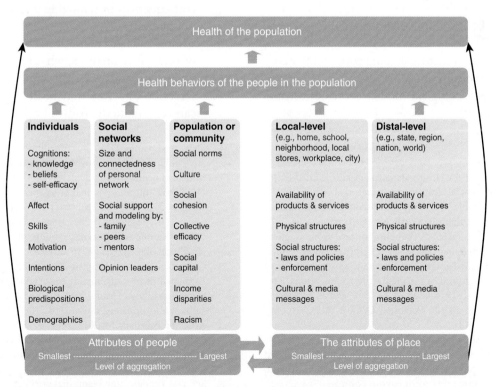

FIGURE 1-12 People and places framework.

Reproduced from Maibach EW, Abroms LC, Marosits M. Communication and marketing as tools to cultivate the public's health: a proposed "people and places" framework. *BMC Public Health*. 2007;7:88. https://doi.org/10.1186/1471-2458-7-88.

communication promote voluntary behavior change based on information, motivation, and self-efficacy, among other psychological processes, and are more effective at changing people fields. A health communicator can use this information to develop an overarching intervention strategy that will target the desired ecological level(s).

▶ Conclusion

It would be great if staying healthy was everyone's default position. Except for those born with insurmountable obstacles to their health, most children can achieve good health, given a supportive social and physical environment. Health communication can:

- Inform policies and regulations contributing to social determinants
- Educate, motivate, and persuade individuals to choose healthier behaviors

- Assist individuals to access health care, interact with healthcare providers, and follow healthcare instructions
- Work with healthcare providers to be better communicators

This text is designed to provide you with a foundation for appreciating, understanding, and applying health communication methods in educational, government, worksite, and healthcare settings, and maybe in your own life, family, and community. In the 19th century, public health had enormous impact on population health through infection control. The 20th century brought the power of technology and medicine to improve health through medical treatment. At the outset of the 21st century, health communication—which affects individual knowledge, behaviors, and collective policies—has the power to bring the next major changes in our health and our world.

Key Terms

Affordable Care Act of 2010 (ACA)
Ecological model
Ethnic identity
Gender

Healthy People 2020
Premature death
Quality-adjusted life expectancy
Race
Root cause analysis

Sex
Social determinants of health (SDH)

Chapter Questions

1. What are the differences between sex and gender?
2. Describe how factors shaping your identity contribute to health outcomes.
3. Using the ecological model, describe a health disparity.

4. Discuss femicide. What are some unanticipated consequences of removing girl infants from the population?
5. Choose a health condition. Using the technique of root cause analysis, what are some potential underlying causes for this condition?
6. Describe one way that health communication can contribute to positive health outcomes.

References

1. National Center for Health Statistics. Health, United States, 2015: with special feature on racial and ethnic health disparities. Table 15. http://www.cdc.gov/nchs/data/hus/hus15.pdf#015. Published 2016. Accessed February 14, 2018.
2. Squires, D, Anderson C. U.S. health care from a global perspective: spending, use of services, prices, and health in 13 countries. The Commonwealth Fund website. http://www.commonwealthfund.org/~/media/files/publications/issue-brief/2015/oct/1819_squires_us_hlt_care_global_perspective_oecd_intl_brief_v3.pdf. Published October 2015. Accessed February 14, 2018.
3. A guide to your genome. NIH Publication No. 07-6284. National Human Genome Research Institute website. https://www.genome.gov/pages/education/allaboutthehumangenomeproject/guidetoyourgenome07_vs2.pdf. Published 2007. Accessed February 14, 2018.
4. Stewart ST, Cutler DM. The contribution of behavior change and public health to improved US population health. National Bureau of Economic Research website. NBER Working Paper No. 20631. http://www.nber.org/papers/w20631. Published October 2014. Accessed February 14, 2018.
5. Singh GK, Siahpush M, Kogan MD. Neighborhood socioeconomic conditions, built environments, and childhood obesity. *Health Aff*. 2010;29(3):503-512.
6. Galea S, Tracy M, Hoggatt KJ, DiMaggio C, Karpati A. Estimated deaths attributable to social factors in the United States. *Am J Public Health*. 2011;101(8):1456-1465. http://ajph.aphapublications.org/doi/abs/10.2105/AJPH.2010.300086. Accessed February 14, 2018.
7. Social determinants of health. World Health Organization website. http://www.who.int/social_determinants/en/. Accessed July 29, 2016.
8. Sex and gender: how being male or female can affect your health. NIH News in Health. U.S. Department of Health and

Human Services website. https://newsinhealth.nih.gov/issue/may2016/feature1. Published May 2016. Accessed February 14, 2018.

9. Rosario VA. The history of aphallia and the intersexual challenge to sex/gender. In: Haggerty GE, McGarry M, eds. *A Companion to Lesbian, Gay, Bisexual, Transgender, and Queer Studies.* Wiley-Blackwell; Malden, MA: 2007:262-281. http://dx.doi.org/10.1002/9780470690864.ch13.

10. Kinsey A, Pomeroy W, Martin C, Gebhard P. *Sexual Behavior in the Human Female.* Philadelphia, PA and London, UK: W.B. Saunders; 1953. Cited by: American Psychological Association. Guidelines for psychological practice with lesbian, gay, and bisexual clients. *Am Psychol.* 2012;67(1): 10-42. doi:10.1037/a0024659.

11. Snow RC. *Sex, Gender and Vulnerability.* Population Studies Center Research Report 07-628. Ann Arbor, MI: Population Studies Center, University of Michigan; 2007.

12. Murthy P, Smith CL, eds. *Women's Global Health and Human Rights.* Sudbury, MA: Jones and Bartlett; 2010.

13. Hudson VM, den Boer AM. *Bare Branches: The Security Implications of Asia's Surplus Male Population.* Cambridge, MA: MIT Press; 2004:62. Cited by: Hudson VM, den Boer AM. Missing women and bare branches: gender balance and conflict. Environmental Change and Security Program report. 2005;11:20-24.

14. Substance Abuse and Mental Health Services Administration. *Top Health Issues for LGBT Populations Information & Resource Kit.* HHS Publication No. (SMA) 12-4684. Rockville, MD: Author; 2012:23.

15. Park H, Mykhyalyshyn I. L.G.B.T. people are more likely to be targets of hate crimes than any other minority group. *The New York Times.* June 16, 2016. http://www.nytimes.com/interactive/2016/06/16/us/hate-crimes-against-lgbt.html. Accessed June 16, 2016.

16. Barsh GS. What controls variation in human skin color? *PLoS Biol.* 2003;1(1):e27.

17. Jablonski NG. *Living Color: The Biological and Social Meaning of Skin Color.* Oakland, CA: University of California Press; 2014.

18. Impaired driving: get the facts. Centers for Disease Control and Prevention website. http://www.cdc.gov/motorvehiclesafety/impaired_driving/impaired-drv_factsheet.html. Updated April 15, 2016. Accessed July 25, 2016.

19. Center for Behavioral Health Statistics and Quality. Behavioral health trends in the United States: results from the 2014 National Survey on Drug Use and Health. HHS Publication No. SMA 15-4927, NSDUH Series H-50. Retrieved from http://www.samhsa.gov/data/sites/default/files/NSDUH-FRR1-2014/NSDUH-FRR1-2014.pdf. Published September 2015. Accessed February 14, 2018.

20. Lipari RN, Jean-Francois B. A day in the life of college students aged 18 to 22: substance use facts. *The CBHSQ Report.* Center for Behavioral Health Statistics and Quality website. http://www.samhsa.gov/data/sites/default/files/report_2361/ShortReport-2361.html. Published May 26, 2016. Accessed February 14, 2018.

21. Mapping life expectancy: short distances to large gaps in health. Robert Wood Johnson Foundation website. http://www.rwjf.org/en/library/articles-and-news/2015/09/city-maps.html. Published September 11, 2015. Accessed February 14, 2018.

22. Davison KK, Birch LL. Childhood overweight: a contextual model and recommendations for future research. *Obes Rev.* 2001;2(3):159-171.

23. Maibach EW, Abroms LC, Marosits M. Communication and marketing as tools to cultivate the public's health: a proposed "people and places" framework. *BMC Public Health.* 2007;7:88. https://doi.org/10.1186/1471-2458-7-88.

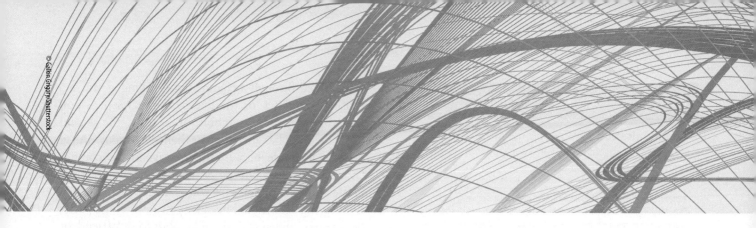

CHAPTER 2

Communication 101: What's Health Got to Do with It?

Sarah Bauerle Bass and Claudia Parvanta

LEARNING OBJECTIVES

By the end of this chapter, the reader will be able to:

- Define *communication* and *health communication*.
- Describe how the perceptual process affects communication.
- Identify key principles of information processing theory used in communication.
- Describe the factors that go into how people make decisions based on communication cues.
- Recognize factors influencing how nonscientific audiences process and understand scientific information.
- Describe how health communication is used to address different levels of health behavior.
- Identify numerous contexts in which health communication occurs.
- Describe how risk perception affects communication effects.

▶ Introduction

Communication is something we do every day, even if we are not talking. We are communicating when we stand quietly in an elevator with other people, when we go to the movies and scream during a horror film, when we are talking with our friend about an assignment that is due, when we are texting or posting to social media, and yes, when we phone home. Although we take these everyday occurrences for granted, our communication follows culturally specific principles of which we are mostly unaware. In this chapter, we will provide an overview of communication, describe some of the cognitive processes that allow us to communicate, and then discuss the basics of health communication.

▶ Communication

Think about all the times you have had a failure to communicate with someone: You order food and it does not come the way you asked for it, or you ask your friend to do something and they do not do what you asked. Often the problem is that you do not think the person responded "appropriately" to your instructions. These communication failures illustrate the point that communication travels back and forth between a sender and a receiver. The recipient's response is how we know that a message has been understood as intended. If the response resembles our expectations, we believe our communication was successful.

At its core, communication is how people perceive and use messages to generate common meaning (**BOX 2-1**). The term *meaning* is where we usually get into trouble. Meaning can change according to the context, the culture, and the channel used to convey a message. Think about this example:

> You meet someone new who does not make eye contact. The person only responds to your questions and does not initiate any communication. Later, you may think of that encounter and, judging from your own experience, decide this person was not interested in you, or was even being rude.
>
> Now consider that this encounter happened in a federal Special Supplemental Nutrition Program for Women, Infants, and Children clinic where you were the dietitian and the other person was a young Vietnamese mother meeting you for the first time. In her culture, it is a sign of respect to not make eye contact and not speak unless asked a question. The same situation could occur if you were a teacher and the individual was a young student from a culture with similar societal rules. How would you feel now about the interaction?

The Transactional Model of Communication

In communication, the devil is in the details, and often the details are misunderstood due to a breakdown in what is referred to as the **transactional model of communication**. As Barnlund emphasized in his original presentation of the transactional communication model, communication "…is not a reaction to something, nor an interaction with something, but a transaction in which man invents and attributes meaning to realize his purposes."[1] To simplify greatly, the way this meaning is generated is through a process of encoding and decoding. A first individual (the sender) puts thoughts into words, symbols, or gestures. This process is called *encoding*. The encoded message is then transmitted through a channel by speaking, gesturing, writing, signaling, or the like to the recipient. Upon receiving the words, symbols, or gestures, the second individual applies meaning to them—*decoding*. But it is not that simple, because the message may encounter "noise." Noise is any type of distortion or distraction. Some examples of noise for you as the recipient include not hearing the message because you are at a loud party; being preoccupied with thoughts about a sick friend; or not speaking the same language as the sender. Another example could be that in your country a raised middle finger means something rude and not "hi there". In addition, encoding and decoding are occurring simultaneously, meaning on both the sender side and the receiver side, making it more complicated. These barriers may then prevent the message from being received or fully understood, and miscommunication occurs.

Communication can be viewed as the transfer of symbolic information within a common symbol system. And that means that a symbol must be understood in the same way for those communicating. This can be difficult if the symbols change or are used differently. Think about slang language or texting language—they may mean different things to different people. Writing with ALL CAPS can be used for emphasis, but in social media the writer may be perceived to be angry or yelling. Ogden and Richards proposed the "semantic triangle" (**FIGURE 2-1**) to illustrate this issue.[2] It indicates that the concept evoked by a word may be different depending on the receiver. If you hear the word *mustang*, do you first think of an animal or a car? It really depends on the context in which the word is communicated and whether you even know that a mustang could also be the name of a car. The essential point is that if people do not share a common symbol system, communication will be difficult.

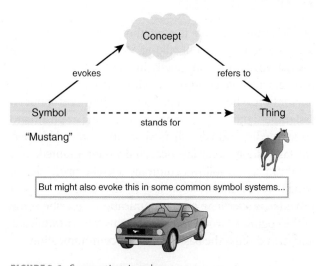

FIGURE 2-1 Semantic triangle.

It's All in Your Head

The field of communication has benefited from discoveries in psychology and neurology, but also extensively from artificial intelligence and information technology. The way we attend to and process stimuli—our perceptions—and the way we remember and assign meaning to these stimuli all have a bearing on our communication abilities.

Perceptual Process and Attribution Theory

Anaïs Nin, referring to an ancient religious text, penned, "We do not see things as they are, we see them as we are."[3] We can imagine two lovers looking at the Seine river flowing through Paris, and one sees a shimmering path and the other sees only dead fish and garbage. We can imagine that one was feeling happy and the other, maybe not so much. Mood is one of many factors that influence our ability to use our senses to take in information. **FIGURE 2-2** illustrates the **perceptual process** and the factors that operate to shape and sometimes distort perception.

Our perceptions are influenced by our internal attitudes, motives, experiences, and expectations. However, characteristics of the object being perceived (e.g., its motion, sounds, size, novelty) or the context of the situation (e.g., time, place, ambient conditions) can also influence perception. In fact, as we are in the act of perceiving an event or a behavior, we also are attempting to determine what brought it about, or its cause. The social psychological term for this calculation is *attribution*.

Attribution theory, which was developed by Weiner,[4] posits that when an individual observes an event or a behavior, the thought process goes something like this: Was what I just saw intentional? Is it caused by something internal to the individual or external to the individual? Weiner classified the mental calculations we make in this manner:

- *Distinctiveness:* Does this person behave in this manner in other situations?
- *Consensus:* Do other people behave in the same manner?
- *Consistency:* Does this person behave in the same manner at other times?

Here is an example: You are at a party and see your friend, James, smoking a cigarette. Your thoughts might go like this: Have I ever seen James smoking before (distinctiveness)? Is James with a group of other people who are smoking (consensus)? Have I been at other parties where I've seen James smoke (consistency)?

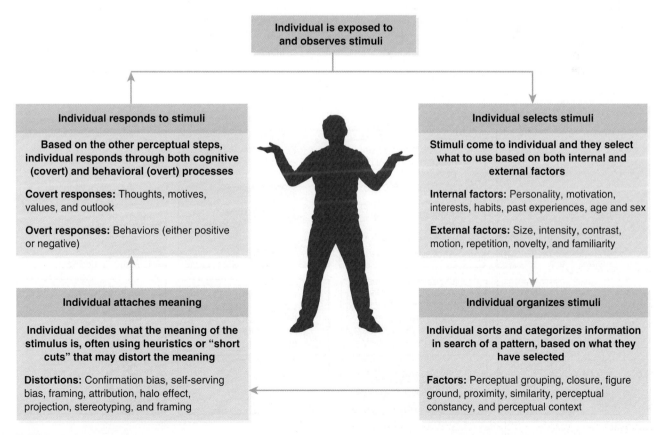

Individual is exposed to and observes stimuli

Individual responds to stimuli

Based on the other perceptual steps, individual responds through both cognitive (covert) and behavioral (overt) processes

Covert responses: Thoughts, motives, values, and outlook

Overt responses: Behaviors (either positive or negative)

Individual selects stimuli

Stimuli come to individual and they select what to use based on both internal and external factors

Internal factors: Personality, motivation, interests, habits, past experiences, age and sex

External factors: Size, intensity, contrast, motion, repetition, novelty, and familiarity

Individual attaches meaning

Individual decides what the meaning of the stimulus is, often using heuristics or "short cuts" that may distort the meaning

Distortions: Confirmation bias, self-serving bias, framing, attribution, halo effect, projection, stereotyping, and framing

Individual organizes stimuli

Individual sorts and categorizes information in search of a pattern, based on what they have selected

Factors: Perceptual grouping, closure, figure ground, proximity, similarity, perceptual constancy, and perceptual context

FIGURE 2-2 Perceptual process.

(See **FIGURE 2-3**.) If you come to the decision that your friend James only smokes when others are smoking at a party, you would decide that his smoking was intentional but "externally attributed," meaning that it was the party that contributed to him smoking. If instead you have seen James smoking in other environments, and not just at parties, the smoking is intentional, but "internally attributed," meaning that it is something he does all the time and is not being caused by some external factor.

Here is a second example, same party: You see your friend Amy, whom you have known to be a "goody two shoes" since childhood, very intoxicated. This is completely inconsistent with your concept of Amy. You look around and do not see others behaving in this manner (lack of consensus), but you notice that Amy is drinking something pink and sweet. You conclude that either Amy did not realize how much alcohol was in her drink, or worse, that somebody put something in her drink to make her so drunk or possibly drugged. So, you consider this behavior to be unintentional on Amy's part and externally attributed.

Cognitive Dissonance

You are still shaking your head over Amy and James, right? This is in part explained by a concept put forth by Leon Festinger called **cognitive dissonance**.[5] Humans tolerate inconsistencies poorly. We feel most comfortable when our affect (emotion), cognition (reasoning), and behavior are in harmony.[6] Misalignment of our thoughts, feelings, and behaviors results in an uncomfortable state—cognitive dissonance. To restore a state of comfort, we try to change the condition that is out of line with the others—change our attitudes and beliefs to align with our behavior, or change our behavior to align with our attitudes and beliefs (**FIGURE 2-4**).[7] James may experience cognitive

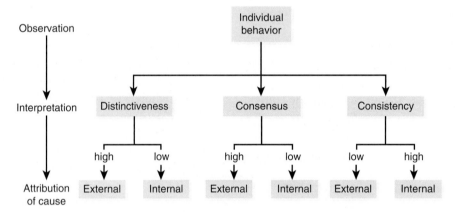

FIGURE 2-3 Attribution theory.

Robbins SP, Judge TA. *Organizational Behavior*. 15th ed. Upper Saddle River, NJ: Prentice Hall; 2013. Reprinted by permission of Pearson Education, Inc., New York, NY.

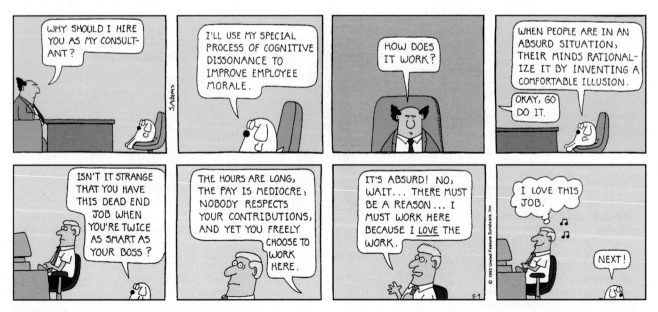

FIGURE 2-4 Cognitive dissonance.

dissonance if he enjoys smoking but also knows that smoking is bad for him. To reduce this dissonance, he can either change his behavior (stop smoking) or change his attitudes/beliefs about smoking ("I can get away with this because I'm still young and, besides, the risks are exaggerated"). A growing field of counseling psychology focuses on aligning self-identity with healthier behaviors (e.g., I'm the kind of person who loves fresh air), more than trying to modify behavior without an attitudinal adjustment. This approach has been adopted in communication efforts, as discussed later in this chapter.

Information Processing Theory

The preceding concepts (perception, attribution theory, and cognitive dissonance) have been a lot to take in. No wonder, because humans are limited in how much information they can process at one time. As infants, we learn to associate word units of sound (phonemes) and meaning (morphemes). Throughout our lives, there are millions of bits of new information passing by our sensory system daily—that is, all the sights, sounds, smells, tastes, and textures we either recognize as "information" or ignore. We also learn to pay attention and attach significance to some of those sights, smells, tastes, textures, and nonverbal sounds. By the time we reach adulthood, our brains have been literally reshaped by stimuli that underlie our knowledge, attitudes, and beliefs as well as by unrecognized cultural and environmental stimuli.

There are thousands of words, numbers, and other organized packets of information that reach us every day, some of which we are capable of processing for memory or action and some of which we are not. On top of our inherent human limitations, *individual* limitations also affect the ability to use complex information to varying degrees. One way the brain deals with information overload is by simplifying and linking new information to old. Once we have managed to learn something, we tend to rely on it as a kind of "shortcut" to interpret new information.

There is extensive literature on these shortcuts for decision making—logical rules or heuristics.[8] When faced with a complex problem, we tend to focus on one piece of information and draw inferences from it instead of analyzing an entire set of factors—most notably ignoring probability (the likelihood of an event) and denominators (the size of the population in which it is occurring). Some of these heuristics include the following:

- *Selective perception:* Interpretation of what we see based on our own interests, background, experiences, and attitudes and the tendency to overlook information that contradicts those beliefs. (Some

news channels and an increasing number of apps are designed from this perspective.)

- *Halo effect:* A general impression about someone/ something based on a single characteristic (e.g., eye color ["Scandinavian"] or height ["You must play basketball"]).
- *Contrast effect:* The comparative evaluation of a person, object, or characteristic as better, or worse, than our own (e.g., "They have a better smile than I do").
- *Projection:* Attribution of our own characteristics to others (e.g., "If I'm nice, they must be nice, too").
- *Representativeness:* How much a new perception resembles something that we have seen before, again based on a limited set of characteristics. This is a little complicated but works like this: We have a prototype in our head, attribute this to a class, consider whether the new perception belongs to this class, and then ascribe the prototype's characteristics to it (e.g., thinking every fresh herb will taste like mint). Recognition is based on similarity to a class prototype.
- *Stereotyping:* A form of representativeness based on our perception of the group to which we believe someone belongs (e.g., gender, profession, religion, or ethnicity).
- *Availability:* The use of only readily available information to make a decision. This happens when you estimate your chance of having a problem or condition by counting only how many of your friends have had something similar.
- *Anchoring and adjustment:* In quantitative situations, people start with a "ballpark" figure (the anchor) and adjust up or down to reach an estimate. These estimates can be wildly inaccurate and influenced by context. Tversky and Kahneman[9] gave the example of two groups of high school students given 5 seconds to estimate the product of either $8 \times 7 \times 6 \times 5 \times 4 \times 3 \times 2 \times 1$ or $1 \times 2 \times 3 \times 4 \times 5 \times 6 \times 7 \times 8$. The students who started with the higher numbers had a mean product estimate of 2250, whereas those who started at the lower end came up with 512. (The correct answer is 40,320.)

Heuristics help us, but they can also lead us to make decisions based on false or inadequate estimates.

Elaboration Likelihood Model

Building on the previous models, our ability to pay attention to new information is also affected by how much we care about it. The **elaboration likelihood model (ELM)**[10] suggests that if you are already engaged in an issue, you will pay more attention to new information about it. Women who are hoping to get pregnant will pay a lot of attention to information (e.g., advertising) about pregnancy or baby care, whereas women not interested in getting pregnant or who do not have a baby will not look twice at ads for diapers.

Without engagement, other stimuli are needed to grab our attention. An example is the use of appealing images to sell things like cologne or personal care products. Most of these ads are aimed at men who do not spend a lot of time thinking about shampoo and body wash. Appealing models may grab their awareness and cause them to pay attention to and "elaborate" the product information presented by the advertiser. **FIGURE 2-5** shows the model developed by Petty and Cacioppo,[10,11] which posits two routes by which we process and are persuaded by information: a *central route* and a *peripheral route*. In the central route, we are actively engaged in the topic and think about the information carefully (i.e., "elaborate" it), as we decide. In the peripheral route, we are less engaged in the topic, if at all. Other cues, usually culturally specific spokespersons, images, languages, sounds, and the like, are necessary to both get our attention and perhaps persuade us about the merits of a position. In the peripheral route, the cues may have no logical connection to the subject matter, but they help to form an emotional bridge to the information. The ELM suggests that most people will read the pamphlets their doctors give them if they have been diagnosed with a disease but will throw away materials that they feel do not pertain to them. A good example of this model is its use in the national folic acid campaign. The Centers for Disease Control and Prevention (CDC) and the March of Dimes have collaborated in a long-running campaign to prevent birth defects due to a lack of folic acid at the time of conception.[12] The original campaign segmented women of child-bearing age into two groups: women actively contemplating pregnancy and women who felt they were not ready to think about having children. Using ELM, the "pregnancy contemplators" were motivated to pay attention and elaborate on persuasive messages pertaining to childbirth because they were highly involved with the issue. Those who were "not ready" would tune out information pertaining to pregnancy. Ads featuring cute babies made no impression on them. To reach these women, a peripheral route would be necessary that featured other cues (images, music, role models) and messages that resonated with their attitudes toward being young and healthy. **FIGURE 2-6** shows the different communication strategies.

So, before knowing anything else about an individual or a group, and before concerning ourselves with a specific topic, what we have learned from our study of cognition and information processing theory suggests that the most successful communication will:

- Be simple
- Be brief
- Show clear lines of cause and effect
- Grab attention
- Take advantage of decision rules and heuristics

Perception, how we process information, and heuristics all influence not only how a message is received, but also whether someone chooses to act on that message. We will now look at how these basic principles are applied to *health* communication.

▶ Communicating About Health

We communicate all the time in our daily life (except, arguably, when we are asleep) and encounter health communication nearly as often. **BOX 2-2** shows examples of when and how we might encounter health communication.

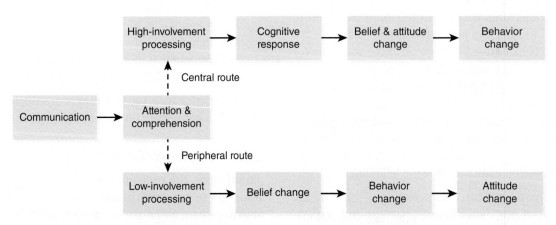

FIGURE 2-5 Elaboration likelihood model.

Modified from Petty RE, Cacioppo JT. The elaboration likelihood model of persuasion. *Adv Exp Soc Psychol*. 1986;19:123-205.

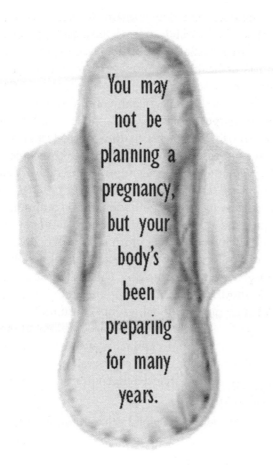

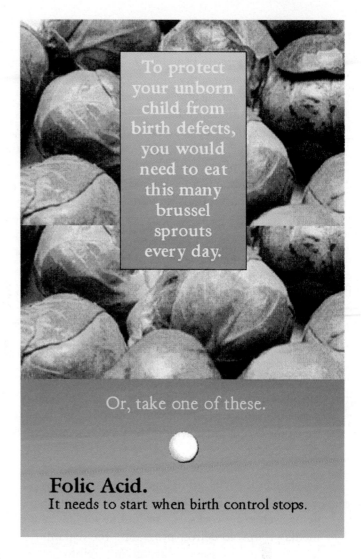

FIGURE 2-6 CDC and March of Dimes folic acid campaign.

Reproduced from Centers for Disease Control and Prevention. CDCynergy, Micronutrients Edition, Folic Acid Case Study. https://www.cdc.gov/healthcommunication/cdcynergy/editions.html

---

BOX 2-2 Examples of Health Communication in Daily Life

- Calling your mom on the phone for advice about your sore throat
- Seeing posters in the pharmacy to get your flu shot now
- Searching for information on the internet about symptoms you are experiencing
- Reading the flyer that came with your medications about how to take them correctly
- Noticing signs in the cafeteria that show the number of calories in each dish
- Hearing emergency TV or radio broadcasts from a local public health official about what to do during a hurricane, flood, or snowstorm
- Looking at advertising in magazines that shows "responsible drinking"
- Engaging in a social media platform that discusses contraceptive choices
- Signing up for health insurance or a clinical trial
- Finding your way in a hospital or clinic to your provider's office
- Seeing a television show or movie where someone flourishes through good health behavior or perishes due to poor health behavior choices
- Reading tweets from a celebrity about her special needs child and his progress
- Using an internet connection and camera to show your doctor the rash on your arm, from a rural location (i.e., telehealth)
- Participating in a worksite program to quit smoking
- Using a vending machine at school that offers water, low-calorie beverages, and fruit instead of junk food

Practitioners of health communication use what we know about strategic communication in its various forms to *engage* people in thinking about their health, to *inform* them about healthy choices, and to *persuade* them to adopt safe and healthy behaviors. A basic definition of health communication is "The study and use of communication strategies to inform and influence individual and community decisions that enhance health."[13] **BOX 2-3** offers other useful definitions of health communication from various experts.

Health communication functions on multiple levels.

- *Individual:* Effective health communication can raise an individual's awareness of health risks and solutions, provide motivation and skills, link one to a network of support, and create or strengthen positive attitudes. Health communication varies on where we are in what is called a continuum of care relative to disease: prevention (where we hope to stay for as long as possible), but if not, then diagnosis, treatment, hopefully survivorship, but also compassionate and effective end-of-life care. Often this type of communication is done in the context of a patient/individual and a healthcare provider.

- *Group:* Increasingly, health communication takes advantage of social groupings, such as religious congregations, beauty or barber shop clientele, gyms, schools, worksites, or online or social media groups, to deliver programs. The dynamics of group message sharing and reinforcement of positive behaviors make this approach particularly effective. Organizational partners, such as clubs or civic groups, businesses, government, or national organizations, also amplify the efforts of health communicators to reach larger numbers of people.

- *Community:* Effective health communication can influence policymakers and public opinion to make positive changes in the physical environment, increase the availability of healthy choices in the marketplace, and improve the delivery of healthcare services.

- *Society:* By influencing individual and community values and attitudes, health communication eventually helps create new norms for behavior and standards for quality that affect populations. Laws concerning indoor smoking, child safety seat use, and littering all came about through changing norms at the individual, group, community, and eventually societal level. Global opinions about climate change and national, state, and community standards for energy conservation and recycling also demonstrate health communication at a societal level.

The overarching role of health communication is to support the translation of science into practice and connect information about problems with potential solutions. This can occur at many levels (e.g., intrapersonal, interpersonal, group or organizational, societal), across many channels (e.g., face to face, mass media, social media, written), and in diverse social contexts (e.g., homes, schools, workplaces, hospitals, community groups, population).

BOX 2-3 Definitions of Health Communication

"Health communication is the study of messages that create meaning in relation to physical, mental, and social well-being."[14(p9)]

"Health communication encompasses the study and use of communication strategies to inform and influence individual and community decisions that enhance health. It links the domains of communication and health and is increasingly recognized as a necessary element of efforts to improve personal and public health. Health communication can contribute to all aspects of disease prevention and health promotion and is relevant in a number of contexts, including (1) health professional–patient relations, (2) individuals' exposure to, search for, and use of health information, (3) individuals' adherence to clinical recommendations and regimens, (4) the construction of public health messages and campaigns, (5) the dissemination of individual and population health risk information, that is, risk communication, (6) images of health in the mass media and the culture at large, (7) the education of consumers about how to gain access to the public health and health care systems, and (8) the development of telehealth applications."[15(p11-3)]

"Public health communication: The scientific development, strategic dissemination, and critical evaluation of relevant, accurate, accessible, and understandable health information communicated to and from intended audiences to advance the health of the public."[16]

Harrington, NG. Health communication: an introduction to theory, method and application. In: Harrington NG, ed. *Health Communication: Theory, Method and Application*. New York, NY: Routledge; 2015; U.S. Department of Health and Human Services. Health communication. In: *Healthy People 2010, Volume 1: Understanding and Improving Health*. 2nd ed. Washington DC: U.S. Government Printing Office; 2000:11.0-11.25; Healthpeople.gov website. Bernhardt JM. Communication at the core of effective public health. *Am J Public Health*. 2004;94(12):2051-2053.

Communicating About Health Using the Ecological Model

Remember that our health is affected by our physical environment, the limiting or enabling factors created by our society, as well as our own behavior and biology. Reciprocally, our physical condition and behavior affect the health and social welfare of others, and we obviously affect the physical environment. This is called the ecological model. Evidence has shown that interventions conducted on multiple levels of the ecological model are more effective than those focusing solely on one level. A good example of this multilevel approach is how communities have addressed the problem of smoking through a combination of taxes on cigarettes, national advertising, worksite cessation and education programs, community-based interventions, and the availability of medical cessation aids (e.g., nicotine gum, patches). **TABLE 2-1** illustrates how health

TABLE 2-1 Communication Interventions in the Ecological Model

Ecological Model Level	Primary Intervention	Communication Support
State, national, global	Policies, laws, treaties, "movements," emergencies **Examples:** Global tobacco and traffic safety efforts (WHO and Bloomberg Foundation), U.S. seat belt law, food fortification or enrichment regulations, smallpox or polio vaccination programs, border closing or quarantine to control epidemiologic outbreaks	Advocacy to create or maintain policy or law, national- and state-specific reinforcement advertising, incentive programs, package warnings and labels, government educational campaigns, social mobilization (e.g., national immunization days), multimedia emergency information campaign to advise and calm public
Living and working conditions	Environmental conditions, hours, policies **Examples:** Worker safety, time off and vacation policies, creation of walking paths, elimination of lead in gasoline and paint, availability of healthy food choices and healthcare services	Citizen or worker advocacy (multimedia) to improve conditions, awareness and promotion campaigns for improved facilities and services, state or local lead education campaigns, private-sector advertising for healthy food choices and services
Social, community, family	Social norms, elimination of social disparities, provision of community health and social services, cultural "rules" for group behavior **Examples:** Community Watch, day care, church ministries of health, volunteers	Social media campaigns; radio-, TV-, internet-, print-, or locale- (e.g., church, bar) based social marketing or promotional campaigns; opinion leaders and role models; public service announcements; health fairs; small media educational materials; reinforcement of norms through group processes
Individual behavior	Acquisition of beliefs, attitudes, motivation, self-efficacy, products, and services through social marketing, behavior change communications, paid advertising, or psychological counseling **Examples:** Individual wants to change behavior (e.g., stop smoking, lose weight) or gain knowledge about health (e.g., how to protect self from flu).	Multimedia decision aids; educational materials; guidelines; promotional advertising; reinforcement through home, healthcare providers, and the community
Individual biology, physiology	Prevention or treatment of illness **Examples:** Individual wants to prevent or treat illness (e.g., screening testing, visiting healthcare provider).	Behavior change communication to maintain or establish good health habits, reminders for screening, healthcare provider communication during office visits

communication strategies can be applied at different levels of the ecological model.

An ecological approach to health communication suggests that all factors affecting a situation should be explored and that upstream factors be considered prior to efforts to change individual behavior. This applies to healthcare provider communication in clinical settings as much as to health-related media campaigns. Obviously, communication alone cannot change some systemic determinants of poor health, such as toxic waste, a poor social environment, limited healthcare resources, or poverty. Even though health communicators are not all-powerful, our responsibilities run deeper than we might think. If individuals who need critical information to protect their health are not seeking or receiving it, understanding it, or being moved to action, we can use health communication to change the situation. This can be done on multiple levels, from the clinical encounter to community-based or media-based messaging. If policymakers who determine national, state, and local laws, regulations, and public services have not received crucial information or been moved to action, we can use policy communication and advocacy to promote change.

Challenges to Effective Health Communication

Designing information to be "clear, compelling, actionable, and available to all who need it…" (personal communication, Katherine Lyon Daniel, Associate Director for Communication, CDC) is hard work! We face many challenges in being effective health communicators.

We previously mentioned several of the psychological processes that determine whether we even notice new information, as well as how quickly, or completely, we process it. Equally educated and linguistically competent individuals will still process information in their own order, speed, and time span. So, even when communicating with audiences we believe to be homogenous, we may need to create multiple versions of messages and materials, and extend the time we allow for communication activities.

There are many at-risk consumers who have limited access to relevant health information, including the elderly, immigrants, and those with low socioeconomic status, limited literacy, and disabilities. These groups may have barriers to accessing information, especially if online, or understanding information because of cognitive deficits or linguistic abilities.

Finally, we need to pay special attention to culture and belief systems. As noted earlier, communication can occur only if people share a common symbol system. If beliefs, values, and expectations are not shared, a shared meaning of health communication messages is less likely. Many people are simply not motivated to seek out health information, deliberately ignore it when it is presented to them, and possibly negate it when forced to confront it. Some of this behavior is externally attributed, such as belonging to social groupings that demand unhealthy or risky behavior for membership. In this case, the health communicator must work at the group or community level to shift societal norms and attitudes.

A growing challenge is the multitudes of information sources, from traditional media to an almost inexhaustible amount on the internet and social media. Too many people accept individual anecdotes as "trends" and rumors as facts when they see them repeated frequently. In contrast to the flood of dubious information, healthcare providers lament the lack of time they now have available to educate patients. As one primary care physician remarked, "The days when I would have said a patient's best source of information is their personal physician are long gone. Other healthcare providers might have more time to spend, but physicians are really on a clock these days" (Danine Fruge, MD, personal communication, September 12, 2016). So, choosing an amount of information that can be relayed during a healthcare appointment and ensuring it is appropriate to the patient's needs also require thought.

Risk and Risk Perception

We previously laid out many of the information-processing foibles that affect communication, including the fact that most people do not consider computed probabilities and population size when thinking about risk. This has a critical bearing on health communication, both when we are trying to gain attention for prevention messages and particularly when we are dealing with presentation of risk. This is called **risk perception**. We use risk comparisons in health care for patients to evaluate the relative value of different procedures or treatments, to explain the likelihood of contracting chronic illness, and to estimate the dangers of environmental contaminants. Presenting these risks during an emergency is one of the most challenging aspects of health communication, engendering an entire field (crisis and risk communication).

Most health risk discussions concern causality (Does A [thing] cause B [disease]?) or risk (If you are exposed to A, what is your likelihood of contracting disease B?). The Environmental Protection Agency (EPA) developed a framework for distinguishing among hazard and risk, exposure, and toxicity, as shown in **BOX 2-4**.

The distinctions in Box 2-4 are important. Toxicity is innate to a substance, whereas hazard, risk, and exposure are situation specific. For example, chlorine

BOX 2-4 EPA Framework for Risk

Hazard: Any source of potential damage or harm or adverse outcome. For example, a substance (such as benzene), source of energy (e.g., electricity), process (e.g., crossing the street) or condition (e.g., wet floor).
Risk: The chance or probability that a person will be harmed or experience an adverse outcome if exposed to the hazard.
Exposure: Contact with a hazard. Exposure varies by the manner of exposure (breathing in, skin contact, whole body) and the quantity of time spent in an exposed condition.
Toxicity: The intrinsic ability of a substance to cause adverse health effects.

Reproduced from U.S. Environmental Protection Agency. *Risk Assessment Guidance for Superfund (RAGS)*. Washington, DC: Environmental Protection Agency; 1989.

is a gas that was used in warfare as a poison. In much smaller doses, we use it to keep our water safe and whiten our wash. Many in risk assessment use the criteria developed by Hill[17] to demonstrate a causal association between environmental risks and disease, as shown in **TABLE 2-2**.

Scientists make the distinctions outlined in Table 2-2 concerning hazards and risks, and apply the criteria defined by Hill when assessing actual risk probabilities. The public, on the other hand, uses little of this thinking when considering risk. In some cases, the public greatly overestimates the risk and demands costly and difficult interventions. In other cases, the public may greatly underestimate the risk and ignore recommendations that might have a substantial impact on their health. A good example of this is the flu and getting vaccinated. Most people greatly underestimate their risk of getting the flu, or believe that if they do get it, it is not a big deal. But the CDC estimates that between 10 and 35 million people get the flu every year, 200,000 are hospitalized, and 12,000 to 56,000 die.[18] Yet less than half of adults and just 60% of children get vaccinated.

We have learned a great deal about how the public at large, which has not studied statistics or probabilities, responds to risk information. To begin, people tend to believe that the members of their own community are all above average but that others are not. An example comes from a survey conducted for the Allstate insurance company. Of the 885 licensed U.S. drivers surveyed, 64% rated themselves as "excellent" or "very good" drivers. In the same survey, more than 70% admitted that "as a result of being distracted while driving, I have slammed the brakes or swerved to avoid an accident, missed a traffic signal, or actually caused an accident."[19] The clear majority of respondents (91%) did not connect that the fact they texted, listened to music with headphones, ate, put on makeup, or engaged in other distractions while driving might mean they were less than a "very good driver." By the way, only 29% thought their friends were excellent or very good drivers. This positive self-opinion in the language of risk is called **optimism bias**.

As we described in our discussion of information-processing heuristics, we use another set of rationalizations to manage what might be an overwhelming number of potential hazards in our everyday life. The *more we know* about a risk, the *less likely* we believe it will happen to us. For example, we know now that smoking causes lung cancer, but among smokers, few believe they will get the disease. A form of cognitive dissonance, we *attenuate* or lessen the risk because this allows us to cope with the many risks and events we encounter every day.

Peter Sandman, a specialist in risk perception and risk communication, says, "The risks that kill you are not necessarily the risks that anger and frighten you."[20] Fear is a basic human emotion, grounded in a biological necessity to protect ourselves from danger. What this means is that if a risk occurs that we do not know a lot about, and about which we are likely to feel "outrage," our perception of that risk is higher because we are fearful, even if the real or actual risk is low. A good example of this is the Ebola outbreak of 2014.

Ebola is a life-threatening infection that has a high mortality rate, but before 2014, outbreaks were contained in rural locations in central Africa. However, the 2014 outbreak occurred in large urban centers in Western Africa, such as Monrovia, Liberia, and affected more than 28,000 people, killing over 11,000.[21] In the United States, just four people were infected, all of whom contracted the virus either in West Africa or when they cared for a patient who was infected in West Africa. Despite an estimate of contracting Ebola in the United States of 1 in 13.3 million,[22] a significant portion of the U.S. public viewed Ebola as a real health threat. An October 2014 Pew Research Center survey found that 41% of respondents were worried that they or someone in their family would be exposed to the virus, including 17% who said they were very worried.[23] As a result, some of the reactions included airline cleaners walking off the job for fear of contamination, parents pulling children out of school because the principal had visited Zambia (which is not located in West Africa, and had no Ebola cases), healthcare workers quarantined against their will in

TABLE 2-2 Important Considerations for Assessing Causality: Hill's Criteria

Label	Meaning	Rules of Evidence
Strength of association	What is the magnitude of relative risk?	The probability of a causal association increases as the summary relative risk estimate increases. Hill himself was suspicious of relative risks less than two. Others have set the limits higher; however, a relative risk less than two does not rule out the possibility of causality.
Dose–response	Does a correlation exist between exposure and effect?	A regularly increasing relationship between dose and magnitude is indicative of a causal association. This works for bad things, such as the greater the exposure to radiation, the worse your symptoms (usually). It also works for things we are trying to measure in behavior change, such as if you are exposed to 10 advertisements as opposed to 1, will your behavior be any different?
Consistency of response	How many times has this effect been reported in various populations under similar conditions?	The probability of a causal association increases as the proportion of studies with similar (e.g., positive) results increases.
Temporally correct association	Does the exposure precede the effect, or does the occurrence of the disease show the appropriate latency?	Exposure to a causal factor *must* precede the effect. This is an *immutable requirement* that is often ignored.
Specificity of the association	How specific is this effect? Do many things influence the effect?	For uncommon health effects (e.g., liver cancer), this evidence can be useful. For diseases with many causes, it is of little use.
Biological plausibility	Is the mechanism of action known or reasonably postulated?	Although a mechanism of action is not a requirement for determining causality, the finding of causality should not be biologically implausible. In contrast, a plausible mechanism of action or other supportive evidence increases the probability of a causal association.
Coherence	Does the cause–effect interpretation seriously conflict with generally known facts of the natural history and biology of the disease?	See the previous entry for biological plausibility.
Experimental evidence	Do laboratory animals show a similar effect?	As in the previous two criteria, findings in laboratory animals are supportive of a causal association. However, materials such as cigarettes, benzene, and arsenic that are notably carcinogenic to humans have all tested negative in animal studies.
Analogy	Do structurally similar chemicals cause similar effects?	For some classes of compounds, such as nitrosamines, structure-activity predictions can be supportive of a causal association. In contrast, materials such as organotins do not lend themselves to cross-class extrapolations.

Data from Friis RH, Sellers TA. *Epidemiology for Public Health Practice*. Gaithersburg, MD: Aspen Publishers; 1999; U.S. Department of Health, Education, and Welfare, Public Health Service. *Smoking and Health: Report of the Advisory Committee to the Surgeon General of the Public Health Service*. PHS Publication No. 1103. Washington, DC: Government Printing Office; 1964; 1103.; Hill AB. The environment and disease: association or causation? *Proc R Soc Med*. 1965;58:295-300.

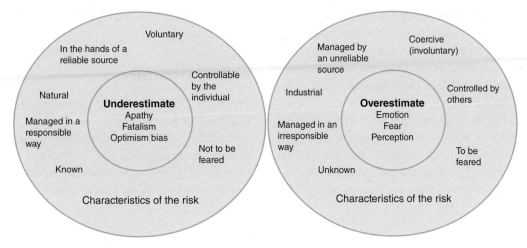

FIGURE 2-7 Public estimation of hazards and risk.
Modified from Slovic P. Perception of risk. *Science.* 1987;236:280–285.

spite of negative (i.e., no exposure) test results, and the U.S. government appointing an "anti-Ebola czar" to oversee U.S.-based efforts to prevent an outbreak.[24] One CNN commentator called the public reaction "fear-bola."[25] So why this response to something that would be so unlikely? The answer is risk perception. **FIGURE 2-7** shows how the public perceives various hazards.

People tend to *underestimate* their risk if the hazard is:

- *Voluntary/chosen:* A risk that we choose to take seems less hazardous than one imposed upon us. For example, you may be angry about people texting or looking at their cell phones while driving, but when you do it, it is "different" because you believe you do it safely and are less likely to suffer negative consequences of the action. You are choosing to text and drive, and this allows you to think it is less risky.
- *Natural:* If the hazard comes from a natural event, we think it is less likely to hurt us. Compare the radiation we are exposed to from the sun vs. radiation that we may be exposed to from a cell phone. Although the sun causes the highest number of cancer cases a year (skin), we may fear radiation from a cell phone because it seems scarier, even though there is little evidence that it causes brain cancer.
- *Known:* Risks that are known and we have experience with are less likely to be concerning to us than new or "exotic" risks, even if the known risk is more hazardous. As mentioned previously, few people worry about getting the flu, despite it causing up to 12,000 deaths a year in the United States.[26] Compare that to the reaction to Ebola in the United States, which caused only one death.

- *Trusted:* The more confidence we have in those who are responsible for our protection, the less we feel worried about the effect on us. As trust of government and public officials goes down, the more we feel we might be personally impacted.
- *Controlled:* The more we think that the response to the risk is being managed well and the agencies responsible are being honest, the less at-risk we feel.

On the other hand, people tend to *overestimate* risk if the risk is perceived as opposite of these characteristics. Other things that cause overestimation of risk include the following:

- *Dread:* Which idea frightens you more: being eaten by a shark or dying of heart disease? Your risk of being bitten by a shark in your lifetime is 1 in 3,748,067,[27] whereas your risk of dying of heart disease is 1 in 4.[28] Heart disease is, in fact, the number one killer of people in the United States. Despite this, often the most feared deaths are the ones that worry us the most, despite the low odds of them happening.
- *Childhood impact:* The survival of the species depends on the survival of its offspring; risks to children appear to be more serious than the same risks to adults. For example, finding asbestos in the walls of a school will cause more outrage and fear than finding asbestos in a workplace.
- *Personal impact:* Any risk can seem greater to us if we or others close to us are the victims. If a close friend has had colon cancer, we think that our risk of having colon cancer is higher, despite there being no evidence of this.
- *Previous exposure:* When we can remember a previous risk, the future risk is easier to imagine and seems greater. If we have had a fire in our house, we may fear it happening again and think our risk is higher than it is.

■ *Rarity:* Unusual events, such as a nuclear accident, are perceived as riskier than more commonplace risks, such as a car accident. Such unusual events are more fear-producing than everyday occurrences, even though our chances of being in a car accident are far higher.

■ *Fairness:* People who feel that they are at higher risk because of who they are or where they live may believe that things are not "fair." For example, if a chemical plant is in a poor neighborhood, the residents may feel they are at a higher risk to develop cancer, even if evidence does not support that fear.

▶ Conclusion

We have discussed what communication is, what might affect it, and how it relates to health. The evolution of the health communication field has produced numerous approaches for practitioners to engage, inform, and persuade individuals about personal-, group-, and community-level health.

Key Terms

Attribution theory
Cognitive dissonance
Elaboration likelihood model (ELM)

Optimism bias
Perceptual process
Risk perception

Transactional model of communication

Chapter Questions

1. Using the transactional model of communication, describe the process of message exchange among communicators.
2. Why do actual risk and risk perception tend to differ from one another?
3. What characteristics of risk affect the perception of a particular risk?
4. What is health communication, and how is it used?
5. Give an example of effective health communication for the individual and for the greater community.
6. What are the implications of failing to consider the ecological model when shaping interventions health communicators consider and choose?

References

1. Barnlund DC. A transactional model of communication. In: Akin J, Goldberg A, Myers G, Stewart J, eds. *Language Behavior: A Book of Readings in Communication*. Paris: Mouton; 1970:47-57.
2. Ogden CK, Richards IA. *The Meaning of Meaning*. New York: Harcourt, Brace; 1923.
3. Nin A. *Seduction of the Minotaur*. Chicago, IL: Swallow Press; 1961:124.
4. Weiner B. Attribution theory, achievement motivation, and the educational process. *Rev Educ Res*. 1972;42(2):203-215.
5. Festinger L. *A Theory of Cognitive Dissonance*. Stanford, CA: Stanford University Press; 1957.
6. Kendrick DT, Neuberg SL, Cialdini RB. *Social Psychology: Goals in Interaction*. 5th ed. Boston, MA: Allyn & Bacon; 2010:167.
7. McLeod SA. Cognitive dissonance. Simply Psychology website. http://www.simplypsychology.org/cognitive-dissonance.html. Updated 2014. Accessed February 16, 2018.
8. Kahneman D, Slovic P, Tversky A. *Judgment Under Uncertainty: Heuristics and Biases*. Cambridge, UK: Cambridge University Press; 1982.
9. Tversky A, Kahneman D. Judgment under uncertainty: heuristics and biases. *Science*. 1974;185(4157):1124-1131.
10. Petty RE, Cacioppo JT. The elaboration likelihood model of persuasion. *Adv Exp Soc Psychol*. 1986;19:123-205.
11. Petty RE, Cacioppo JT. Source factors and the elaboration likelihood model of persuasion. *Adv Consum Res*. 1984;11:668-672.
12. Centers for Disease Control and Prevention. Media campaign implementation kit. http://www.cdc.gov/ncbddd/folicacid/documents/mediacampaignkit.pdf. Revised April 2002. Accessed February 16, 2018.
13. U.S. Department of Health and Human Services, National Institutes of Health, National Cancer Institute. Making health communication programs work. http://www.cancer.gov/publications/health-communication/pink-book.pdf. Published 2004. Accessed February 16, 2018.
14. Harrington, NG. Health communication: an introduction to theory, method and application. In: Harrington NG, ed. *Health Communication: Theory, Method and Application*. New York, NY: Routledge; 2015.
15. U.S. Department of Health and Human Services. Health communication. In: *Healthy People 2010, Volume 1: Understanding and Improving Health*. 2nd ed. Washington DC: U.S. Government Printing Office; 2000:11.0-11.25.
16. Bernhardt JM. Communication at the core of effective public health. *Am J Public Health*. 2004;94(12):2051-2053.
17. Hill AB. The environment and disease: association or causation? *Proc R Soc Med*. 1965;58:295-300.
18. Centers for Disease Control and Prevention. Disease burden of influenza. CDC website. https://www.cdc.gov/flu/about

/disease/burden.htm. Published May 16, 2017. Accessed February 16, 2018.

19. Allstate. New Allstate survey shows Americans think they are great drivers—habits tell a different story. Allstate Newsroom website. https://www.allstatenewsroom.com/news /new-allstate-survey-shows-americans-think-they-are -great-drivers-habits-tell-a-different-story/2011. Published August 2, 2011. Accessed February 16, 2018.

20. Sandman P. Risk communication: facing public outrage. *EPA J.* 1987;13(9):21-22.

21. Centers for Disease Control and Prevention. 2014–2016 Ebola outbreak in West Africa. Ebola (Ebola Virus Disease) webpage. http://www.cdc.gov/vhf/ebola/outbreaks/2014-west -africa/. Updated June 22, 2016. Accessed February 16, 2018.

22. Doucleff M. What's my risk of catching Ebola? NPR Goats and Soda website. http://www.npr.org/sections /goatsandsoda/2014/10/23/358349882/an-answer-for -americans-who-ask-whats-my-risk-of-catching-ebola. Published October 23, 2014. Accessed February 16, 2018.

23. Pew Research Center. Ebola worries rise, but most are 'fairly' confident in government, hospitals to deal with disease. Pew Research Center website. http://www.people-press .org/2014/10/21/ebola-worries-rise-but-most-are-fairly -confident-in-government-hospitals-to-deal-with-disease. Published October 21, 2014. Accessed February 16, 2018.

24. Huang Y. Are Americans overreacting to the Ebola virus? Forbes website. http://www.forbes.com/sites/yanzhonghuang /2014/10/21/are-americans-overreacting-to-the-ebola -virus/#103adeaa1b46. Published October 21, 2014. Accessed February 16, 2018.

25. Ford S, Thurman S. Fear-bola: Experts say Ebola hysteria is an epic overreaction. WJLA website. http://wjla.com/news /health/fear-bola-experts-say-ebola-hysteria-is-an-epic -overreaction-108262. Published October 20, 2014. Accessed February 16, 2018.

26. Centers for Disease Control and Prevention. Estimating seasonal influenza-associated deaths in the United States. Influenza (Flu) website. http://www.cdc.gov/flu/about /disease/us_flu-related_deaths.htm. Published May 26, 2016. Accessed February 16, 2018.

27. Gleason M. Nat Geo WILD: what are the odds? Some surprising shark attack stats. National Geographic website. http://voices.nationalgeographic.com/2011/11/22/nat-geo -wild-what-are-the-odds-some-surprising-shark-attack -stats/. Published November 22, 2011. Accessed February 16, 2018.

28. Centers for Disease Control and Prevention. Heart disease facts. Heart Disease website. http://www.cdc .gov/heartdisease/facts.htm. Updated November 28, 2017. Accessed February 16, 2018.

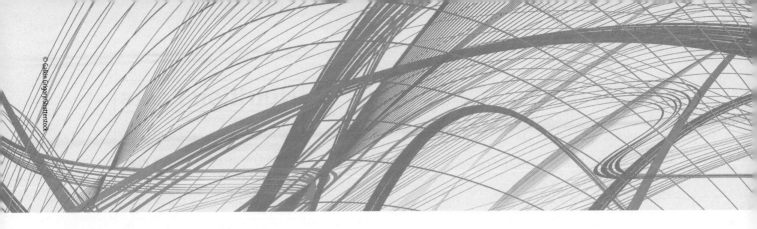

CHAPTER 3

Getting It Right: Words, Numbers, and Meaning

Claudia Parvanta

LEARNING OBJECTIVES

By the end of this chapter, the reader will be able to:

- Explain how the ability to read and understand information affects health decision making.
- Explain how cultural views define meaning.
- Define basic literacy, health literacy, and numeracy.
- Describe the factors that affect health literacy.
- Define the current state of health literacy in the United States.
- Discuss health literacy policy initiatives in the United States.
- Describe tools for assessing health literacy in research and practice.
- Apply readability tools.
- Understand how to use the Clear Communication Index to rate and revise materials.

▶ Introduction

Scenario 1

*H*ello, Patient X. Time for a test. Please take a look at this card and follow these directions:

Le voy a mostrar tarjetas con tres palabras en ellas. Primero, me gustaría que usted leyera la palabra arriba en voz alta. Entonces, yo leeré las dos palabras debajo a usted y me gustaría que usted me dijera cuál de las dos palabras es más similar a la palabra arriba. Si usted no sabe la respuesta, por favor diga, "No sé." No adivine.

Oh, wait. The instructions are in Spanish and you don't speak Spanish. (Lucky you, if you do.) OK, here they are in English:

I'm going to show you cards with three words on them. First, I'd like you to read the top word out loud. Next, I'll read the two words underneath, and I'd like you to tell me which of the two words is more similar to or has a closer association with the top word. If you don't know, please say, "I don't know." Don't guess.

So, here are the words on the first card:

<u>**Empleo**</u>

Trabajo

Educación

Which word, *trabajo* or *educación*, is most like empleo?

Oh, darn. They're still in Spanish. But that one was pretty easy, you should be able to figure it out. No? OK, let's see if we can find something that works better for you. How about this:

雇用

工作

教育

That's not any better, huh? I suppose you have some problems reading, so we'll just note that you have low health literacy in your patient record. OK, the doctor will see you now.

Scenario 2

Please look at the food labels in FIGURE 3-1 and answer this question: You are trying to be healthy and get the most nutrition out of everything you eat. You're also trying not to eat too much fat, sugar, or salt these days. You have two products available to eat with the food labels shown in Figure 3-1A and 3-1B. You're also really hungry and are going to eat half the box of whichever product you choose. Which one is the "healthier" choice, and why?

Comparison of Scenario 1 and Scenario 2

The first example is obviously exaggerated to give you the feeling of having limited proficiency in a language and being asked to complete a standard assessment of **health literacy** in your doctor's office. In fact, the "Short Assessment of Health Literacy,"[1] on which this question is modeled, can be used to determine if you need additional resources to understand your medical information. It can be administered in several different languages. Your healthcare provider might also just ask you if you want some help reading medical

A

Nutrition Facts

8 servings per container
Serving Size 2/3 cup (55g)

Amount per serving
Calories 230

	% Daily Value*
Total Fat 8g	**10%**
Saturated Fat 1g	**5%**
Trans Fat 0g	
Cholesterol 0mg	**0%**
Sodium 160mg	**7%**
Total Carbohydrate 37g	**13%**
Dietary Fiber 4g	**14%**
Total Sugars 12g	
Includes 10g Added Sugars	**20%**
Protein 3g	
Vitamin D 2mcg	10%
Calcium 260mg	20%
Iron 8mg	45%
Potassium 235mg	6%

* The % Daily Value (DV) tells you how much a nutrient in a serving of food contributes to a daily diet. 2,000 calories a day is used for general nutrition advice.

B

Nutrition Facts

Serving Size 2/3 cup (55g)
Servings Per Container About 8

Amount Per Serving

Calories 230	Calories from Fat 72
	% Daily Value*
Total Fat 8g	**12%**
Saturated Fat 1g	**5%**
Trans Fat 0g	
Cholesterol 0mg	**0%**
Sodium 160mg	**7%**
Total Carbohydrate 37g	**12%**
Dietary Fiber 4g	**16%**
Sugars 12g	
Protein 3g	
Vitamin A	10%
Vitamin C	8%
Calcium	20%
Iron	45%

*Percent Daily Values are based on a 2,000 calorie diet. Your daily values may be higher or lower depending on your calorie needs:

		Calories:	2,000	2,500
Total Fat	Less than		65g	80g
Sat Fat	Less than		20g	25g
Cholesterol	Less than		300mg	300mg
Sodium	Less than		2,400mg	2,400mg
Total Carbohydrate			300g	375g
Dietary Fiber			25g	30g

FIGURE 3-1 **A.** The new nutritional label. **B.** The old nutritional label.

instructions, or what grade in school you completed, but neither of these approaches is best, as we will discuss in this chapter.

In the case of the food label, this is the kind of challenge you encounter when grocery shopping or, increasingly, when you dine out. It assesses not only your ability to interpret the information on the food label, but also what you think is a healthy diet, which is culturally constructed. The test also measures your computational skills, which is referred to as **numeracy**.

You can probably think of many examples when your concepts about health as well as your abilities to process complex information are tested. Even watching TV or seeing an internet ad with the latest weight loss miracle tests more than your gullibility. The simplest health message assumes a common reference frame for what is desirable, as well as a shared vocabulary. But often neither of these two conditions is true, causing a lack of understanding and potentially fatal mistakes.

This chapter describes how individuals use language, math, and culturally derived frames of reference and knowledge to navigate a complex world of health-related decisions. We also discuss how health communicators can make navigating that world easier and more meaningful for their patients, clients, or the public.

▶ Health Literacy Basics

What Is Health Literacy?

Health literacy is a combination of capacity and skills to access and use information to make decisions affecting health. As described in **BOX 3-1**, individuals require a certain amount of linguistic and numeric skill in order to accomplish their goals to be healthy, take care of others (such as children or elderly parents), or seek health care.

Box 3-1 also asserts that it is up to communicators, whether working in a hospital, a pharmacy, a grocery store, or an organization, to skillfully use audiovisual or other media and their own words to help their audiences understand and use health information. After years of research, we have developed the philosophy that health literacy is not an individual "deficit," but it is the right of individuals to understand and be understood in the health arena.[2] As such, it requires a system-wide approach.

The **Affordable Care Act of 2010**[3] adopted the National Library of Medicine's definition of health literacy (in Box 3-1), and contains provisions that identify four areas to be addressed[4]:

1. Healthcare delivery system research and quality improvement
2. Facilitation of shared decision making (SDM) between patients and providers
3. Presentation of prescription drug benefits and risk information
4. Training of practitioners across all healthcare fields

In response to these direct provisions, as well as numerous indirect references in the law, the U.S. Department of Health and Human Services created the National Action Plan to Improve Health Literacy

---

BOX 3-1 Definition of Health Literacy

The Patient Protection and Affordable Care Act of 2010, Title V, defines *health literacy* as the degree to which an individual has the capacity to obtain, communicate, process, and understand basic health information and services to make appropriate health decisions.

Anyone who *needs* health information and services also needs health literacy skills to:

- Find information and services
- Communicate their needs and preferences and respond to information and services
- Process the meaning and usefulness of the information and services
- Understand the choices, consequences, and context of the information and services
- Decide which information and services match their needs and preferences so they can act

Anyone who *provides* health information and services to others, such as a doctor, nurse, dentist, pharmacist, or public health worker, also needs health literacy skills to:

- Help people find information and services
- Communicate about health and health care
- Process what people are explicitly and implicitly asking for
- Understand how to provide useful information and services
- Decide which information and services work best for different situations and people so they can act

Reproduced from What is health literacy? Centers for Disease Control and Prevention website. http://www.cdc.gov/healthliteracy/learn/index.html. Updated December 13, 2016. Accessed February 17, 2018.

1. Develop and disseminate health and safety information that is accurate, accessible, and actionable
2. Promote changes in the healthcare system that improve health information, communication, informed decision making, and access to health services
3. Incorporate accurate, standards-based, and developmentally appropriate health and science information and curricula in child care and education through the university level
4. Support and expand local efforts to provide adult education, English language instruction, and culturally and linguistically appropriate health information services in the community
5. Build partnerships, develop guidance, and change policies
6. Increase basic research and the development, implementation, and evaluation of practices and interventions to improve health literacy
7. Increase the dissemination and use of evidence-based health literacy practices and interventions

(NAP) in 2010.[5] The plan encourages a cross-section of society to work together to improve health literacy. The NAP is based on two core principles:

- All people have the right to health information that helps them make informed decisions.
- Health services should be delivered in ways that are easy to understand and that improve health, longevity, and quality of life.

The NAP has seven goals, which can be seen in **BOX 3-2**.

We will discuss application of the NAP's goals in various domains in the following sections. But first, why did the U.S. government make health literacy such a high priority in the delivery of health care?

Why Health Literacy Matters

Good health literacy allows us to have a greater understanding of our own health status as well as how to prevent illness. Those with adequate health literacy are more likely to:

- Participate in preventive healthcare measures
- Understand the need for early detection and management of disease
- Use healthcare services more efficiently
- Comply better with our treatment plans

Negative Effects of Poor Health Literacy

Mortality rates are higher among persons with lower health literacy. Why? Because they tend to[6-8]:

- Be less likely to get preventive screenings, such as for colon, breast, and cervical cancer
- Be less likely to immunize themselves against seasonal flu, pneumonia (for the elderly), and preventable diseases in children

- Have difficulty taking medications properly or interpreting labels and health messages
- Misunderstand or not respond appropriately to public health emergencies
- Have more trouble accessing health insurance

In addition, compared to those with proficient health literacy, adults with low health literacy tend to:

- Make more frequent use of the emergency department
- Incur 4 times higher annual healthcare costs ($13,000 vs. $3000)
- Have 6% more frequent hospital visits
- Spend 2 days longer in the hospital

The total costs of poor health literacy in the United States are estimated to be as high as $238 billion, which includes the increased cost in care, loss of wages, and compromised public health.[8] Poor health literacy is dangerous and expensive to those who have it and creates costs across the healthcare system. Poor reading ability is a factor in poor health literacy, but the two are not identical, as we will explain.

▶ What Creates Good or Poor Health Literacy?

Basic Literacy vs. Health Literacy

Basic literacy refers to an individual's ability to make sense of information in any form in which it is presented. The Educational Testing Service (ETS) (the same company that handles the SATs and GREs) defines and routinely measures different forms of literacy in the United States. Its most basic definition of *literacy* is task-based: "Using printed and written information to function in society, to achieve one's goals, and to develop one's knowledge and potential."[9]

ETS distinguishes three types of literacy scales:

- **Prose literacy**: The ability to read sentences and paragraphs.
- **Document literacy**: The ability to interpret tables, forms, graphs, or other structured formats.
- **Quantitative literacy**: The ability to use information that requires a mathematical operation for interpretation. Quantitative literacy is a subset of numeracy.

These areas are assessed through different challenges on the ETS test.

How Literate Is the U.S. Public?

The U.S. Department of Education conducted the last *strictly national* survey of literacy in 2003. The National Assessment of Adult Literacy tested a representative sample of U.S. adults on prose, document, and quantitative literacy. In 2003, about 93 million Americans, or 43%, read at what was defined as below the *basic* level

of literacy. People tended to have more difficulty with what ETS refers to as document literacy, using graphs and tables, as well as numeracy, than with basic prose.[10]

In 2012, the United States participated in an *international* effort to measure adult competencies across literacy and numeracy areas. This assessment allows the United States to compare its results with other countries that participate in the Program for the International Assessment of Adult Competencies (PIAAC). PIAAC examined four domains: literacy, reading components, numeracy, and problem solving in technology-rich environments. The report compiled information for the United States from a nationally representative sample of 5000 adults aged 16 to 65 years old. These were compared to samples from other partner countries from the Organization for Economic Cooperation and Development. PIAAC used a scale from 0 to 500, with six levels from Below Level 1 to Level 5. **TABLE 3-1** shows the levels and literacy tasks assessed.

In a second survey run to supplement the first, the U.S. average literacy score was just below Level 3, at 272. (This was indistinguishable from the first-round score.)

TABLE 3-1 PIAAC Proficiency Levels on the Literacy Scale

Proficiency Levels and Cut Scores for Literacy	Literacy Task Descriptions
Level 5 (Score of 376–500)	At this level, tasks may require the respondent to search for and integrate information across multiple, dense texts; construct syntheses of similar and contrasting ideas or points of view; or evaluate evidence-based arguments. Application and evaluation of logical and conceptual models of ideas may be required to accomplish tasks. Evaluating reliability of evidentiary sources and selecting key information is frequently a key requirement. Tasks often require respondents to be aware of subtle, rhetorical cues and to make high-level inferences or use specialized background knowledge.
Level 4 (Score of 326–375)	Tasks at this level often require respondents to perform multiple-step operations to integrate, interpret, or synthesize information from complex or lengthy continuous, noncontinuous, mixed, or multiple type texts. Complex inferences and application of background knowledge may be needed to perform successfully. Many tasks require identifying and understanding one or more specific, noncentral ideas in the text in order to interpret or evaluate subtle evidence-claim or persuasive discourse relationships. Conditional information is frequently present in tasks at this level and must be taken into consideration by the respondent. Competing information is present and sometimes seemingly as prominent as correct information.
Level 3 (Score of 276–325)	Texts at this level are often dense or lengthy, including continuous, noncontinuous, mixed, or multiple pages. Understanding text and rhetorical structures becomes more central to successfully completing tasks, especially in navigation of complex digital texts. Tasks require the respondent to identify, interpret, or evaluate one or more pieces of information, and often require varying levels of inference. Many tasks require the respondent to construct meaning across larger chunks of text or perform multistep operations in order to identify and formulate responses. Often tasks also demand that the respondent disregard irrelevant or inappropriate text content to answer accurately. Competing information is often present, but it is not more prominent than the correct information.

(continues)

TABLE 3-1 PIAAC Proficiency Levels on the Literacy Scale	*(continued)*
Proficiency Levels and Cut Scores for Literacy	**Literacy Task Descriptions**
Level 2 (Score of 226–275)	At this level, the complexity of text increases. The medium of texts may be digital or printed, and texts may be composed of continuous, noncontinuous, or mixed types. Tasks at this level require respondents to match text and information, and may require paraphrasing or low-level inferences. Some competing pieces of information may be present. Some tasks require the respondent to cycle through or integrate two or more pieces of information based on criteria, compare and contrast or reason about information requested in the question, or navigate within digital texts to access and identify information from various parts of a document.
Level 1 (Score of 176–225)	Most of the tasks at this level require the respondent to read relatively short digital or print continuous, noncontinuous, or mixed texts to locate a single piece of information that is identical to or synonymous with the information given in the question or directive. Some tasks may require the respondent to enter personal information onto a document, in the case of some noncontinuous texts. Little, if any, competing information is present. Some tasks may require simple cycling through more than one piece of information. Knowledge and skill in recognizing basic vocabulary, evaluating the meaning of sentences, and reading of paragraph text are expected.
Below Level 1 (Score of 0–175)	The tasks at this level require the respondent to read brief texts on familiar topics to locate a single piece of specific information. Only basic vocabulary knowledge is required, and the reader is not required to understand the structure of sentences or paragraphs or make use of other text features. There is seldom any competing information in the text, and the requested information is identical in form to information in the question or directive. Although the texts can be continuous, the information can be located as if the text were noncontinuous. As well, tasks below level 1 do not make use of any features specific to digital texts.

Data from Goodman M, Finnegan R, Mohadjer L, Krenzke T, Hogan J. Literacy, *Numeracy, and Problem Solving in Technology-Rich Environments Among U.S. Adults: Results from the Program for the International Assessment of Adult Competencies 2012: First Look* (NCES 2014-008). U.S. Department of Education. Washington, DC: National Center for Education Statistics; 2013. http://nces.ed.gov/pubs2014/2014008.pdf. Accessed February 17, 2018.

Twelve countries participating in the PIAAC had higher national averages, and five were below the United States.[11] We have a long way to go to bring our overall literacy levels in the United States up to international standards.

It is important to stress that persons with limited literacy often feel ashamed of their lack of skills and take pains to hide their difficulty reading or understanding information. For this reason, and because all of us can use simpler, clearer information, we take a "universal precautions" approach to health literacy, as described later in this chapter. But basic literacy and numeracy are only part of what determines comprehensive health literacy.

▶ Determinants of Health Literacy

Knowledge and Organizational Skills

Because humans have evolved to have limited capacity to take in new information and keep it organized in their brain, we tend to pay attention to things that matter most to us, and ignore the rest. This is usually good because we are bombarded with thousands of pieces of information daily; if we treated each piece as equally important, we would be exhausted if not dead from missing an important warning.

There are many ways to keep information organized in our heads, and good educators build on these natural tendencies to help students add new information to old. The core concept is to use what someone already knows as a scaffolding or framework for adding, remembering, and using new information. Diagrams and concept maps (also known as mind maps) are ways to visualize how individual facts fit together. Concept maps are drawings that link together ideas, represented as words or pictures, through boxes, circles, and directional arrows. They allow us to see hierarchical levels or other relationships among what might at first seem to be unrelated pieces of information. Seeing patterns and constructing mental models, and then being able to incorporate new information into the model, are one of the hallmarks of meaningful learning, in contrast to rote memorization.[12] Perhaps you have created your own concept maps when trying to assimilate new information from a course. **BOX 3-3** features a concept map for health literacy.

BOX 3-3 Concept Mapping and Health Literacy

FIGURE 3-2 diagrams sources of determinants of health literacy (on the left), the contexts and way in which it functions (in the middle), and some of the outcomes associated with it (on the right). There are arrows indicating that health literacy is acquired over a lifetime and that the context occurs on the individual and population level. Someone who made this diagram would have a good overview of health literacy and possibly remember more of its components. If you had a picture like this in your head of health literacy, you would have a way of characterizing and organizing new facts and references as you acquired them (e.g., this is a determinant, this is an outcome, this is a process).

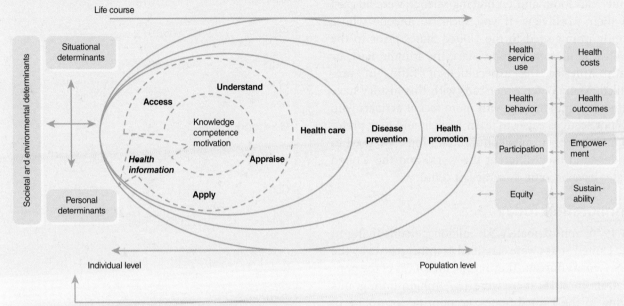

FIGURE 3-2 Sørensen et al.'s integrated model of health literacy.

Reproduced from Sørensen K, Van den Broucke S, Fullam J, Slonska Z, Brand H. Health literacy and public health: a systematic review and integration of definitions and models. *BMC Public Health.* 2012;12:80. http://www.biomedcentral.com/1471-2458/12/80

One of the challenges of health literacy is that the ability to make mental models is socially and culturally determined. Those with more exposure to health and science are more likely to create mental models and integrate scientific knowledge about health more easily. Others have difficulty with mental modeling because they have not been taught how or because they use a different culturally determined model of how things work.

For example, when a healthcare provider explains that a drug must be taken with the morning meal, some people will think they need to eat a whole breakfast; some will eat a cracker; and some will skip it because they do not normally eat breakfast. There is no common understanding of why and how the drug interacts with food in the body. Similarly, providers may tell diabetic patients that they have high blood sugar and need to cut out carbohydrates. Besides not being familiar with the term *carbohydrate*, many patients will not think that something that is not sweet, such as a potato or bread, could be problematic for diabetes because it is not *sugar*.

The ability to use a shared scientific perspective on health (cause and effect, the scientific method) to integrate new information into a mental model is an important determinant of health literacy. This capacity is far more important than a lack of knowledge about specific subjects or vocabulary, which can be acquired more easily.

Cultural and Linguistic Differences

For many of us, "Dr. Mom" is our first expert on whether we are healthy or sick, for example, too sick to go to school. In my case, I went to school unless I had a temperature above 99°F. Sticking the thermometer into a cup of hot water did not fool mom. My mom would call our pediatrician, or her own father (a doctor), if anything seemed beyond her capacities. Her mother was often consulted by neighbors because she was "Frau Doctor" (i.e., married to my grandfather, the doctor). My grandmother's advice for most ailments was, "Take two (buffered) aspirin and be quiet." Our family's culture of health was based in an Austrian approach to cleanliness, science, and a little bit of expected suffering thrown in.

My mother and her parents escaped Nazi-occupied Austria in the late 1930s, and my mom went to U.S. schools from the age of seven onward. The public attitude held by refugees and immigrants in those days was to do everything possible to assimilate into U.S. culture. Learning English, eating so-called American food, and embracing science were all part of their worldview. If you speak to anyone whose family immigrated to the United States prior to the 1960s, be it from Europe, Asia, the Middle East, or Latin America, this expectation of "fitting in" prevailed. Many older Americans with this history have difficulty empathizing with more recent arrivals who do not seem as eager to learn English and may prefer to maintain their own cultural traditions. We need to understand how different the world and the United States have become over the last century.

Immigration Today

In 1970, approximately 9.6 million persons living in the United States were classified as **immigrants** by the U.S. Census Bureau. They represented 4.7% of the population. In 2016, there were 43.7 million immigrants living in the United States, accounting for 13.5% of the population.[13] In 2014, nearly half (47%) of these persons were naturalized U.S. citizens; the remaining 53% percent was made up of "lawful permanent residents, unauthorized immigrants, and legal residents on temporary visas (such as students and temporary workers)."[13] **TABLE 3-2** shows the countries of origin for those representing 1% or more of our total immigrant population based on data from the U.S. Census Bureau's American Community Survey conducted between 2010 and 2014.

In 2016, the United States planned to accept 85,000 refugees, chiefly from Syria, Afghanistan, and Somalia and 100,000 in 2017.[14] Compared to our total population of more than 324 million, as well as the estimated 20 million people displaced globally, 85,000–100,000 is not that large a number. The United States is already the world's top resettlement country, followed by Canada, Australia, Germany, and Scandinavian countries. Still, a coalition of organizations that created the Embrace Refugees Campaign offers a different perspective, "An individual is 13 times more likely to gain admission to Harvard than to the U.S. as a refugee."[15] The United Nations High Commission for Refugees referred only 0.7% of all refugees for resettlement in 2015. Of this group, 50% were children.[16] Although children are remarkably quick

TABLE 3-2 Country of Birth of U.S. Immigrant Population in 2014 for Countries Representing 1% or More of Total Foreign-Born Population

Country	Number	Percentage of Immigrant Population
Mexico	11,710,013	27.7
China	2,505,197	5.9
India	2,181,604	5.2
Philippines	1,923,075	4.6
El Salvador	1,322,893	3.1
Vietnam	1,298,268	3.1
Cuba	1,175,936	2.8
Korea	1,082,173	2.6
Dominican Republic	995,755	2.4
Guatemala	909,267	2.2
Canada	794,355	1.9
Jamaica	710,572	1.7
Colombia	697,002	1.7
Haiti	616,631	1.5
Germany	584,234	1.4
Honduras	569,027	1.3
Peru	442,217	1.0
Poland	432,069	1.0
Ecuador	418,951	1.0

Data from The U.S. Bureau of the Census, 2014 American Community Survey.

to learn English (or any new language), adults have more difficulty.

Language Use in the United States

In 2015, the U.S. Census Bureau reported that at least 382 languages were spoken across the United States.

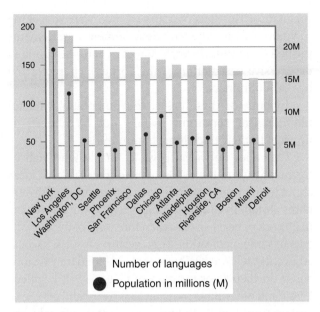

FIGURE 3-3 Number of languages spoken in the 15 largest metropolitan areas of the United States.

Reproduced from U.S. Department of Commerce Economics and Statistics Administration, U.S. Census Bureau. Number of languages spoken in the 15 largest metro areas. U.S. Census Bureau website. https://www.census.gov/content/dam/Census/newsroom/releases/2015/cb15-185_graphic.pdf.

FIGURE 3-3 shows the number of languages spoken in the 15 largest metropolitan areas of the United States.

Although this amazing diversity of languages can seem overwhelming, as shown in **TABLE 3-3**, the vast majority of the population that speaks a language other than English speaks Spanish.

Depending on your location in the United States, there will be a core group of immigrant populations and languages in use. For example, in Philadelphia, many healthcare facilities provide language resources in addition to Spanish, including Chinese, Vietnamese, and French. Some health centers will also provide information in Arabic, Polish, and Russian. Northern California has large populations of Chinese, Japanese, Korean, and other Asian language users. Minnesota was long the "home away from home" for Hmong speakers from highland Southeast Asia, and so on. You can access the U.S. Census Bureau maps to see which languages are the most used in your region.

Cultural Meanings

As mentioned previously, my mother embraced a modern and western view of health due to her family upbringing, her community, and the times in which she lived. But people from different backgrounds, different walks of life, and different parts of the world often have vastly different views of what constitutes good health and what causes illness.

TABLE 3-3 Origins, Languages, and English Language Proficiency	
World Region of Birth of Foreign Born	
Foreign-born population, excluding population born at sea	40,917,701
Europe	11.8%
Asia	29.2%
Africa	4.3%
Oceania	0.6%
Latin America	52.2%
Northern America	2.0%
Language Spoken at Home	
Population 5 years and older	293,913,098
English only	79.1%
Language other than English	20.9%
Speak English less than "very well"	8.6%
Spanish	13.0%
Speak English less than "very well"	5.5%
Other Indo-European languages	3.7%
Speak English less than "very well"	1.2%
Asian and Pacific Islander languages	3.3%
Speak English less than "very well"	1.6%
Other languages	0.9%
Speak English less than "very well"	0.3%

Reproduced from U.S. Census Bureau. Comparative social characteristics in the United States. 2011-2013 American Community Survey 3-year estimates. American FactFinder website. http://factfinder.census.gov/faces/tableservices/jsf/pages/productview.xhtml?pid=ACS_13_3YR_CP02&prodType=table. Accessed February 18, 2018.

Brokering cultural differences can be an even bigger challenge than identifying the best language to use with a client.

On a global basis, anthropologists have described two primary ways of viewing illness causation:

- *Personalistic disease theory:* Illness is due to the purposeful intervention of a supernatural being (e.g., a god), a nonhuman being (e.g., a ghost or evil spirit), or a person who has supernatural powers (e.g., a witch).
- *Naturalistic disease theory:* A person's health is closely connected to the environment, with natural conditions or biologic materials impacting a person's health; disease occurs impersonally.[17]

A Western-trained doctor believing an illness to be the result of biological processes, such as bacteria, may prescribe penicillin as a cure. A traditional or folk healer who believes that an illness is the result of supernatural causes will use other means to bring about a cure. Some people seek out both forms of treatment, which may bring them comfort and some benefit. Anne Fadiman's *The Spirit Catches You and You Fall Down* poignantly describes such a situation.[18]

In the late 1980s, five-year-old Lia Lee had what her Hmong family called *qaug dab peg*, caused by the separation of her soul from her body. The traditional cure required a shaman to make a spiritual journey, find the soul, lure it back, and retie it to the sufferer's body. The doctors treating Lia in northern California called this condition *epilepsy* and tried to get Lia's parents to follow a prescribed regime of medications. Lia lived most of her life in a persistent vegetative state caused by the brain damage she sustained after a very long-lasting seizure. It is possible that the seizure might have been prevented if communication between Lia's parents and her doctors had been better.

The Lees and their doctors all suffered terribly due to this miscommunication. On the positive side, thousands of students have read Fadiman's book, and many have come to appreciate cultural differences in health beliefs. Those who go on to become health professionals may show more sensitivity and respect for other traditions in medicine.

Differences in cultural beliefs may also lead one group to see a condition as a disease or illness, whereas another perceives it to be a natural progression in life. For instance, schistosomiasis was widespread in Egypt in the early twentieth century. Boys would join their fathers in fishing in the rivers and would soon see blood in their urine. This "male menstruation" was considered a rite of passage to manhood. But by the early twentieth century, schistosomiasis was known to be a parasitic infection, acquired from wading in rivers where the parasite was present. If left untreated, it leads to liver damage and kidney failure.[19]

In a similar vein, villagers in rural Mali (West Africa) believed that night blindness, called "chicken eye" in the local language, was an early indicator of pregnancy. The diets of many women were so lacking in vitamin A that the fetal development requirements pushed them into the early stages of xerophthalmia (a progressive destruction of the cornea), characterized by night blindness.[20]

In both of these cases, the potentially harmful physiological conditions would not be noticed as unusual in their traditional communities.

One does not have to go as far away as Mali or Egypt, or back to the 1980s, to encounter different ideas about health or illness. Religious practitioners of several faiths abstain from consuming specific animal products (e.g., pork or beef) and are therefore wary of the ingredients in some medications (e.g., gelatin capsules, vaccine adjuvants). Jehovah's Witnesses avoid blood transfusions based on their interpretation of Genesis 9:4, Leviticus 17:10, and other Bible passages that command people to abstain from blood. As they state on their official website, they "avoid taking blood in obedience to God and out of respect for God as the Giver of Life."[21]

Culturally competent health care includes knowing about issues where there might be different views, and trying to identify ways to provide optimal care in the least objectionable manner. The Tanenbaum Center for Interreligious Understanding has produced a number of resources for healthcare students and professionals describing how to work with patients from religiously diverse backgrounds. **TABLE 3-4** lists and briefly describes what Tanenbaum terms *trigger topics* in health care. These are situations in which a patient's religious values, beliefs, or practices might need to be addressed in order to deliver the best health care.

Culturally and Linguistically Appropriate Services

To respond to the needs of clients with different languages and world views, the U.S. Office of Minority Health developed a set of voluntary **Culturally and Linguistically Appropriate Services (CLAS)** that all healthcare providers are encouraged to employ. These were revised in 2013 after more than a decade of use and public comment. **BOX 3-4** lists these revised standards.

The principal standard is to "Provide effective, equitable, understandable, and respectful quality care and services that are responsive to diverse cultural health beliefs and practices, preferred languages, health literacy, and other communication needs." The remaining standards fall under three large groupings[22]:

1. *Governance, Leadership, and Workforce:* Emphasizes that the responsibility for CLAS implementation rests at the highest levels of organizational leadership.

TABLE 3-4 Trigger Topics in Health Care

Trigger Topic	Description
Dietary requirements	The patient/client has religiously motivated food restrictions that impact meals and/or medication.
Dress and modesty	The patient/client wears religious garb or symbols that need to be removed for examination and/or treatment, and/or the patient's/client's religious beliefs dictate specific behavior relating to modesty.
Hygiene	The patient/client has religious practices relating to washing prior to prayers and mealtimes or has religious concerns pertaining to maintaining a beard or other grooming needs.
Informed consent	The patient/client requires the consultation and/or consent of a family member or religious leader to approve a course of treatment.
Observance of holy days and rituals	The patient/client observes certain holy days or performs religious rituals that require accommodations around scheduling of procedures or modifying treatments for fasting.
Complementary and alternative medicine	The patient/client uses religiously or culturally indicated alternative remedies or seeks the assistance of a traditional healer.
Organ transplants and donations	The patient/client and/or their family have religious beliefs that influence their willingness to accept a donor organ or agree to donate an organ.
Reproductive health	The patient/client has religious views on contraception, abortion, or fertility procedures such as in vitro fertilization or sterilization.
Pregnancy and birth	The patient/client has religion-specific practices associated with labor and birth, such as particular foods, rituals, or traditional remedies.
End-of-life	The patient's/client's religious beliefs require performing particular rituals before or after death or dictate particular perspectives on withdrawing care or prolonging life.
Acceptance of drugs and procedures	The patient/client refuses specific drugs and procedures due to various religious restrictions such as fasting, exhibits a preference to use alternative medicine, or has religious dietary objections.
Blood and blood products	The patient/client has religious beliefs that restrict the use of blood or blood products.
Conscience rules	The religious beliefs of the healthcare provider conflict with the needs or requests of the patient/client.
Prayer with patient	The patient/client and/or family of the patient requests that a member of their healthcare team pray with them.
Proselytizing	The patient/client experiences inappropriate religious expression from staff in a healthcare setting.

Reproduced from Tanenbaum. *Religious and Cultural Competence: Advancing Patient-Centered Care: Trigger Topics*. New York, NY: Tanenbaum Center for Interreligious Understanding; 2014.

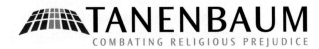

BOX 3-4 National Standards for Culturally and Linguistically Appropriate Services (CLAS) in Health and Health Care

The CLAS standards are intended to advance health equity, improve quality, and help eliminate health care disparities by establishing a blueprint for health and health care organizations:

Principal Standard

1. Provide effective, equitable, understandable, and respectful quality care and services that are responsive to diverse cultural health beliefs and practices, preferred languages, health literacy, and other communication needs.

Governance, Leadership, and Workforce

2. Advance and sustain organizational governance and leadership that promotes CLAS and health equity through policy, practices, and allocated resources.
3. Recruit, promote, and support a culturally and linguistically diverse governance, leadership, and workforce that are responsive to the population in the service area.
4. Educate and train governance, leadership, and workforce in culturally and linguistically appropriate policies and practices on an ongoing basis.

Communication and Language Assistance

5. Offer language assistance to individuals who have limited English proficiency or other communication needs, at no cost to them, to facilitate timely access to all health care and services.
6. Inform all individuals of the availability of language assistance services clearly and in their preferred language, orally and in writing.
7. Ensure the competence of individuals providing language assistance, recognizing that the use of untrained individuals or minors as interpreters should be avoided.
8. Provide easy-to-understand print and multimedia materials and signage in the languages commonly used by the populations in the service area.

Engagement, Continuous Improvement, and Accountability

9. Establish culturally and linguistically appropriate goals, policies, and management accountability and infuse them throughout the organization's planning and operations.
10. Conduct ongoing assessments of the organization's CLAS-related activities and integrate CLAS-related measures into measurement and continuous quality-improvement activities.
11. Collect and maintain accurate and reliable demographic data to monitor and evaluate the impact of CLAS on health equity and outcomes and to inform service delivery.
12. Conduct regular assessments of community health assets and needs and use the results to plan and implement services that respond to the cultural and linguistic diversity of populations in the service area.
13. Partner with the community to design, implement, and evaluate policies, practices, and services to ensure cultural and linguistic appropriateness.
14. Create processes for conflict and grievance resolution that are culturally and linguistically appropriate to identify, prevent, and resolve conflicts or complaints.
15. Communicate the organization's progress in implementing and sustaining CLAS to all stakeholders, constituents, and the general public.

2. *Communication and Language Assistance:* Suggests that organizations provide language assistance in a manner appropriate to the organization's size, scope, and mission. (Healthcare facilities and practitioners receiving federal funding at any level must provide free language assistance per Title VI of the Civil Rights Act of 1964, which states, "No person in the United States shall, on ground of race, color, or national origin, be excluded from participation in, be denied the benefits of, or be subjected to discrimination under any program or activity receiving federal financial assistance.")

3. *Engagement, Continuous Improvement, and Accountability:* Underscores the importance of quality improvement, community engagement, and evaluation.

Context

A clinical setting or medical encounter can make anyone feel fearful, stressed, and confused. Think about your own experience making an appointment with a healthcare provider. Where do you start? The process is not at all obvious and usually involves multiple layers. Internet portals, meant to simplify patient communications, are rarely easy to navigate. Even persons with a high degree of self-confidence and education may become less able to process information when faced with bad medical news or a stressful setting. The health literacy burden is increased in the context of the intense emotions associated with being sick, finding and paying for health services, and even the location where health care takes place.

In sum, health literacy is created from:

- Our core background abilities in reading and math, and the ways we mentally organize, retain, and integrate new information
- Our linguistic skills
- Our cultural beliefs and attitudes that shape our perceptions
- The time and place context in which we find ourselves facing new health information

There has been considerable research to understand how these factors engender health literacy skills, as well as what interventions lead to the best health outcomes.[23,24]

▶ Tools to Enhance Health Literacy

Assessment of an Individual's Health Literacy Skills

For the past two decades, researchers have been developing tools to identify different components of health literacy and ways to measure them. The **Health Literacy Tool Shed** was constructed by Boston University with funding from the National Library of Medicine. It has more than 100 tools for specific applications and allows users to access specific instruments by health literacy domain, health context, administration time, modality of administration, language (there are many available), and more. Users are invited to submit validated tools to the site for fellow researchers and practitioners. All of the tools listed here, and their validation publications, can be found at this site.

It is important to ensure that research or survey participants consent to assessments of health literacy, which may be time consuming and may cause participants to feel ashamed of their skill level.[25]

There are three benchmarks, and several new instruments that can be used to measure health literacy across a range of research and practice contexts. These are the REALM, TOFHLA, and NVS, and the newer eHEALS, NUMI, and HLSI.

REALM

The Rapid Estimate of Adult Literacy in Medicine (REALM)[26] is a word recognition test consisting of 66 medical words. It is one of the oldest and most widely used health literacy assessment tools. It starts with easy words (e.g., fat, flu, pill) and moves to difficult words (e.g., osteoporosis, impetigo, potassium). Patients are asked to pronounce each word out loud. The test makes no attempt to determine if patients actually understand the meaning. REALM can be administered in about three minutes, and it is available only in English. The number of correctly pronounced words is used to assign a grade-equivalent reading level.

The REALM-R[27] is a quick version of the REALM consisting of the following 11 words:

Fat	Osteoporosis	Anemia	Colitis
Flu	Allergic	Fatigue	Constipation
Pill	Jaundice	Directed	

Fat, flu, and pill are not scored and are positioned at the beginning of the REALM-R to decrease test anxiety and enhance confidence. Unlike the REALM, which must be purchased, all materials related to the REALM-R may be downloaded without charge from the American Society on Aging and American Society of Consultant Pharmacists Foundation (http://www.adultmeducation.com/assessmenttools_1.html).

TOFHLA

The Test of Functional Health Literacy in Adults (TOFHLA)[28] has been the instrument of choice when a detailed evaluation of health literacy is needed for research purposes. It is available in both English and Spanish. The full-length form requires 20 minutes; the short version requires about 12 minutes. The TOFHLA uses multiple-choice as well as fill-in-the-blank questions. A testing kit may be ordered from the distributor, Peppercorn Books.

NVS

The Newest Vital Sign (NVS) features an ice cream label challenge in English or Spanish. It can typically be completed by patients who read in either language in about three minutes. Many patients find the ice cream label challenge acceptable as part of standard medical care, with more than 98% of patients agreeing to undergo the assessment during a routine office visit.[29] A toolkit to administer the NVS can be obtained online at no cost from Pfizer, Inc. (http://www.pfizer .com/health/literacy/public_policy_researchers /nvs_toolkit).

eHEALS

The eHealth Literacy Scale (eHEALS)[30] is an eight-item measure of electronic health literacy that assesses an individual's knowledge, skills, and perceived comfort in finding, evaluating, and applying electronic health information to health problems. It has been used in several studies to evaluate ehealth literacy and communications programs. This instrument also may be downloaded free of charge (http://www.jmir .org/2006/4/e27/).

NUMi

The Numeracy Understanding in Medicine instrument (NUMi)[31] was developed by Schapira and colleagues at the University of Pennsylvania. It is a 20-item pencil-and-paper test that measures most of the quantitative challenges a patient may face in health care. Items include reading the numbers on a digital thermometer, interpreting an icon array and a simple bar chart and line graph, and multiple-choice questions pertaining to reading labels and estimating probability. The NUMi has been validated with 1000 patients. An eight-item version is available at no charge.

HLSI

The Health Literacy Skills Instrument (HLSI)[32] was developed by McCormack and a team of other national health literacy experts. It measures print literacy as well as numeracy, oral skills, and internet-based information-seeking skills that U.S.-based adults are likely to face in the context of health care. The 25-item HLSI can be self-administered via a computer in approximately 12 minutes. A 10-item version is also available.[33] Both tests are free of charge.

Assessment in Clinical Practice

It can be important to assess a patient's health literacy in order to:

- Comply with quality of care standards within a profession or facility

- Select appropriate educational materials (e.g., video, foreign language)
- Rule out other complications, such as cognitive impairment, hearing, or vision loss

Some of the measures developed for research may be used cautiously in practice, as can specific measures posted at the Health Literacy Tool Shed online. One- or two-question tests have been found to work well in the healthcare setting.[34] These include the following questions:

1. How often do you have problems learning about your medical condition because of difficulty understanding written information?
    Response choices: Always, often, sometimes, occasionally, or never
2. How often do you have someone help you read hospital materials?
    Response choices: Always, often, sometimes, occasionally, or never
3. How confident are you filling out medical forms by yourself?
    Response choices: Extremely, quite a bit, somewhat, a little bit, or not at all

It is best to assume that anyone who does not select the most proficient choice (i.e., Question 1, "never," Question 2, "never," Question 3, "extremely") should be given materials that are more simply written. However, as we will explain in the following section, few people will be insulted by receiving clear and simple materials in a healthcare setting.

Health Literacy Universal Precautions[35]

The number one precaution about health literacy (we could say, "in life,") is that you cannot judge a book by its cover. People go to great pains to hide what they perceive to be deficient educational backgrounds, and others who are highly educated might give a false impression. So, in practice, you should:

- Not judge anyone by appearance
- Strive to communicate clearly with everyone
- Confirm understanding with everyone

We recommend that all healthcare providers use plain language (e.g., "high blood pressure" instead of "hypertension") and focus on the two or three most important concepts during an interaction. It helps to prepare a message map to accomplish this.

Message Mapping

Message mapping is used to manage talking points during public health emergencies,[36] but "maps" are also used to organize information when more than one person needs to deliver information, and it is important to keep the message consistent. In addition, message maps help you make sure you are focusing on the most important information. People tend to remember about three pieces of information—usually the first and last thing you said, and maybe something in the middle. Message maps help you chunk what you want to say into these units. Messages are presented in three short sentences that convey three key messages in about 27 words. Those familiar with Twitter can think of them as tweetable units.

Message maps should be written at about a sixth-grade reading level. Each primary message has three supporting messages that can be used when and where appropriate to provide context for the issue being mapped. **BOX 3-5** shows a message map template as well as a filled-in map for avoiding Zika virus.

All providers should confirm patient understanding using a "teach-back" or "ask-educate-ask" method. In patient–provider interactions, it is the provider who is responsible for clear and effective communication. The purpose of the teach-back is to verify that the *provider* is communicating clearly, not to test the patient's ability to understand.[37] **BOX 3-6** explains teach-back in greater detail.

▶ Developing and Assessing Materials

As in all health communication, understanding the intended user is essential when creating materials that are easier to understand. Audience inputs will determine how you create your materials and which channels you choose for dissemination. It will also be important to test your materials with the intended users and revise them as needed based on this feedback.

The Centers for Disease Control and Prevention (CDC) updated its guide, *Simply Put*, which provides many tips on writing simply and clearly about health (http://www.cdc.gov/healthliteracy/pdf

---

BOX 3-5 Message Mapping

Message Mapping Template

Key Message 1	Key Message 2	Key Message 3
Supporting Message 1 a	Supporting Message 2a	Supporting Message 3a
Supporting Message 1 b	Supporting Message 2b	Supporting Message 3b
Supporting Message 1 c	Supporting Message 2c	Supporting Message 3c

Avoiding Zika Message Map

Zika is a virus that may harm unborn babies or adults	You can prevent Zika by avoiding mosquitoes or people bitten by mosquitoes with Zika	You can protect children from Zika
Unborn babies may develop birth defects if the mother is bitten by a mosquito with Zika	Know if mosquitoes with Zika are in your community	Stay in places with screens on windows and doors
Adults may have no symptoms, feel like they have the flu, or have more serious problems	Use insect repellent and wear long sleeves and pants when outside	Keep air conditioning or fans on at all times
Find out if there is Zika in your area	Use condoms to avoid passing Zika during sex	Do not use insect repellents on babies younger than 2 months old

---

BOX 3-6 Using Teach-Back to Check Patient Understanding of Information

- *Keep in mind this is not a test of the patient's knowledge.* It is a test of how well you explained the concept.
- *Plan your approach.* Think about how you will ask your patients to teach back the information. For example:
  - "We covered a lot today and I want to make sure that I explained things clearly. So let's review what we discussed. Can you please describe the three things you agreed to do to help you control your diabetes?"
  - "Tell me what you will tell your significant other [as appropriate, spouse, partner, child, friend] about what we just discussed."
- *Chunk and check.* Don't wait until the end of the visit to initiate teach-back. Chunk out information into small segments and have your patient teach it back. Repeat several times during a visit.
- *Clarify and check again.* If teach-back uncovers a misunderstanding, explain things again using a different approach. Ask patients to teach back again until they are able to correctly describe the information in their own words. If they parrot your words back to you, they may not have understood.
- *Start slowly and use consistency.* At first, you may want to try teach-back with the last patient of the day. Once you are comfortable with the technique, use teach-back with everyone, every time!
- *Practice.* It will take a little time, but once it is part of your routine, teach-back can be done without awkwardness and does not lengthen a visit.
- *Use the show-me method.* When prescribing new medicines or changing a dose, research shows that even when patients correctly say when and how much medicine they'll take, many will make mistakes when asked to demonstrate the dose. You could say, for example: "I've noticed that many people have trouble remembering how to take their blood thinner. Can you show me how you are going to take it?"
- *Use handouts along with teach-back.* Write down key information to help patients remember instructions at home. Point out important information by reviewing written materials to reinforce your patients' understanding. You can allow patients to refer to handouts when using teach-back, but make sure they use their own words and are not reading the material back verbatim.
- *Train nonclinical staff.* Nonclinical staff members who interact with patients should also use teach-back. For example, staff making appointments may use it to ensure the patients understand what is required of them at the next visit such as arrival time, insurance documentation, bringing medicines, fasting, and details about referrals to other clinicians.
- *Share teach-back stories.* Ask one person at each staff meeting to share a teach-back "Aha!" moment. This serves as a reminder of the importance of using teach-back consistently.

Adapted with permission from Use the teach-back method: tool #5. Agency for Healthcare Research and Quality website. http://www.ahrq.gov/professionals/quality-patient-safety/quality-resources/tools/literacy-toolkit/healthlittoolkit2-tool5.html. Accessed February 18, 2018.

/Simply_Put.pdf). In addition, the Centers for Medicare and Medicaid Services (CMS) has an excellent toolkit for writing for audiences with basic and below-basic literacy levels (https://www.cms.gov/Outreach-and-Education/Outreach/WrittenMaterialsToolkit/Downloads/ToolkitPart01.pdf). CMS defines "clear and effective" written material as being able to:

- Attract the reader's attention
- Hold their attention
- Make them feel respected and understood
- Help them understand the messages in the material
- Move them to action[38]

These are goals you would want to accomplish in any writing for any audience. These resources are free and easy to access, so we will not reiterate their content here. Instead, we will discuss how to assess the clarity of communications materials using several tools. By seeing what matters, this should help you also plan and prepare materials more effectively.

Readability

Thanks to word processing packages that incorporate the measures, it has become very easy to check the readability of prose using some "old school" approaches to determining reading level. These tools provide a quick and easy way to assess word choice, sentence length, and some other factors that make text harder to understand. They can be used as a first pass over your materials, allowing you to simplify your language before moving on to layout, visual images, numeric representations, and more.

The **Flesch-Kincaid Grade Level Readability Test**[39] uses words per sentence and syllables per word as part of a formula to determine the "reading grade level" of the text. The formula is calculated as (0.39 × Average Sentence Length) + (11.8 × Average Number of Syllables per Word) − 15.59. A score of 8.3, for example, would indicate an 8th-grade reading level. Electronic calculators are available through the Internet. The formula is also built into Microsoft Word; however, the Word version is not able to determine any grade above 12.

The **SMOG** (Simple Measure of Gobbledygook)[40] provides an estimate of the number of years of education needed to understand prose material, including website copy. It is a rigorous assessment that focuses on word length and sentences. The SMOG tool is available online (https://library.med.utah.edu/Patient_Ed/workshop/handouts/smog_formula.pdf).

Both of these measures refer to a school grade level to represent readability. This approach has fallen out of favor with professionals, and it does not match up with the levels now in use to describe literacy as "basic," "below basic," and so on. However, following our own principles, saying that an informed consent document needs to be written at a 6th-grade level will be clearer to most lawyers, who usually approve such documents, than saying it needs to be at the "basic" level.

Making Numbers Clear

Given the difficulty that many people have in interpreting graphs, charts, and mathematical concepts, the first decision to make is to determine if you really need to use numbers to get your message across, or if another approach is better. For example, you may be able to explain the scale of a problem using a common metaphor rather than an accurate but often incomprehensible numeric relationship. Antismoking advocates have long described the annual number of smoking deaths in the

United States as equivalent to two jumbo jets crashing every day for a year with no survivors. Another popular analogy is, "College students consume enough alcohol each year to fill an Olympic-sized swimming pool on every campus in the United States." Choose your metaphor wisely; select something familiar but not ridiculous. Metaphors are not useful when people misunderstand, or choose to not recognize, scale. Think about how many people buy lottery tickets even though the chance of winning big is less than being struck by lightning—twice. As many a hopeful player has thought, "If the chance is 1 in 9 million, I've got as good a chance as anyone else. And, to double my chances, I'll buy two tickets."

Because most people never knew, or have forgotten, how probability works, it is very difficult to explain risk both accurately and clearly. Unless the concept is very simple (e.g., "Nine out of ten dentists prefer sugarless gum" [the other one wants more business]), it helps to have visual aids. The University of Michigan's Visualizing Health project (http://www.vizhealth.org) is a great resource for this. With funding from the Robert Wood Johnson Foundation, University of Michigan scientists and their artist colleagues created and tested graphs, charts, and images to explain complex numeric concepts that occur quite commonly in health communication. A gallery of the tested images is available at the University of Michigan website together with a "wizard" tool to generate your own. **BOX 3-7** shows two examples from this site as well as an icon array generated from another site created by University of Michigan scientists.

BOX 3-7 Risk Visualizations

1. Comparing the side effects of different treatments

This simple table supplements the individual risk numbers with a color coding system designed to highlight which treatments are more vs. less likely to result within each side effect row. It also includes a very subtle bar graph feature within each cell (the height of the darker color is proportionate to the risk). The large numbers should facilitate numeric recall. People recalled risk numbers more accurately for this graphic than for other graphics.

	A	B	C	D
MILD PAIN	30%	60%	45%	45%
DIARRHEA	15%	10%	8%	20%

EACH OPTION RANKED: **LOWEST** TO **HIGHEST**

Treatment option chart.

(continues)

BOX 3-7   Risk Visualizations

2. Explaining the relationship of a biomarker, such as high blood pressure, to risk of an event, such as a heart attack or stroke

This variant of a bar graph uses circle size/area to represent elevations in risk as blood pressure increases. Because the circles are aligned at the base, the circle edges create an upwardly curving exponential shape that helps evoke a sense of increasing risk. The overlapping circles at the higher levels convey an additional sense of being "large" that may help viewers recognize that further elevations in blood pressure result in particularly large levels of risk. People who viewed this graphic were more likely to perceive and classify their blood pressure risk as slightly above normal vs. way above normal.

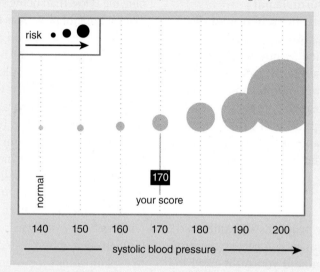

Translating test results into risk.

Reproduced from Translating test results into risk. Visualizing Health website. http://www.vizhealth.org/gallery/assets/38/. Accessed February 18, 2018.

3. Icon array

Icon arrays use a matrix of icons (usually 100 to 1000) to represent the at-risk population in the context of the rest of the unaffected population. As a result, icon arrays have some advantages: (1) The icons can be counted, making them easier to understand than a pie or bar chart; and (2) they show the part–whole relationship clearly.

Icon arrays are particularly useful for explaining risks, for example, of procedures or treatments. You can say something like, "If 100 people just like you had this operation, we would expect that 1 might not survive, 2 might have a temporary paralysis, and 97 will return to full health."

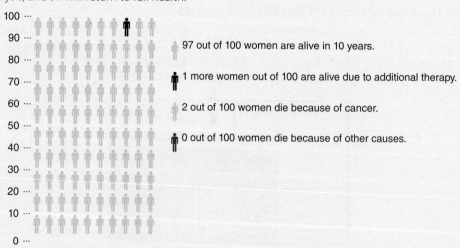

Risks of surgical procedure.

Reproduced from Iconarray.com. Risk Science Center and Center for Bioethics and Social Sciences in Medicine, University of Michigan. http://www.iconarray.com. Accessed August 21, 2016.

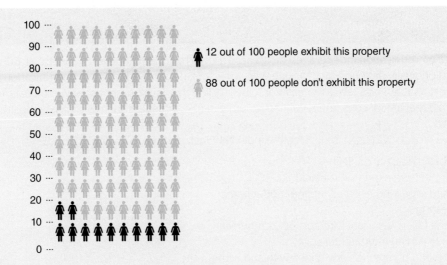

Icon array to show *lifetime* risk of developing breast cancer for an "average risk" woman who lives to age 70.

Reproduced from Iconarray.com. Risk Science Center and Center for Bioethics and Social Sciences in Medicine, University of Michigan. http://www.iconarray.com. Accessed August 21, 2016.

Now note the distinction in imagery made by the Worldwide Breast Cancer Organization to emphasize the role of aging in the lifetime risk calculation.

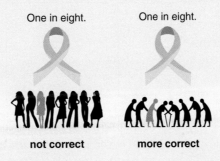

Breast cancer statistics.

Reproduced from Breast cancer statistics worldwide. Worldwide Breast Cancer website. http://www.worldwidebreastcancer.com/learn/breast-cancer-statistics-worldwide/. Accessed February 18, 2018.

A Focus on Patient Decision Aids

When faced with choosing a medical treatment or intervention, many of us just want to ask our health-care provider to choose what is best for us. But, health care is increasingly moving to a position of SDM. Making decisions through SDM is the hall-mark of patient-centered care; however, many of us are frustrated by this idea. We realize that we do not have the knowledge or experience of our providers but, at the same time, we do want to have a say in our care or the care of our loved ones. Patient decision aids (PDAs) make use of best practices in health literacy and patient engagement to provide patients with the clearest understanding of their choices. Ideally, PDAs help patients clarify and communicate to physicians the personal value they associate with different features of the treatment options. They are not meant to persuade patients to choose one option over another, nor are they meant to replace practitioner consultation. Instead, they prepare patients to make informed, values-based decisions with their practitioner.[41]

An entire literature and practice area has grown up around PDAs, spearheaded by the International Patient Decision Aid Standards Collaborative.[42] In the United States, funding from the Agency for Healthcare Research and Quality (AHRQ) and the Patient-Centered Outcomes Research Institute has led to the development of hundreds of decision tools to aid in SDM. **APPENDIX 3A** provides an overview of how the Nationwide Children's Hospital in Columbus, Ohio, developed a tablet-based tool using health literacy best practices for parents to decide between surgery or antibiotic treatment for children experiencing appendicitis.

BOX 3-8 CDC Clear Communication Index

The CDC Clear Communication Index is a research-based tool to help people develop and assess public communication materials. It was originally designed for CDC staff who write, edit, design, and review communication products, but anyone can use it to assess and revise materials or to help guide the development of new materials. The index can be used for materials that are for consumers, patients, or professional audiences such as clinicians, health department staff, or policymakers.

An extensive process was used to develop the index that included the following:

- Reviewing health literacy guidelines
- Obtaining input from experts in the field
- Searching and reviewing research findings about items
- Cognitive testing
- Review by the CDC's Associate Directors of Communication
- User testing including interrater reliability
- Consumer testing of materials developed with and without the index

The end result of this process is a 20-item index. All items are supported by research, expert review, and testing. In addition, they represent the most important characteristics that can enhance and aid people's understanding of information. The index assesses materials in six areas:

1. Main Message and Call to Action Language (7 items)
2. Information Design (3 items)
3. State of the Science (1 item)
4. Behavioral Recommendations (3 items)
5. Numbers (3 items)
6. Risk (3 items)

A unique component of the index is the initial the cover sheet, containing four open-ended questions before you begin scoring, which help *identify your primary audience* and their health literacy skills, motivation, beliefs, and current behaviors. Knowing your audience and the challenges they face in accessing health information is critical to developing materials they can understand and use in health decision making. Formative research can provide insights about the audience's knowledge attitudes, beliefs, and behaviors. If you are unable to conduct formative research, assume your audience has limited skills.

The worksheet also asks you to write out your *primary communication objective*. A communication objective is what you want your audience to think, feel, or do after they receive the message or material. The primary communication objective will guide development of the material's main message. The *main message* is the one thing you would like audience members to remember after reading, viewing, or using the material.

Using the Index to Guide Materials Development

The index can also be used to guide the development of a communication product from its inception. The CDC has provided an online user guide that defines and explains the 20 items comprising the index and how to score them (http://www.cdc.gov/ccindex/pdf/clear-communication-user-guide.pdf).

Modified Version of the Clear Communication Index

There is also a version of the index that has only 13 items. It was created for shorter materials, like social media messages, podcast and call center scripts, and infographics: http://www.cdc.gov/ccindex/pdf/modified -index-scoresheet.pdf.

Data from The CDC Clear Communication Index: frequently asked questions. Centers for Disease Control and Prevention website. https://www.cdc.gov/healthliteracy/pdf/clear-communication -user-guide.pdf.

Comparing Your Own Work Against Best Practices

The CDC's **Clear Communication Index (CCI)** is a key tool to evaluate a draft material and see if it is working on several levels. See **BOX 3-8** for a description of the origins and development of the CCI, and APPENDICES 3B and 3C for before and after examples of how to use the CCI. The guidelines that go with the index are also useful for creating materials from scratch, be they meant for print, website, or mobile applications.

Health-Literate Organizations

As discussed earlier, the healthcare setting itself can present barriers for those with low health literacy. The Institute of Medicine's Health Literacy Roundtable identified 10 features that healthcare organizations can embrace to promote patient understanding and the use of health information, that is, to become a health-literate organization.[43] Kripalani and colleagues then performed an extensive literature review (the final analysis included nearly 2000 original articles as well as toolkits and other items) to develop measures for assessing these factors within organizations.[44] The factors and examples are found in **TABLE 3-5**.

This is also a good source for identifying resources to build capacity within various healthcare settings, including an audit tool that can be used to determine how difficult it is for a patient to become oriented and to locate specific personnel and locations within a healthcare facility.[45,46]

▶ Conclusion

Health literacy goes beyond basic skills and refers to an individual's personal knowledge base, as well as the ability to add new information that is necessary to make informed health-related decisions. As we have discussed, social disparities in education leave far too many adults unequipped to manage complex health information. We have an increasing number of immigrant, refugee, and asylum-seeking families that cannot use English to navigate health care or who have different cultural beliefs and values about health. It is up to us as communicators to do all we can to ensure that individuals can find, understand, and use health information to make optimal health decisions. Health literacy has moved from being thought of solely as an individual competency to becoming an institutional philosophy—one that must be embraced to move health care forward.

TABLE 3-5 Attributes and Examples of Health-Literate Organizations

A Health-Literate Organization:	Examples
Has leadership that makes health literacy integral to its mission, structure, and operations	<ul><li>Develops and implements policies and standards</li><li>Sets goals for health literacy improvement, establishes accountability, and provides incentives</li><li>Allocates fiscal and human resources</li><li>Redesigns systems and physical space</li></ul>
Integrates health literacy into planning, evaluation measures, patient safety, and quality improvement	<ul><li>Conducts health literacy organizational assessments</li><li>Assesses the impact of policies and programs on individuals with limited health literacy</li><li>Factors health literacy into all patient safety plans</li></ul>
Prepares the workforce to be health literate and monitors progress	<ul><li>Hires diverse staff with expertise in health literacy</li><li>Sets goals for training of staff at all levels</li></ul>
Includes populations served in the design, implementation, and evaluation of health information and services	<ul><li>Includes individuals who are adult learners or have limited health literacy</li><li>Obtains feedback on health information and services from individuals who use them</li></ul>
Meets needs of populations with a range of health literacy skills while avoiding stigmatization	<ul><li>Adopts health literacy universal precautions, such as offering everyone help with health literacy tasks</li><li>Allocates resources proportionate to the concentration of individuals with limited health literacy</li></ul>
Uses health literacy strategies in interpersonal communications and confirms understanding at all points of contact	<ul><li>Confirms understanding (e.g., using the teach-back, show-me, or chunk-and-check methods)</li><li>Secures language assistance for speakers of languages other than English</li><li>Limits to two to three messages at a time</li><li>Uses easily understood symbols in way-finding signage</li></ul>

(continues)

TABLE 3-5 Attributes and Examples of Health-Literate Organizations   *(continued)*

A Health-Literate Organization:	Examples
Provides easy access to health information and services and navigation assistance	▪ Makes electronic patient portals user-centered and provides training on how to use them ▪ Facilitates scheduling appointments with other services
Designs and distributes print, audiovisual, and social media content that is easy to understand and act on	▪ Involves diverse audiences, including those with limited health literacy, in development and rigorous user testing ▪ Uses a quality translation process to produce materials in languages other than English
Addresses health literacy in high-risk situations, including care transitions and communications about medicines	▪ Prioritizes high-risk situations (e.g., informed consent for surgery and other invasive procedures) ▪ Emphasizes high-risk topics (e.g., conditions that require extensive self-management)
Communicates clearly what health plans cover and what individuals will have to pay for services	▪ Provides easy-to-understand descriptions of health insurance policies ▪ Communicates the out-of-pocket costs for healthcare services before they are delivered

Key Terms

Affordable Care Act of 2010
Clear Communication Index (CCI)
Culturally and Linguistically Appropriate Services (CLAS)

Document literacy
Flesch-Kincaid Grade Level Readability Test
Health literacy
Health Literacy Tool Shed
Immigrant

Numeracy
Prose literacy
Quantitative literacy
SMOG

Chapter Questions

1. What are some examples of how health literacy is used?
2. Compare and contrast the effects of low health literacy and high health literacy.
3. How do cultural differences play a role in an individual's health literacy?
4. Describe an experience you have had with health literacy at the doctor's office.
5. Explain how two of the health literacy assessments measure an individual's health literacy.
6. Discuss the differences between basic literacy and health literacy.

References

1. Health literacy measurement tools (revised). Agency for Healthcare Research and Quality website. http://www.ahrq .gov/professionals/quality-patient-safety/quality-resources /tools/literacy/index.html. Revised February 2016. Accessed February 19, 2018.
2. Rudd R. Improving Americans' health literacy. *N Engl J Med*. 2010;363(24):2283-2285.
3. The Patient Protection and Affordable Care Act. Pub. Law No. 111-148. 124 Stat. 119. https://www.gpo.gov/fdsys/pkg /PLAW-111publ148/pdf/PLAW-111publ148.pdf. March 23, 2010. Accessed February 19, 2018.

4. The Patient Protection and Affordable Care Act. Sections 3501, 3506, 3507, and 5301. Pub. Law No. 111-148. 124 Stat. 119. https://www.gpo.gov/fdsys/pkg/PLAW-111publ148/pdf /PLAW-111publ148.pdf. March 23, 2010. Accessed February 19, 2018.
5. U.S. Department of Health and Human Services, Office of Disease Prevention and Health Promotion. National action plan to improve health literacy. Health.gov website. https:// health.gov/communication/initiatives/health-literacy -action-plan.asp. Published 2010. Accessed February 17. 2018.
6. Berkman ND, Sheridan SL, Donahue KE, et al. Health literacy interventions and outcomes: an updated systematic review. *Evidence Rep Tech Assess*. 2011;199:1-941.

7. Scott TL, Gazmararian JA, Williams MV, Baker DW. Health literacy and preventive health care use among Medicare enrollees in a managed care organization. *Med Care*. 2002;40(5):395-404.

8. Vernon JA, Trujillo A, Rosenbaum S, DeBuono B. Low health literacy: implications for national health policy. The George Washington University Public Health website. https://publichealth.gwu.edu/departments/healthpolicy/CHPR/downloads/LowHealthLiteracyReport10_4_07.pdf. Published 2007. Accessed February 19, 2018.

9. Baer J, Kutner M, Sabatini J, White S. Basic reading skills and the literacy of America's least literate adults: results from the 2003 National Assessment of Adult Literacy (NAAL) supplemental studies. NCES 2009-481. National Center for Education Statistics, Institute of Education Sciences website. https://nces.ed.gov/pubs2009/2009481.pdf. Published February 2009. Accessed February 19, 2018.

10. Kutner M, Greenberg E, Baer J. A first look at the literacy of America's adults in the 21st century. National Center for Education Statistics, Institute of Education Sciences website. https://nces.ed.gov/pubsearch/pubsinfo.asp?pubid=2006470. Published December 15, 2005. Accessed February 19, 2018.

11. Rampey BD, Finnegan R, Goodman M, et al. Skills of U.S. unemployed, young, and older adults in sharper focus: results from the Program for the International Assessment of Adult Competencies (PIAAC) 2012 /2014: first look. NCES 2016-039. U.S. Department of Education website. https://nces.ed.gov/pubsearch/pubsinfo.asp?pubid=2016039rev. Published March 2016. Accessed February 19, 2018.

12. Novak JD, Cañas AJ. The theory underlying concept maps and how to construct and use them. Technical Report IHMC CmapTools 2006-01 Rev 01-2008. BetterEvaluation website. http://www.betterevaluation.org/en/resources/guides/concept_mapping/theory_underlying_concept_maps. Published 2008. Accessed February 19, 2018.

13. Zong J, Batalova J, Hallock J. Frequently requested statistics on immigrants and immigration to the United States. http://www.migrationpolicy.org/article/frequently-requested-statistics-immigrants-and-immigration-united-states. Published March 8, 2017. Accessed March 27, 2017.

14. Associated Press. John Kerry: U.S. to accept 85,000 refugees in 2016, 100,000 in 2017. https://www.nbcnews.com/storyline/europes-border-crisis/john-kerry-u-s-accept-85-000-refugees-2016-100-n430576. Published September 20, 2015.

15. Embrace Refugees. Embrace Refugees website. http://embracerefugees.org. Accessed February 19, 2018.

16. Embrace Refugees. The long search for a new home. http://www.embracerefugees.org/resettlement/#. Published July 20, 2016. Accessed February 19, 2018.

17. Foster GM, Anderson BG. *Medical Anthropology*. New York, NY: John Wiley & Sons; 1978.

18. Fadiman A. *The Spirit Catches You and You Fall Down*. New York, NY: Farrar, Straus & Giroux; 1997.

19. Kloos H, David R. The paleoepidemiology of schistosomiasis in ancient Egypt. *Hum Ecol Rev*. 2002;9:14-25.

20. Dettwyler K. *Qualitative Research in Mali*. Washington, DC: Nutrition Communication Project, AED/USAID; 1985.

21. Why don't Jehovah's Witnesses accept blood transfusions? Jehovah's Witnesses website. https://www.jw.org/en/jehovahs-witnesses/faq/jehovahs-witnesses-why-no-blood-transfusions/. Accessed February 19, 2018.

22. Koh HK, Gracia JN, Alvarez ME. Culturally and linguistically appropriate services—advancing health with CLAS. *N Engl J Med*. 2014;371:198-201.

23. Squiers L, Peinado S, Berkman N, Boudewyns V, McCormack L. The health literacy skills framework. *J Health Comm*. 2012;17(suppl 3):30-54.

24. Sørensen K, Van den Broucke S, Fullam J, Slonska Z, Brand H. Health literacy and public health: a systematic review and integration of definitions and models. *BMC Public Health*. 2012;12:80. http://www.biomedcentral.com/1471-2458/12/80

25. Abrams MA, Earles B. Developing an informed consent process with patient understanding in mind. *N C Med J*. 2007;68(5):352-355.

26. Davis TC, Long SW, Jackson RH, et al. Rapid estimate of adult literacy in medicine: a shortened screening instrument. *Fam Med*. 1993;25(6):391-395.

27. Bass PF, Wilson JF, Griffith CH. A shortened instrument for literacy screening. *J Gen Intern Med*. 2003;18(12): 1036-1038.

28. Baker D, Williams M, Nurss J. The test of functional health literacy in adults: a new instrument for measuring patients' literacy skills. *J Gen Intern Med*. 1995;10:537-541.

29. Weiss BD, Mays MZ, Martz W, et al. Quick assessment of literacy in primary care: the newest vital sign. *Ann Fam Med*. 2005;3(6):514-522.

30. Norman CD, Skinner HA. eHEALS: the ehealth literacy scale. *J Med Internet Res*. 2006;8(4):e27. http://www.jmir.org/2006/4/e27/. Accessed February 19, 2018.

31. Schapira MM, Walker CM, Cappaert KJ, et al. The numeracy understanding in medicine instrument: a measure of health numeracy developed using item response theory. *Med Decis Making*. 2012;32(6):851-865. doi:10.1177/0272989X12447239.

32. McCormack L, Bann C, Squiers L, et al. Measuring health literacy: a pilot study of a new skills-based instrument. *J Health Commun*. 2010;15(S2):51-71.

33. Bann CM, McCormack LA, Berkman ND, Squiers LB. The health literacy skills instrument: a 10-item short form. *J Health Commun*. 2012;17(suppl 3):191-202. doi: 10.1080/10810730.2012.718042.

34. Wallace LS, Rogers ES, Roskos SE, Holiday DB, Weiss BD. Brief report: screening items to identify patients with limited health literacy skills. *J Gen Intern Med*. 2006;21(8):874-877.

35. Brega AG, Barnard J, Mabachi NM, et al. *Health Literacy Universal Precautions Toolkit*. 2nd ed. Rockville, MD: Agency for Healthcare Research and Quality; 2015. AHRQ Publication No. 15-0023-EF.

36. Covello VT. Risk communication and message mapping: a new tool for communicating effectively in public health emergencies and disasters. *J Emerg Manag*. 2006;4(3):25-40.

37. DeWalt DA, Broucksou KA, Hawk V, et al. Developing and testing the health literacy universal precautions toolkit. *Nurs Outlook*. 2011;59(2):85-94.

38. Toolkit for making written material clear and effective. Centers for Medicare and Medicaid Services website. https://www.cms.gov/Outreach-and-Education/Outreach/WrittenMaterialsToolkit/index.html?redirect=/WrittenMaterialsToolkit/. Updated March 16, 2012. Accessed February 19, 2018.

39. Kincaid JP, Fishburne Jr RP, Rogers RL, Chissom BS. *Derivation of New Readability Formulas (Automated Readability Index, Fog Count and Flesch Reading Ease Formula) for Navy Enlisted Personnel.* Millington, TN: DTIC Document; 1975.

40. McLaughlin GH. SMOG grading: a new readability formula. *J Reading.* 1969;12(8):639-646.

41. What are patient decision aids? International Patient Decision Aid Standards Collaboration website. http://ipdas.ohri.ca/what.html. Updated June 20, 2012. Accessed February 19, 2018.

42. Elwyn G, O'Connor AM, Bennett C, et al. Assessing the quality of decision support technologies using the International Patient Decision Aid Standards instrument (IPDASi). *PLoS ONE.* 2009;4(3):e4705. doi:10.1371/journal.pone.0004705.

43. Brach C, Keller D, Hernandez LM, et al. *Ten Attributes of Health Literate Health Care Organizations.* Discussion paper. Washington, DC: Institute of Medicine; 2012. https://nam.edu/wp-content/uploads/2015/06/BPH_Ten_HLit_Attributes.pdf

44. Kripalani S, Wallston K, Cavanaugh KL, et al. Measures to assess a health-literate organization. The National Academies of Sciences, Engineering, and Medicine website. http://www.nationalacademies.org/hmd/Activities/PublicHealth/HealthLiteracy/~/media/Files/Activity%20Files/PublicHealth/HealthLiteracy/Commissioned-Papers/Measures_to_Assess_HLO.pdf. Accessed February 19, 2018.

45. Literacy audit for healthcare settings. National Adult Literacy Agency website. https://www.nala.ie/sites/default/files/publications/literacy_audit_for_healthcare_settings.pdf. Published 2009. Accessed February 19, 2018.

46. AHRQ health literacy tools for use in pharmacies. Agency for Healthcare Research and Quality website. http://www.ahrq.gov/professionals/quality-patient-safety/pharmhealthlit/tools.html. Updated November 2015. Accessed February 19, 2018.

Appendix 3A

Use of a Patient Activation Tool for Shared Decision Making in Pediatric Appendicitis

Dani O. Gonzalez, Katherine J. Deans, and Peter C. Minneci

We developed a patient activation tool (PAT) to determine if it could improve decision making and patient-centered outcomes in pediatric patients with appendicitis and their caregivers. We conducted a randomized controlled trial of standard surgical consultation alone compared to standard surgical consultation plus a PAT in patients with appendicitis choosing operative or non-operative management for appendicitis. In addition to comparing medical outcomes between the groups, we compared decision making and patient-centered outcomes utilizing questionnaires, including *the Pediatric Quality of Life Inventory™ (PedsQL™) 4.0 Generic Core Scales—Child and Parent Report, PedsQL™ 3.0 Healthcare Satisfaction Generic Module—Parent Report, Decision Self-Efficacy Scale, Decision Regret Scale, Parent Patient Activation Measure®*, and a knowledge recall quiz.

The PAT encouraged active involvement in the treatment choice, outlined the two treatment options with the attendant risks and benefits, elucidated the caregiver's values and decisional support, and taught patient–caregiver dyads how to communicate decisional uncertainty. The PAT was provided as a computer tablet–based application that was tailored for a Flesch-Kincaid reading level between the 5th and 6th grade. It was narrated to ensure that both children and low-literacy adults were able to understand the tool. In addition, we attempted to minimize the effects of differences in numeracy by presenting numbers, percentages, and proportions graphically using figures to facilitate understanding. At the beginning of the PAT, each patient–caregiver dyad was given the opportunity to choose a "guide" to take them through the PAT. The character options included both cartoons and people representing both genders and various races/ethnicities. The goal of this process was to allow each patient–caregiver dyad to personalize the PAT experience.

Select screenshots from the PAT on an iPad tablet are shown in FIGURE 3A-1 through FIGURE 3A-17.

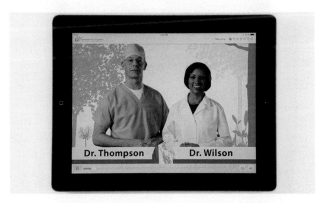

FIGURE 3A-1 The PAT is introduced to patient–caregiver dyads.

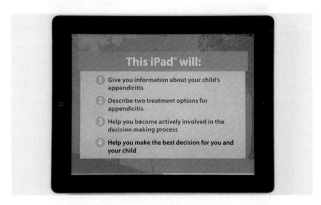

FIGURE 3A-2 The objectives of the PAT are highlighted.

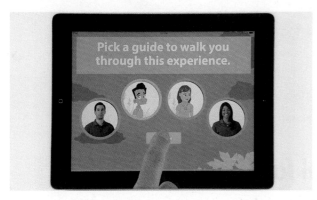

FIGURE 3A-3 Patient–caregiver dyads then select a "guide" to walk them through the experience.

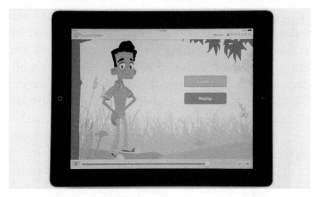

FIGURE 3A-4 Patient–caregiver dyads are instructed on how to use the PAT and its features, including pause, play, rewind, replay, and closed captioning.

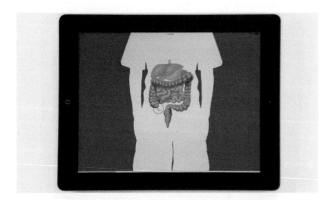

FIGURE 3A-5 The definition and pathophysiology of appendicitis are explained to users.

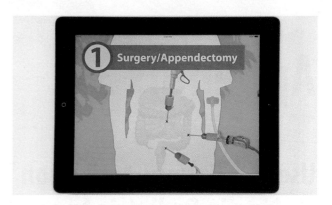

FIGURE 3A-6 The two treatment options are reviewed. The surgical option (appendectomy) is reviewed and explained.

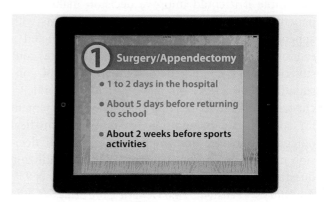

FIGURE 3A-7 The postoperative course is reviewed.

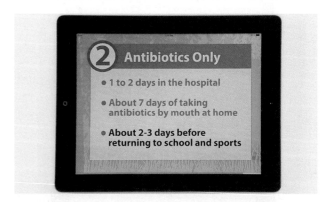

FIGURE 3A-8 The nonoperative option (antibiotics only) is reviewed.

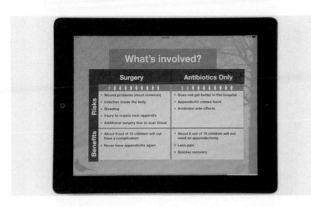

FIGURE 3A-9 The risks and benefits of both management options are reviewed.

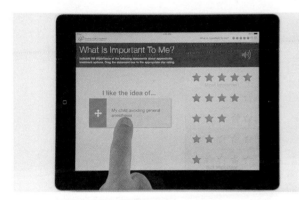

FIGURE 3A-10 Users then participate in an exercise to weigh the risks and benefits of both management options. In this exercise, they rank the importance of each of the risks and benefits.

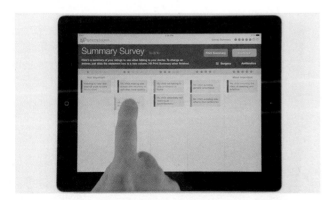

FIGURE 3A-11 Once they have ranked each risk and benefit, users are given a summary of their choices. They can change the ranking by dragging and dropping each statement to its corresponding level of importance. They are encouraged to use these summaries to guide the discussion with their physician after they have completed the PAT.

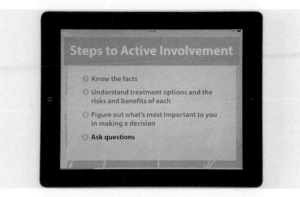

FIGURE 3A-12 The steps involved in active engagement for clinical decision making are described and reviewed. Patient–caregiver dyads are encouraged to ask questions now that they know the facts, understand the treatment options and their risks and benefits, and have decided what factors are most important to them when making a decision. They are encouraged to complete the final step, which is to ask questions about any additional concerns they have.

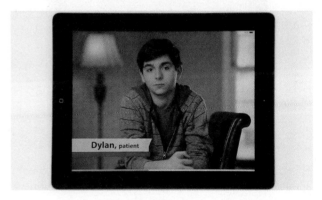

FIGURE 3A-13 Actors portraying patients and parents then share their experiences with making the decision about a treatment option and encourage parents to discuss the questions they may have with their physicians.

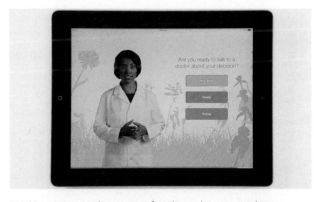

FIGURE 3A-14 At that point, families who are ready to discuss their decision with the physician have the option to do so and exit the PAT. Families who are not ready to discuss the decision with their physician have the option to listen to additional information.

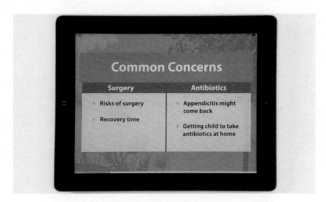

FIGURE 3A-15 Families who choose to hear additional information are given summaries of common concerns of other patient–caregiver dyads faced with the same decision.

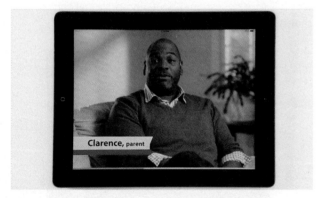

FIGURE 3A-16 In addition, they watch vignettes of actors portraying families faced with the same decision, describing why they made their decisions.

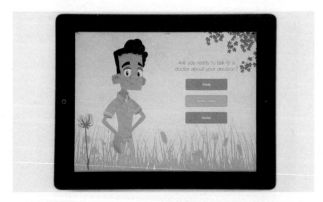

FIGURE 3A-17 At that point, the PAT has concluded. Families can speak with their physician, review specific videos within the PAT, or replay the entire PAT experience.

All figures courtesy of Katherine J. Deans.

Appendix 3B

Vaccine Safety: Original Fact Sheet

A-Z Index A B C D E F G H I J K L M N O P Q R S T U V W X Y Z #

Vaccine Safety

Vaccine Safety
- Vaccines Safety Basics
- Addressing Common Concerns
  - Adjuvants
  - Autism
  - CDC Statement on Pandemrix
  - Fainting (Syncope)
  - Febrile Seizures
  - GBS
  - IOM Assessment of Studies on Childhood Immunization Schedule
  - IOM Report on Adverse Effects of Vaccines
  - Pregnancy and Influenza Vaccine Safety
  - Sudden Infant Death Syndrome (SIDS)
  - Thimerosal
    - Vaccines & Immunoglobins & Risk of Autism
    - Infant & Environmental Exposures to Thimerosal
    - ▶FAQs about Thimerosal
    - Timeline: Thimerosal in Vaccines (1999-2010)
    - Publications
- FAQs about Multiple Vaccines and the Immune System
- FAQs about Vaccine Recalls
- FAQs about Vaccine Safety
- Vaccine Monitoring
- Activities
- Special Populations
- Resource Library

Vaccine Safety > Addressing Common Concerns > Thimerosal

[f Recommend] 88 [y Tweet] 16 [+] Share

Frequently Asked Questions About Thimerosal (Ethylmercury)

There are two, very different, types of mercury which people should know about: **methylmercury** and **ethylmercury**.

Mercury is a naturally occurring element found in the earth's crust, air, soil, and water. Since the earth's formation, volcanic eruptions, weathering of rocks and burning coal have caused mercury to be released into the environment. Once released, certain types of bacteria in the environment can change mercury into **methylmercury**. Methylmercury makes its way through the food chain in fish, animals, and humans. At high levels, it can be toxic to people. For more information about methylmercury: please read "What You Need to Know about Mercury in Fish and Shellfish " from the Environmental Protection Agency (EPA).

Thimerosal contains a different form of mercury called **ethylmercury**. Studies comparing ethylmercury and methylmercury suggest that they are processed differently in the human body. Ethylmercury is broken down and excreted much more rapidly than methylmercury. Therefore, ethylmercury (the type of mercury found in the influenza vaccine) is much less likely than methylmercury (the type of mercury in the environment) to accumulate in the body and cause harm.

On this Page
- What is thimerosal?
- Why is thimerosal used as a preservative in vaccines?
- How does thimerosal work in the body?
- Is thimerosal safe?
- What are the possible side-effects of thimerosal?
- Does thimerosal cause autism?
- Do MMR vaccines contain thimerosal?
- Do all flu vaccines contain thimerosal?
- How can I find out if thimerosal is in a vaccine?

What is thimerosal?
Thimerosal is a mercury-based preservative that has been used for decades in the United States in multi-dose vials (vials containing more than one dose) of medicines and vaccines.

Top of page ⓖ

Why is thimerosal used as a preservative in vaccines?
Thimerosal is added to vials of vaccine that contain more than one dose to prevent the growth of could cause severe local reactions, serious illness or death. In some vaccines, preservatives are added during the manufacturing process to prevent microbial growth.

Top of page ⓖ

How does thimerosal work in the body?
Thimerosal does not stay in the body a long time so it does not build up and reach harmful levels. When thimerosal enters the body, it breaks down, to ethylmercury and thiosalicylate, which are easily eliminated.

Top of page ⓖ

Is thimerosal safe?
Thimerosal has a proven track record of being very safe. Data from many studies show no convincing evidence of harm caused by the low doses of thimerosal in vaccines.

Top of page ⓖ

What are the possible side-effects of thimerosal?

The most common side-effects are minor reactions like redness and swelling at the injection site. Although rare, some people may be allergic to thimerosal. Research shows that most people who are allergic to thimerosal will not have a reaction when thimerosal is injected under the skin (Wattanakrai, 2007; Heidary, 2005).

Top of page ⊕

Does thimerosal cause autism?

Research *does not* show any link between thimerosal in vaccines and autism, a neurodevelopmental disorder. Although thimerosal was taken out of childhood vaccines in 2001, autism rates have gone up, which is the opposite of what would be expected if thimerosal caused autism.

Top of page ⊕

Do MMR vaccines contain thimerosal?

No, measles, mumps, and rubella (MMR) vaccines do not and never did contain thimerosal. Varicella (chickenpox), inactivated polio (IPV), and pneumococcal conjugate vaccines have also never contained thimerosal.

Top of page ⊕

Do all flu vaccines contain thimerosal?

No. Influenza (flu) vaccines are currently available in both thimerosal-containing and thimerosal-free versions. The total amount of flu vaccine without thimerosal as a preservative at times has been limited, but availability will increase as vaccine manufacturing capabilities are expanded. In the meantime, it is important to keep in mind that the benefits of influenza vaccination outweigh the theoretical risk, if any, of exposure to thimerosal.

Top of page ⊕

How can I find out if thimerosal is in a vaccine?

For a complete list of vaccines and their thimerosal content level, you may visit the U.S. Food and Drug Administration. ⊡ Additionally, you may ask your health care provider or pharmacist for a copy of the vaccine package insert. It lists ingredients in the vaccine and discusses any known adverse reactions.

Top of page ⊕

References

Please see References for a list of published articles on thimerosal.

⊠   🖶   ☑
Email   Print   Updates

Page last reviewed: March 1, 2010
Page last updated: October 14, 2011
Content source: Centers for Disease Control and Prevention
National Center for Emerging and Zoonotic Infectious Diseases (NCEZID)
Division of Healthcare Quality Promotion (DHQP)

Home   A-Z Index   Site Map   Policies   Using this Site   Link to Us   All Languages   CDC Mobile   Contact CDC

Centers for Disease Control and Prevention   1600 Clifton Rd. Atlanta, GA 30333, USA
800-CDC-INFO (800-232-4636) TTY: (888) 232-6348 - Contact CDC-INFO

Appendix 3C

Vaccine Safety: Revised Fact Sheet

A-Z Index A B C D E F G H I J K L M N O P Q R S T U V W X Y Z #

Vaccine Safety

Vaccine Safety > Addressing Common Concerns > Thimerosal

[f] Recommend   106   [t] Tweet   9   [+] Share

Email page link
Print page

Thimerosal: You asked. We answered.

Some parents have questions about the safety of ingredients – like thimerosal ("THY-mayr-uh-sal") – in children's shots (vaccines).

We want you to know that thimerosal is no longer used in children's shots, except the flu shot. You can ask for a flu shot without thimerosal.

Check out these answers to common questions about thimerosal.

What is thimerosal?

Thimerosal is added to some shots to prevent germs (like bacteria and fungi) from growing in them.

If germs grow in vaccines, they can cause illness — or even death.

Why do some people worry about thimerosal in vaccines?

You may have heard that thimerosal has mercury in it. Not all types of mercury are the same. Some types of mercury, like mercury in some kinds of fish, can stay in the human body and make us sick. Thimerosal is a different type of mercury. It doesn't stay in the body, and is unlikely to make us sick.

Is thimerosal safe?

Yes. Thimerosal has been used safely in vaccines for a long time (since the 1930s).

Scientists have been studying the use of thimerosal in vaccines for many years. They haven't found any evidence that thimerosal causes harm.

Is thimerosal still used in vaccines for children?

No. Thimerosal hasn't been used in vaccines for children since 2001.

However, thimerosal is still used in some flu vaccines. The flu vaccine is recommended for all children. If you are worried about thimerosal, ask for a flu vaccine without it.

Does thimerosal cause autism?

No. Research does not show any link between thimerosal and autism.

Read more about vaccines and autism.

Remember: Shots help protect your kids from dangerous diseases. The benefits of vaccines outweigh any possible side effects. Find out which shots your children need.

Are there side effects from thimerosal?

Most people don't have any side effects from thimerosal. The most common reactions are usually mild (like redness and swelling at the place where the shot was given) and only last 1 to 2 days. It's very unlikely that you will have an allergic reaction to thimerosal.

How can I find out if thimerosal is in a vaccine?

1. Ask your doctor or pharmacist.
2. Ask to see the vaccine's list of ingredients. All vaccine packages come with information (called an insert) that lists the ingredients.
3. Check out this complete list of vaccines to see which ones contain thimerosal.

References

See references for a list of scientific articles on thimerosal.

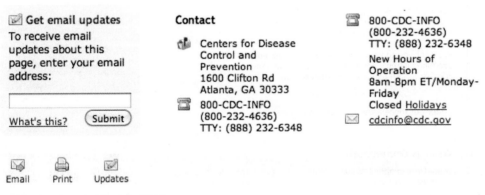

☑ **Get email updates**
To receive email updates about this page, enter your email address:

[   ]

What's this?   (Submit)

Contact

🏛 Centers for Disease Control and Prevention 1600 Clifton Rd Atlanta, GA 30333

☎ 800-CDC-INFO (800-232-4636) TTY: (888) 232-6348

☎ 800-CDC-INFO (800-232-4636) TTY: (888) 232-6348

New Hours of Operation 8am-8pm ET/Monday-Friday Closed Holidays

✉ cdcinfo@cdc.gov

✉   🖨   ☑
Email   Print   Updates

Page last reviewed: March 1, 2010
Page last updated: October 19, 2012
Content source: Centers for Disease Control and Prevention
Office of the Associate Director for Communication

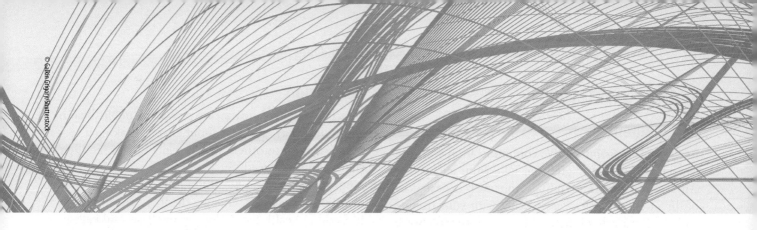

CHAPTER 4

Health Communication Practice Strategies and Theories

Claudia Parvanta

LEARNING OBJECTIVES

By the end of this chapter, the reader will be able to:

- Define key differences among health communication strategies used to engage, inform, or persuade.
- Weigh the pros and cons of different practice strategies.
- Grasp the fundamentals of social marketing.
- Explain why theory is used in health communication planning.
- Describe the key theories of behavior change used most commonly in health communication.
- Use two theories to guide media channel selection.

▶ Introduction

There are three basic action words in health communication: *engage*, *inform*, and *persuade*. Regardless of whether we are working with an individual patient, a classroom, a virtual community, or a group of policymakers, or using mass media to reach the public at large, the process begins with engagement. Once an audience begins interacting with us (which can include passive reading or listening), we have an opportunity to inform. In a healthcare setting, this often involves shared decision making (SDM) where the provider truly wants the patient to weigh options without bias. If we feel strongly that what we propose will greatly benefit someone, then we can try to be persuasive. Some approaches mix these strategies together in a seamless way. Entertainment education, the embedding of health topics into dramatic stories, is one such practice strategy that is highly engaging and can be informative and persuasive. Other approaches are more limited, such as signs at the grocery store indicating which foods are the most nutritious (informing) or online communities for patients who share an illness or condition and just want to share their experiences with each other (engaging). However, many people would be persuaded to purchase healthier food based on simple information, and others will find the online community to be their best source of information. So, this distinction is not hard and fast. This chapter discusses why some practice strategies are more effective than others at accomplishing a health communication goal, and the psychological and communication theories on which they are built.

▶ Core Strategies

Engagement

Engagement is interactive communication with the expectation of *timely* give and take from all parties. After your parents and siblings, your early experiences of direct engagement were playing with your friends and going to school. Some of your classmates were highly engaged with the teacher's lesson plan; others were not. Increasingly, we use social media, such as Facebook, Snapchat, and Instagram, to engage with teachers, classmates, family, friends, and more. Health communicators also use social media to "…build and sustain networks, build trust, (and) mobilize communities, … among other benefits."[1]

Ethically, it is worth considering whether a health communicator can ever be just another "friend" in an online community. Consider the motivations. Unless we are engaged as private individuals, why are we reading posts or using social media tools to gather data? Why are we trying to build up trust or respect in a community? Why are we giving encouragement and support, or disagreeing with what others say? Why do we care about the number of followers or friends we have? And if we generate content, where does it come from? If health communicators use social media as a tool for obtaining information and effecting behavior change, then a high level of self-awareness is required to avoid privacy issues in data collection and misrepresentations in communication. (Interestingly, the private sector seems to have no qualms about the use of social media as a deliberate part of marketing strategy.) Engagement is an end in itself but is also the first step in persuading an audience to receive and accept our message.

Informing

The difference between data and information is that information answers questions. Until someone needs to know something, data are like those images from the *Matrix* movie—just strings of numbers cascading down around us out of context. Research in psychology and, increasingly, neuroscience provides much of what we understand to enhance how users can process health information.[2] For example, gain- and loss-framed messaging relies on some of our psychological tendencies, while the best visual displays of numeric information are not only easy to decipher but also provide guidance without unnecessary persuasion. Health communicators can use theory to design patient decision aids and other information materials.

Persuasion

Coaches, teachers, healthcare providers, public health communicators, and just about anyone making a recommendation to others would really like to see their suggestions followed. Such persuasion requires tapping into something meaningful to the object of our attentions. Behavior change theories, mostly from the field of health psychology, provide several keys to motivating people to adopt a new idea or behavior. We will not discuss techniques for individual persuasion (such as motivational interviewing), which are better addressed in psychological texts. But, we will discuss strategies for negotiating change in populations.

▶ Selecting a Practice Strategy: The Behavioral Economics of Choice

A **practice strategy** can be described as an approach or a tactic, as it is a planned process to achieve your overall communication goal of engagement, information, or persuasion. Behavioral economics, and the newer neuro-economics, provide clues about which approach might work best. Older economic models operated on the assumption that individuals make decisions based on the logic of self-interest. However, studies tell us that human behavior is often irrational, inconsistent, and complex.[3] (We often behave like the kid who would rather eat one marshmallow now than wait five minutes for two marshmallows.) Behavioral economics applies information from psychology, neuroscience, and economics to transactions involving goods, services, and wealth and is now trickling into healthcare decision making, especially for choices that involve value-based decisions.

Given any choice, a "rational" decision maker will select the one that benefits them more than it costs; however, as neuroscience demonstrates, we often use a combination of cognitive (rational) and affective (emotional) variables to make decisions.[3] Individual decisions may appear irrational when underlying motivations are not obvious or unseen constraints are at play. In developing health communication messages, we want to start first with the large framework of obvious costs and benefits and then examine the underlying factors that translate into the hidden costs of the suggested behavior. **FIGURE 4-1** illustrates Rothschild's analysis of these parameters.[4]

We can select a basic approach to use depending on where the behavior change falls in the domain of education, law, or marketing (Figure 4-1). Each approach depends on certain conditions being present and can be optimized with certain tactics.

Educational Approaches

When individuals believe they have much more to gain than to lose—including the hidden costs of time, energy, emotional burden, and so forth—then information alone might be sufficient to prompt a change. Educational approaches work best if:

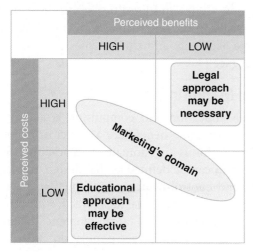

FIGURE 4-1 Interpretation of Rothschild's behavior management model.

■ The recipient of the information has expressed an interest in, or commitment to, the desired behavior.

■ The recipient only needs answers to factual questions such as what, who, where, and how.

■ The information is simple, clear, and unambiguous.

A long-term, nationwide example of a longstanding educational program is the Safe to Sleep campaign, formerly known as Back to Sleep. Since 1994, the campaign has been managed by a collaborative led by the Eunice Kennedy Shriver National Institute of Child Health and Human Development (part of the National Institutes of Health) and the American Academy of Pediatrics. Safe to Sleep materials follow many of the principles of clear health communication, and different culturally targeted versions are available.[5] Many state and local health departments have also customized the materials for their constituents. See **FIGURE 4-2** for examples.

It does not take a lot of persuasion to convince parents to adopt an easily accomplished, no-cost, high-return behavior. Since the start of the campaign, sudden infant death syndrome (SIDS) rates in the

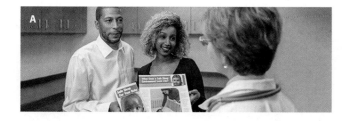

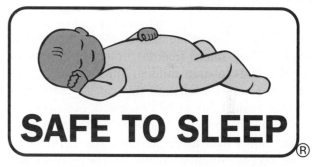

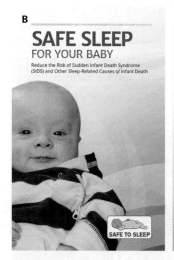

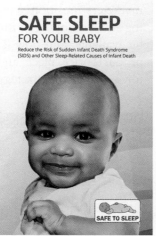

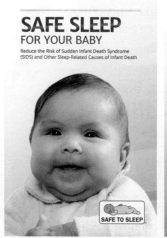

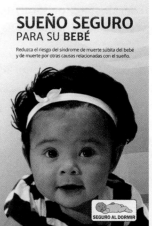

FIGURE 4-2 Safe to Sleep campaign. **A.** The Safe to Sleep® campaign provides clear information to parents about reducing the risk for SIDS and other sleep-related causes of infant death. **B.** Targeted brochures.

A. Used with permission from Safe to Sleep®. https://SafetoSleep.nichd.nih.gov. Safe to Sleep® is a registered trademark of the U.S. Department of Health and Human Services. **B.** Reproduced from National Institutes of Health. Safe to sleep campaign materials. https://www1.nichd.nih.gov/sts/materials/Pages/default.aspx.

United States have decreased by almost 50%, both overall and within various racial and ethnic groups.[6] But SIDS remains the leading cause of death for U.S. infants 1 month to 1 year of age, and it is more prevalent within some populations. The fact that the campaign has been in place for more than 20 years and the death rate has been cut in half, but not more, demonstrates two things about health communication campaigns. First, some believe that health communication campaigns can be run for a while and then stopped because "everyone will have gotten the message." In response, we usually point out that Coke and Pepsi, for example, never stop advertising. On a population level, it takes a very long time for new behaviors to become embedded in the culture—in this case, not letting "granny" cover the baby with a blanket because they might be cold, for example. Second, health communication can address only behavioral risk factors. There are other contributors to SIDS, such as inborn abnormalities.

Policy Approaches

In contrast to low-cost, relatively "easy" behavior changes are those that at first glance appear to be difficult or costly and offer few *individual* benefits, but upon deeper consideration might yield collective population value. Such changes often require enactment of laws or regulations. Most public health hygiene laws, smoke-free restaurant regulations, or requirements to strap children into rear safety seats in motor vehicles fall into this category. For new laws or regulations to be developed, organizations (government agencies, concerned citizen groups) must collect data to demonstrate the harm being done, propose solutions to mitigate the problem, and begin an advocacy effort to convince policymakers (federal, state, or local) to take up the issue. However, laws and regulations aren't always enough; for example, even though there are now laws in many states prohibiting distracted driving, which includes texting and hands-on cell phone use, many people still feel they can "get away with it." One of the more powerful communication approaches is to combine information about a tangible punishment with a persuasive message (e.g., "click-it-or-ticket" for seatbelt use). Many states and localities are using even more persuasive approaches, such as showing the results of horrible accidents and the last messages on smartphones (see **FIGURE 4-3**).

Social Marketing

Between education and compulsion is a gray zone where a cost and a benefit are a matter of negotiated exchange. This is the domain of marketing. **Social marketing** can be defined as the "design, implementation, and control of programs aimed at increasing the acceptability of a social idea, practice [or product] in one or more groups of target adopters. The process actively involves the target population, who voluntarily exchange their time and attention for help in meeting their health needs as they perceive them."[7]

In the world of commercial marketing, people are "consumers" who are trying to solve problems. Sometimes the problems are obvious to them; at other times, their needs are hidden. For example, you probably didn't realize you needed a gadget to turn zucchini, carrots, and other vegetables into noodles, until one was brought to market. But the marketers tapped into the growing trend toward gluten-free eating and people's desire to still eat spaghetti; hence, the spiral vegetable cutter was born.

Social marketers use many of the same tools as commercial marketers use to identify needs and develop products or services to meet them. Social marketers "position" a product or service by researching and developing its image, its price, where it should be available, and how it is promoted. The four Ps—product, price, place, and promotion—form the basis for a marketing strategy. Social marketing involves

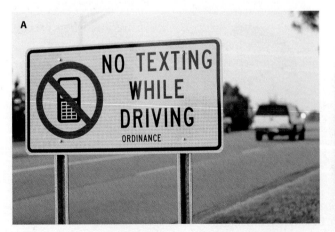

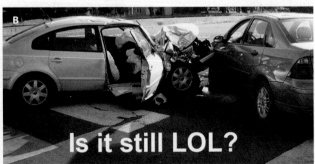

FIGURE 4-3 No texting while driving sign and campaign.

more dimensions than health communication alone. Examples of socially marketed products include condoms to prevent sexually transmitted disease, skim/low-fat milk for children to reduce obesity, and folic acid to prevent birth defects. In low-income countries, social marketing has been used for decades to promote immunization, birth control devices and medications, oral rehydration solution, and mosquito nets, to mention only a few tangible items. Social marketing has also been used extensively to promote intangible "products" (**attitudes** and behaviors), such as acceptance of community-based halfway homes for persons with cognitive impairments, using designated drivers after parties, and eating more fruits and vegetables in our daily diet.

Depending on the degree to which a proposed behavioral change is obvious, easy, or acceptable, a health communicator might choose education, social marketing, or legislative routes as the core strategy. Each of these strategies is built on the work of previous investigators who developed theories related to the problem and to the mechanism of behavioral change.

▶ Working with Theory in Health Communication

In the behavioral and social sciences, theories are systematic ways of understanding what causes an individual or a group to behave in certain ways in specific situations. Theories are made up of "propositions that explain or predict events by illustrating the relationships among variables."[8] We develop theories about causality based on social science and epidemiological research. We tend to use long-standing theories from our discipline to predict how and why change might occur.

When designing a health communication intervention, we start by searching for modifiable risk factors. The word "modifiable" suggests that something has been identified as contributing to a negative outcome, and we believe we can reduce that risk. There will be other risk factors about which we can do nothing. For example, drinking alcohol before driving is a modifiable risk factor for automobile crashes; in contrast, a young person coming of age to drive is a risk factor that is more difficult to modify in most states. To determine the upstream and downstream causes of the problem (e.g., What causes young people to drink alcohol too close to stepping into a car as the driver?), we can use tools from epidemiology and community-based assessment to diagnose what predisposes, enables, or reinforces the problem, and similarly, what factors might contribute to potential solutions. We

build an explanatory model of why the problem exists and which interventions might bring about change.

As in any other scientific enterprise, these hypotheses must be tested systematically in multiple populations and contexts to generate theories of cause and change. Our theories about causality and the best way to effect change then guide our selection of intervention strategies. So, for example, if we see that drunk driving goes down after enacting laws with stiff penalties, we might believe the policy approach with adequate information is sufficient to solve the problem. Or, we might see that persuasive advertising, or a socially marketed ride sharing intervention, are more effective for specific populations and contexts. Any one intervention program might include all of these approaches, or be limited to one. Each approach is grounded in theories about what motivates individuals to form or modify beliefs, attitudes, or behaviors, as well as the best ways to communicate with them in specific contexts.

▶ Theory Used to Guide Informing

"I can explain it to you, but I can't comprehend it for you."
—Attributed to Mayor Ed Koch, New York City.

Information is all around us, and as humans, we are genetically programmed to absorb bits and pieces of information and assemble them into meaningful patterns. Typically, humans lose their sponge-like learning abilities around puberty. Many experience the difficulty of learning a new language in high school or as an adult. But recent studies suggest that it is not the elasticity of our minds that has changed, but our motivation to acquire new information as well as how we go about it.[9]

Findings like this from neuroscience are being translated into new health communication practice strategies. There might be a future time when we can transmit "understanding" and not just information to another being. But for now, we know that being able to comprehend information and caring about it are two keys. This is particularly true in the area of health care, where an SDM model is becoming the dominant model in the United States.

There are several more theories derived from communication study that deepen our understanding of the way we perceive and react to information, which depend largely on the source and the context. We will discuss inoculation theory and the extended parallel process model (EPPM), both of which are also used in persuasion.

Inoculation Theory

Nietzsche's statement, "What does not kill us makes us stronger," is the concept behind vaccines. A weak dose of a virus causes our bodies to create an immune response. McGuire[11,12] applied the concept to what we learned about the brainwashing of Korean War prisoners. Psychological warfare came of age when conceptual inoculation began to be used as defense against it. This theory is one that has been used extensively in communication ever since, with hundreds of applications to not only health, but also politics and advocacy. A very common example of inoculation theory is when your healthcare provider says, "This may hurt a little bit," and you brace yourself for the pain. Often the actual pain is less than what you anticipated, thanks to your body's preparation for a painful sensation.

You might remember health education classes in middle school that told you that other kids would try to convince you that smoking, or taking drugs, was cool. The teachers prepared young students to rehearse how they would react to such peers; for example, "When a role-playing peer called a student 'chicken' for not being willing to try an imaginary cigarette, the student practiced answers such as 'I'd be a real chicken if I smoked just to impress you.'" In a study, Perry and colleagues found that students who were inoculated in this way were about half as likely to become smokers as were students who did not receive this intervention.[13]

For good or for bad, inoculation theory is used extensively in political campaigns when you hear candidates say such things as, "My rival will tell you that I'm a low down dirty dog," or words to that effect. Having heard them first from the candidate him- or herself diffuses some of the impact later. In risk or emergency communication, we use inoculation theory to prepare people that bad news is potentially on the way, such as, "We will learn things in the coming weeks that everyone will wish we had known when we started"[14] or "the death rates will likely go up as we are able to remove more debris." These are population-level applications of saying, "This is going to hurt," and they allow the audience to move with the communicator through difficult times rather than reacting with anger as information changes.

Anticipatory guidance, as used in health care, is almost the reverse of inoculation theory, in that it is meant to make the recipient look forward to, and be ready to learn about, next steps, such as in maternity or pediatric care (e.g., "When you come in for your next prenatal visit, we'll discuss breastfeeding and any questions you might have about how you will feed your newborn").

Extended Parallel Process Model

Humans are motivated to minimize fear. Communications that attempt to scare people into action can backfire due to what Witte[15] described in the extended parallel process model (EPPM). When presented with information about a threat, people undergo two parallel lines of thinking: (1) Am I susceptible to this threat, and how dangerous is it to me? (based on the health belief model), and (2) Is there an action I know that I can take to avoid this threat? This second track is based not only on knowledge of a tactic to avoid the threat, but also on a sense of personal capability (referred to as **self-efficacy**) in performing it. If people do not feel able to side-step the threat, they might justify inaction by telling themselves that the threat does not pertain to them, deciding the threat is not that serious, or ignoring information about the threat altogether (for example, a person might tell you that an aging relative has smoked since childhood and is still in perfect health). EPPM can be used for **audience segmentation** for messages by combinations of perceived fear and self-efficacy, as done by Campo and others[16] in **FIGURE 4-4**.

EPPM AUDIENCE SEGMENTS AND STRATEGIES

	High efficacy Belief in effectiveness of solutions and confidence to practice them	**Low efficacy** Doubts about effectiveness of solutions and about one's ability to practice them
High threat Belief that the threat is harmful and that one is at risk	**Danger control** People take protective action to avoid or reduce the threat. *Strategy: Provide calls to action*	**Fear control** People are too afraid to act, just try to reduce their fear and feel better. *Strategy: Educate about solutions*
Low threat Belief that the threat is trivial and that one is not at risk	**Lesser amount of danger control** People know what to do but are not really motivated to do much. *Strategy: Educate about risk*	**No response** People don't feel at risk and don't know what to do about it anyway. *Strategy: Educate about risk and about solutions*

FIGURE 4-4 Extended parallel process model.

▶ Theory Used to Persuade

We have an almost religious reverence for psychological behavior change theories. However, as R. Schwarzer[17] has pointed out, we rarely test these theories in their entirety, nor subject their constructs to real scrutiny. When our projects do not work, we assume we did something wrong in the delivery and rarely blame the theory on which it was built. Just as Scherer and colleagues have recently challenged the importance of "elaboration" in making decisions, other behavior change researchers are cleaning out our theory tool shed.

The following theories are some of the most established in health communication with decades of effective use. So, although not necessarily tested in and of themselves, the programs on which they have been built have produced positive outcomes.

Health Belief Model

The **health belief model (HBM)** was one of the first theories developed to explain individual health behaviors.[18,19] As suggested by its name, the HBM is all about beliefs and attitudes pertaining to the following:

- *Susceptibility:* The belief that you are at risk
- *Severity:* The belief that the condition is serious
- *Effectiveness:* The belief that the recommended treatment or prevention is effective
- *Self-efficacy:* The belief in one's own capacity to perform a desired behavior
- *Costs:* The perception of monetary, physical, or psychosocial costs needed to perform a behavior

The outbreak of the Zika virus in the southern hemisphere and southern United States provides a recent case of the HBM in action. Most people in the United States are not worried about Zika because (1) they do not live in an area with the *A. aegypti* mosquito, and (2) they've been told it poses few known risks for otherwise healthy individuals (although the risks are mounting as our knowledge of Zika increases). So, there is a low perceived susceptibility and low perceived level of severity. The Centers for Disease Control and Prevention (CDC) has warned women to avoid geographic areas with Zika, or to take extreme precautions either to not get pregnant or to prevent any contact with mosquitoes, due to the risks to the developing fetus.

Health officials have had considerable trouble in Puerto Rico getting individuals to pay attention to these warnings. To quote Sifferlin[20]:

> ...over 80% of adults in Puerto Rico have been infected with dengue, and about a quarter of adults became infected with *chikungunya* (another mosquito borne illness) in less than a year.... since residents are accustomed to mosquitoes spreading diseases, it can be hard to ramp up concern over Zika and mosquito control; to some residents, mosquito-borne diseases are considered a fact of life.

HBM works well with those who believe that they are vulnerable, that proposed interventions will be effective, and that they can perform the interventions. If a population does not feel vulnerable, does not consider the risk of illness to be that serious, or thinks that the preventive steps will be too difficult or costly (e.g., abstinence to avoid pregnancy, or use of insect repellent and wearing long sleeves and pants in over 100°F temperatures), then another approach needs to be used to persuade people to adopt the behavior.

Transtheoretical Model

The awkwardly named **transtheoretical model (TTM)**,[21] also known as the **stages of change (SOC)** model, indicates that individuals move through a specific linear process when deciding to change their behavior and then actually changing their behavior. These SOC are:

- Precontemplation
- Contemplation
- Preparation
- Action
- Maintenance

Different individuals may be at different stages in this process and therefore must receive interventions or communications that are tailored to individual SOC. For example, smokers who are in precontemplation have no intention of quitting smoking in the next 6 months, so information about cessation aids such as nicotine patches will not help them quit. However, smokers in contemplation do plan to quit smoking in the next 6 months; positively reinforcing this goal with enabling information should be effective for them. Descriptions of the stages and appropriate health communication, education, and intervention strategies are listed in **TABLE 4-1**.[8] Many interventions combine TTM with social cognitive theory constructs, or other models, to deliver messages to prompt audiences to take a next step.

Subsequent work[22] that combined the TTM with social cognitive theory (see the next section) eliminated the supposition that the TTM represents a smooth transition from one stage to the next, with different stages being influenced through quantity, not quality, of message.

TABLE 4-1 Transtheoretical or Stages of Change Model Stages

Stage	Definition	Potential Change Strategies
Precontemplation	Has no intention of acting within the next 6 months	Increase awareness of need for change; personalize information about risks and benefits
Contemplation	Intends to act in the next 6 months	Motivate; encourage making specific plans
Preparation	Intends to act within the next 30 days and has taken some behavioral steps in this direction	Assist with developing and implementing concrete action plans; help set gradual goals
Action	Has changed behavior for less than 6 months	Assist with feedback, problem solving, social support, and reinforcement
Maintenance	Has changed behavior for more than 6 months	Assist with coping, reminders, finding alternatives, and avoiding slips/relapses (as applicable)

Reproduced from National Cancer Institute. *Theory at a Glance: A Guide for Health Promotion Practice.* 2nd ed. Bethesda, MD: U.S. Department of Health and Human Services, Public Health Services, National Institutes of Health, National Cancer Institute; 2005. https://cancercontrol.cancer.gov/brp/research/theories_project/theory.pdf. Accessed March 23, 2018.

Social Cognitive Theory

Social cognitive theory (SCT)[22] hypothesizes that individual behavior is the result of constant interaction between the external environment and internal psychosocial characteristics and perceptions. Albert Bandura originally named this social learning theory (1962) and published it as SCT in 1986. "The theory considers a person's past experiences, which factor into whether behavioral action will occur. These past experiences influence reinforcements, and expectations, all of which shape whether a person will engage in a specific behavior and the reasons why a person engages in that behavior."[23] There are many constructs included in SCT (see **TABLE 4-2**). Self-efficacy ("I can do it") is one of them, and has become an end in and of itself for many behavior change interventions (e.g., teens avoiding high-risk behaviors or women negotiating condom use with their partners). **Vicarious (observational) learning** is another well-recognized construct in the SCT model, often used to teach people incremental behavior skills through role modeling. It's hard to overestimate how often SCT has been used explicitly or implicitly in behavior change communication programs. We all owe a huge debt of gratitude to Albert Bandura.

Integrative Model (Theory of Reasoned Action and Theory of Planned Behavior)

The **integrative model (IM)**[24] represents an evolved version of Fishbein and Ajzen's theory of reasoned action (TRA).[25] Ajzen developed the theory of planned behavior[26] as an extension of the TRA. Fishbein and Ajzen worked together to develop the IM, which they also referred to as the *reasoned action approach*.[24] See **FIGURE 4-5** for an illustration of the IM.

The most important assumption of the IM is that the best predictor of behavior is the intention to perform the behavior. This model focuses on the antecedents (predictors) of an individual's intention to perform (or not perform) a behavior. The IM focuses on the following beliefs:

- **Behavioral beliefs** are expectancies about positive or negative outcomes related to performing the behavior. Beliefs lead to formation of attitudes.
- **Normative beliefs** are perceptions about what relevant others think about performing the behavior, or beliefs about what others are doing. Together, these beliefs determine a concept of *perceived normative pressure* related to the behavior.

TABLE 4-2 Social Cognitive Theory

Concept	Definition	Potential Change Strategies
Reciprocal determinism	The dynamic interaction of the person, behavior, and the environment in which the behavior is performed	Consider multiple ways to promote behavior change, including adjusting the environment or influencing personal attitudes.
Behavioral capability	Knowledge and skill to perform a given behavior	Promote mastery learning through skills training.
Expectations	Anticipated outcomes of a behavior	Model positive outcomes of healthful behavior.
Self-efficacy	Confidence in one's ability to act and overcome barriers	Approach behavior change in small steps to ensure success; be specific about the desired change.
Observational learning (modeling)	Behavioral acquisition that occurs by watching the actions and outcomes of others' behavior	Offer credible role models who perform the targeted behavior.
Reinforcements	Responses to a person's behavior that increase or decrease the likelihood of reoccurrence	Promote self-initiated rewards and incentives.

Reproduced from National Cancer Institute. *Theory at a Glance: A Guide for Health Promotion Practice.* 2nd ed. Bethesda, MD: U.S. Department of Health and Human Services, Public Health Services, National Institutes of Health, National Cancer Institute; 2005. https://cancercontrol.cancer.gov/brp/research/theories_project/theory.pdf. Accessed March 23, 2018.

- **Control beliefs** concern **barriers** to and facilitators of the behavior and are directly associated with individually *perceived behavioral control* or *self-efficacy* when performing the behavior.

The IM also takes into account various background factors, which influence the constructs in the model differently. These background factors include race, gender, personality, education, income, past behavior, and so forth. Factors such as media exposure can also be included. This is where health communication messages fit in.

These components of an intervention work together. When performing research subject screening interviews or initial surveys of the intended audience:

- Determine which of the direct antecedents of intention (attitude, perceived norms, self-efficacy) best predict intention.
- Elicit the beliefs underlying the attitudes, norms, and self-efficacy.
- Design your health communication message or messages to influence these antecedent beliefs.

Of course, if, during subject screening and surveys, you determine that your audience already intends to perform the behavior, you need not go through all the steps of the IM. In this case, it is not likely that their beliefs, attitudes, or self-efficacy are preventing them from adopting healthy behaviors. Instead, environmental factors, skills, or knowledge (factors that take *actual control* over the behavior) are likely precluding their behavior change. If environmental barriers exist, for example, rather than designing your communication campaign to change intentions in a population, you might need to focus the campaign on changing policies that affect the population's opportunities to perform the behavior.

Diffusion of Innovations

All the preceding theories and models focus on individual behavior. Although individual factors are important, we must step back and appreciate that individuals perform behaviors within various contexts, groups, and environments. **Diffusion of innovations (DI)**[27] addresses change in a group. Developed by E. M. Rogers in 1962, it is one of the oldest social science theories used in public health. Rogers put it together while studying how new agricultural techniques spread among farmers. The theory

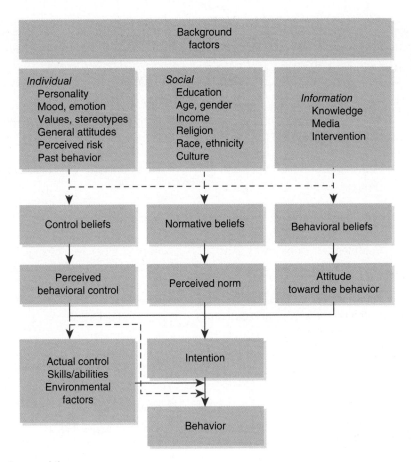

FIGURE 4-5 The integrative model.

describes how new ideas, or innovations, are spread within and among people, organizations, or communities. DI suggests that innovations spread via different communication channels within social systems over a specific period. Health communicators should focus on specific aspects of an innovation, such as the relative advantage, compatibility, complexity, trialability, and observability of the innovation. The innovation should seem better than other leading options, be compatible with its specified audience, and be easy to adopt. People should also be able to try it out before committing to it, and the changes should be obvious enough for measurement.

Successful diffusion often relies on media communication as well as interpersonal communication and social networking. Messages should be targeted to the audience because some audiences are likely to adopt the innovation early, whereas other audiences will do so late. Still other audiences will be the innovators who diffuse the behavior change and will be receptive to very different kinds of messages.

Malcolm Gladwell's popular book, *The Tipping Point*,[28] extends diffusion theory with the suggestion that the "innovators" in Rogers's terminology are indeed trendsetters who can create so much buzz around a new idea that it spreads very rapidly throughout a population. This is reminiscent of the traditional targeting of what Rogers called "early adopters" to lead the majority into adopting a behavior.

▶ Applying Theory to Practice Strategies

The National Cancer Institute emphasizes, "Because different theoretical frameworks are appropriate and practical for different situations, selecting a theory that 'fits' should be a careful, deliberate process."[8(p6)] You might really love social cognitive theory, but that does not mean it works in every situation. Before going forward, you need to ask if the theory is "…logical, consistent with everyday observations, similar to those used in previous successful programs, and supported by research in the same or related areas."[8] It is also essential to apply theories to the correct level of the ecological model: individual (intrapersonal) change, interpersonal change (i.e., dyads or group dynamics), or societal change.

Intervention Mapping

Intervention mapping defines theory-based methods as being derived from empirical studies of behavioral change in individuals or groups. Individual studies then use theory in different ways to create theory-informed methods. One example of a theory-informed method is the use of vicarious learning (learning from another's experience) to promote constructs from SCT.

A practice strategy delivers this method in an intervention. For example, role model stories, a form of **entertainment education (EE)**, are practice strategies built on the construct of vicarious learning from SCT. Finally, practice strategies can be delivered through activities (or channels), in this case, plays mounted by community theater groups, photo-novels, or radio or television soap operas. Specific media (the play, the picture novel, the radio or TV script and production) will then be created to implement these activities. **TABLE 4-3** summarizes some examples of the distinctions among theoretical methods, practice strategies, and activities or channels.

TABLE 4-3 Theoretical Methods, Practice Strategies, and Activities

Theory-Based Method	Practice Strategy	Activities/Channels
Vicarious learning	Entertainment education (Edutainment)	Role-model–narrated stories, photo-novels, TV or radio serial drama, social media posts
Extended parallel process (fear + ease of solution)	Risk communication raising fear of outcome (e.g., skin cancer) and ease of solution (e.g., sunscreen)	TV, radio, and print public service announcements or native advertising in social media
Elaboration likelihood model	Targeting on peripheral cues of images, music, channels, or spokespersons Tailoring to individual criteria	Neighborhood outdoor advertising; targeted print, radio, or TV stations; personalized letters, materials, or interactions; patient navigation, tailoring, and social media channels
Stage-based behavioral adoption	Motivational interviewing; goal setting and rewards	In-person, phone, or online counseling sessions between a trained counselor and client; group meetings (e.g., AA, Weight Watchers); criteria-based texting
Norming (bring attention to actual normative behavior versus perception of minority behavior as norm)—particularly for youth	Edutainment; buzz (viral) marketing	Channel-specific programming (e.g., MTV, VH1, YouTube, Facebook)
Agenda setting (media such as TV) to influence public perception of subject proportional to air time devoted to subject	Media advocacy; public relations	Radio or TV appearances by leaders or personalities; organization of real or phony grassroots demonstrations
Self-efficacy for skills	Breaking complex behavior into steps, breaking it down	Do-it-yourself episodes; youth media channels; online communities; rewards programs
Diffusion of innovation; positive deviance	Target to early adopters; train the trainer models	Agricultural extension; online media; group "sensitization" through community organization partnerships

Entertainment Education

Since the mid-1970s, extensive work has been done with EE,[29] beginning with Miguel Sabido's development of *telenovelas* aired in Mexico based on his analysis of the hugely popular Peruvian television soap opera, *Simplemente María*. Singhal and Rogers defined EE as "the process of purposely designing and implementing a media message both to entertain and educate, in order to increase audience members' knowledge about an educational issue, create favorable attitudes, and change overt behavior."[29] EE seeks to capitalize on the appeal of popular media to show individuals how they can live safer, healthier, and happier lives.[29]

The preponderance of EE was done in international settings until nearly 20 year ago, when the CDC initiated its Hollywood, Health & Society (HH&S) program. The program, managed by the Norman Lear Center of the University of Southern California, has flourished, acquiring a slate of philanthropic leaders (e.g., the Bill and Melinda Gates Foundation, the Barr Foundation) and organizations (National Cancer Institute, Substance Abuse and Mental Health Services Administration, California Endowment, and others) as funding partners.[30] In the spirit of EE, rather than writing out a full explanation, we direct your attention to Norman Lear Center Director and Chair in Entertainment, Media and Society Martin Kaplan's YouTube video, "Tell Me a Science."[31] As Marty says, "You don't bring a data set to a food fight," which is a shorthand way of saying that scientists need to tell our stories more dramatically if we are to capture the hearts and minds of the public.

In public health, EE interventions have ranged from school and community theater productions to embedded storylines in national prime time and daytime dramas, radio drama, and internet serial episodes. This range is represented in the winners of the Sentinel Awards, given out by HH&S annually. Although narrative is at the heart of EE, this has evolved to an *immersive engagement for behavior change model*, shown in **BOX 4-1**.

Note that "immersive engagement" links closely to the uses and gratifications theory (UGT) of media consumption (discussed later)—EE is powerful because people want to be deeply immersed and engaged by a story. Entertainment is an extremely powerful practice strategy for transforming society—perhaps the most enduring one in human civilization.

BOX 4-1 The Immersive Engagement for Change Model

Nedra Weinreich lays out the elements that need to be present for a story to be optimized for behavior change. These components include:

- *Behavior change model:* Start by identifying what action you want the audience to take after being engaged and motivated and how you intend to get there. By using a proven individual or social change model, you will have a framework for what you need to include in the experience to effectively motivate the adoption of the key actions. In a long-term, story-centered project, you can follow the Sabido method, which has been used successfully for decades to drive development of entertainment education content and brings together behavioral, communication, and learning theories. You could also choose to apply other relevant models.
- *Good storytelling:* Engagement starts with a good story; without that element, the rest of the pieces will fall flat. A good story does not just mean an issue that you feel is important for people to know about. Give a lot of thought as to who the key characters are, what the conflict is, how the story arc will play out, and how best to present different parts of the narrative for maximum effect. Otherwise, your audience will lose interest in your project.
- *Ubiquitous media:* By offering your content in the places the audience members are already spending their time, your story can seamlessly integrate into their day. And your selected platforms must work together to support the story strategically and synergistically based on their strengths and weaknesses, and how your audience uses them.
- *Participatory experience:* Design opportunities for the audience to go beyond just consuming what you create, to enable them to participate by interacting with the content or even submitting their own contributions to the story. Though most will likely prefer to watch from the outside, giving those who are most enthusiastic about the project ways to join in will deepen their immersion. This could include activities like playing an online game that moves the narrative forward, interacting with characters, connecting with others via a discussion forum to talk about the project, or sharing their own real stories.
- *Real world:* Ideally, we want the audience to draw the lessons from the story world and apply them to their own lives. This may involve using skills demonstrated in the story, finding local resources such as a medical clinic or community-based organization that provides assistance, or joining a movement to take action on issues portrayed in the story. Your project can connect them to those opportunities.

▶ Media Channel Selection

When planning a multimedia strategy, clearly defining the objective—to inform, to persuade, or to engage—is paramount. Some media channels and formats are best for information, whereas others are more suited to entertainment education. The following contains some guidance on how to select media channels and vehicles depending on the overarching approach.

The Health Communication Capacity Collaborative (HC3), funded by the U.S. Agency for International Development, created the theory-informed media selection (TIMS) framework to guide demand generation for reproductive health products.[18] The framework combines the media richness theory (MRT) and the UGT.

Media Richness Theory

According to HC3, richer communication media, such as face-to-face communication and some emerging technologies, tend to be more effective for conveying ambiguous messages because they allow for discussion and immediate feedback, transmission of both verbal and visual information, and greater personalization. Important richness factors include:

- *Interactivity/feedback:* The ability of communicators to interact directly and rapidly with each other

- *Language variety:* The ability to support natural (conversational or vernacular) language as distinct from more formal language (e.g., formalized business language) or abstract language (e.g., mathematical symbols)
- ***Tailoring:*** The ability to modify the message based on the needs of the recipient in real time
- *Affect:* The ability to transmit feeling and emotion

Uses and Gratifications Theory

UGT considers why and how people use specific media and channels to achieve their own ends (e.g., for information, consensus building, entertainment, or connecting). For the public at large, Facebook is primarily a means of interpersonal communication, a form of entertainment, *and* a source of information. On the other hand, healthcare professionals prefer professional meetings, professional association sites, peer-reviewed journals, Research Gate, and similar sites for connecting, and the National Institutes of Health and CDC websites for their information. Few healthcare professionals would regard a posting on Facebook as a credible, authoritative source (unless the page was managed by a trusted, respected colleague).

FIGURE 4-6 illustrates the TIMS framework's basic idea of choosing a media dissemination strategy using these two principles.

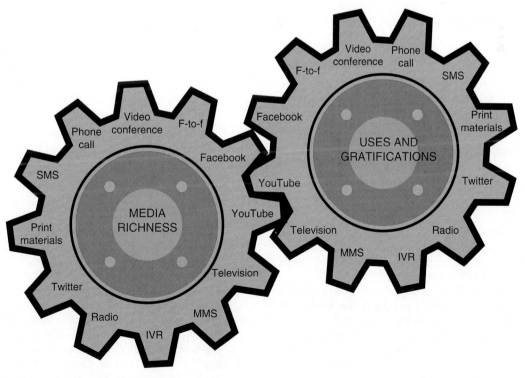

FIGURE 4-6 TIMS framework.

Abbreviation: IVR, interactive voice response; SMS, short message service.

Reproduced from Health Communication Capacity Collaborative (HC3). *A Theory-Based Framework for Media Selection in Demand Generation Programs.* Baltimore, MD: Johns Hopkins Bloomberg School of Public Health Center for Communication Programs; 2014.

TIMS is applied following these steps:

1. Use the MRT criteria (without taking current use or resource availability into consideration) to identify which medium or combination of media can support the necessary level of communication richness. (How complex or ambiguous is the information?)
2. Use the UGT criteria (without considering their specific media richness) to identify which media channels each intended audience uses for the intended type of communication (information, entertainment, engagement, etc.).
3. The best choice of media usually will be where the MRT and UGT choices overlap. If there are no overlapping choices, consider using multiple channels to disseminate less rich media.

If the overall approach is to inform the audience, content needs to appear in the media channels in which consumers have faith. A good indicator for this is where they get their news. If the overall approach is to engage the audience, select channels that the audience presently uses to engage with specific communities. The same is true for entertainment strategies. The next consideration is where and when to present your content.

▶ Conclusion

This chapter describes the theories used most often to predict, persuade, and guide behavior change communication. There are two important take-away messages: (1) health interventions should be grounded in applicable change theories; and (2) behaviors should be addressed systematically, based on health marketing, targeting, and tailoring principles.

Key Terms

Attitudes
Audience segmentation
Barriers
Behavioral beliefs
Control beliefs
Diffusion of innovations (DI)
Engagement

Entertainment education (EE)
Health belief model (HBM)
Integrative model (IM)
Normative beliefs
Practice strategy
Self-efficacy
Social cognitive theory (SCT)

Social marketing
Stages of change (SOC)
Tailoring
Transtheoretical model (TTM)
Vicarious (observational) learning

Chapter Questions

1. Explain why theory is used in health communication planning, citing a specific example from the chapter.
2. How is the integrative model different from the SCT or the TTM?
3. How are theories/models of persuasion in health communication different from behavior change theories/models?

4. Why can communications and interventions designed to scare their intended audience backfire? What types of messages is this approach useful for?
5. Describe the distinctions among theoretical methods, practice strategies, and activities or channels.
6. What can public health communicators learn from the private sector about the perspective of the consumer?

References

1. Heldman AB, Schindelar J, Weaver JB. Social media engagement and public health communication: implications for public health organizations being truly "social." *Public Health Rev.* 2013;35(1):1-18.
2. Elwyn G, Frosch D, Thomson R, et al. Shared decision making: a model for clinical practice. *J Gen Intern Med.* 2012;27(10):1361-1367. doi:10.1007/s11606-012-2077-6.
3. Gazzaniga MS, Ivry RB, Mangun GR. Social cognition. In: Gazzaniga MS, Ivry RB, Mangun GR, eds. *Cognitive Neuroscience: The Biology of the Mind.* 4th ed. New York, NY: W. W. Norton; 2014:559-603.

4. Rothschild ML. Carrots, sticks, and promises: a conceptual framework for the management of public health and social issue behaviors. *J Marketing.* 1999;63:24-37.
5. Safe to sleep® campaign materials. National Institutes of Health website. https://www.nichd.nih.gov/sts/materials/Pages/default.aspx. Accessed February 28, 2018.
6. Trachtenberg FL, Haas EA, Kinney HC, Stanley C, Krous HF. Risk factor changes for sudden infant death syndrome after initiation of back-to-sleep campaign. *Pediatrics.* 2012;129:630-638.
7. Lefebvre RC, Flora JA. Social marketing and public health intervention. *Health Educ Q.* 1988;15:299-315.
8. National Cancer Institute. *Theory at a Glance: A Guide for Health Promotion Practice.* 2nd ed. Bethesda, MD: U.S.

Department of Health and Human Services, Public Health Services, National Institutes of Health, National Cancer Institute; 2005. http://www.sbccimplementationkits.org /demandrmnch/wp-content/uploads/2014/02/Theory-at -a-Glance-A-Guide-For-Health-Promotion-Practice.pdf. Accessed March 23, 2018.

9. Finn AS, Lee T, Kraus A, Hudson Kam CL. When it hurts (and helps) to try: the role of effort in language learning. *PLoS ONE*. 2014;9(7):e101806. https://doi.org/10.1371/journal .pone.0101806]

10. Scherer LD, de Vries M, Zikmund-Fisher BJ, Witteman HO, Fagerlin A. Trust in deliberation: the consequences of deliberative decision strategies for medical decisions. *Health Psychol*. 2015;34(11):1090-1099. doi:10.1037/hea0000203.

11. McGuire WJ. The effectiveness of supportive and refutational defenses in immunizing and restoring beliefs against persuasion. *Sociometry*. 1961;24:184-197.

12. McGuire WJ. Resistance to persuasion conferred by active and passive prior refutation of the same and alternative counterarguments. *J Abnorm Soc Psych*. 1961;63:326-332.

13. Perry CL, Killen J, Slinkard LA, McAlister AL. Peer teaching and smoking prevention among junior high students. *Adolescence*. 1980;15:277-281.

14. Sandman PM, Lanard J. Risk communication recommendations for infectious disease outbreaks. The Peter Sandman risk communication website. http://www.psandman.com /articles/who-srac.htm. Published October 20, 2003. Accessed February 28, 2018.

15. Witte K. Fear as motivation, fear as inhibition: using the extended parallel process model to explain fear appeal successes and failures. In: Anderson PA, Guerrero LK, eds. *Handbook of Communication and Emotion: Research, Theory, Applications, and Contexts*. San Diego, CA: Academic Press. 1998:423-450.

16. Campo S, Askelson NM, Carter KD, Losch M. Segmenting audiences and tailoring messages: using the extended parallel process model and cluster analysis to improve health campaigns. *Soc Mar Q*. 2012;18(2):98-111.

17. Schwarzer R. Life and death of health behaviour theories. *Health Psych Rev*. 2014;8:53-56. doi:10.1080/17437199.2013 .810959.

18. Hochbaum BM. *Public Participation in Medical Screening Programs: A Socio-Psychological Study*. Washington, DC: U.S. Department of Health, Education, and Welfare; 1958.

19. Rosenstock IM. Historical origins of the health belief model. *Health Educ Monogr*. 1974;2:328-335.

20. Sifferlin A. Why Zika is totally out of control in Puerto Rico. *TIME* website. http://time.com/4433359/zika-in-puerto-rico -crisis/. Published August 1, 2016. Accessed February 28, 2018.

21. Prochaska JO, DiClemente CC. Stages and processes of self-change of smoking: toward an integrative model of change. *J Consult Clinical Psych*. 1983;51(3):390-395.

22. Maibach EW, Cotton D. Moving people to behavior change. A staged social cognitive approach to message design. In: Maibach EW, Parrot EL, eds. *Designing Health Messages: Approaches from Communication Theory and Public Health Practice*. Thousand Oaks, CA: Sage; 1995:41-64.

23. Social cognitive theory. Boston University School of Public Health website. http://sphweb.bumc.bu.edu/otlt/MPH -Modules/SB/BehavioralChangeTheories/Behavioral ChangeTheories5.html. Accessed March 21, 2018.

24. Ajzen I, Albarracin D, Hornik R. *Prediction and Change of Health Behavior: The Reasoned Action Approach*. Mahwah, NJ: Lawrence Erlbaum; 2007.

25. Fishbein M, Ajzen I. *Belief, Attitude, Intention, and Behavior: An Introduction to Theory and Research*. Reading, MA: Addison-Wesley; 1975.

26. Ajzen I. The theory of planned behavior. *Organ Behav Hum Decis Process*. 1991;50:179-211.

27. Rogers EM. *Diffusion of Innovations*. 4th ed. New York, NY: Free Press; 1995.

28. Gladwell M. *The Tipping Point. How Little Things Can Make a Big Difference*. New York, NY: Time Warner; 2002.

29. Singhal A, Rogers EM. *Entertainment-Education: A Communication Strategy for Social Change*. Mahwah, NJ: Lawrence Erlbaum; 1999.

30. Hollywood Health and Society website. https:// hollywoodhealthandsociety.org. Accessed December 28, 2015.

31. Kaplan M; USC Annenberg Norman Lear Center. Tell me a science [video]. YouTube website. https://www.youtube .com/watch?v=B2gRlZgqTgE. Published January 22, 2015. Accessed February 28, 2018.

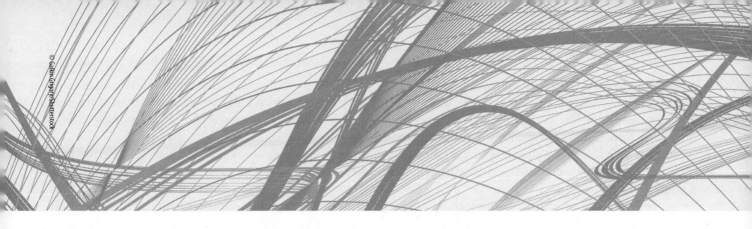

CHAPTER 5

Creating Meaningful Health Communication

Sarah Bauerle Bass and Laurie Maurer

LEARNING OBJECTIVES

By the end of this chapter, the reader will be able to:

- Use segmentation to analyze audience behaviors, cost and benefit beliefs, and motivating factors.
- Distinguish between tailoring and targeting messages and apply these concepts to message creation.
- Describe how framing can be used to craft more effective messages.
- Apply McGuire's hierarchy to the development of effective messages.
- Describe characteristics of effective health messages, including rules for using text, visuals, and quantitative data.

▶ Introduction

Understanding the unique needs of an intended audience is essential for developing meaningful health communication. People approach health with differing beliefs, abilities, and attitudes based on their experiences and culture. These experiences shape the way people accept health messages and whether those messages resonate with their beliefs, attitudes, and values. If you understand your audience and their perspectives, they will be more likely to both pay attention and respond positively to your messages.

▶ Understanding Your Audience

In this section we'll discuss the characteristics of different audiences, as well as a marketing technique called segmentation, which divides a heterogeneous audience into smaller, more homogenous groups, each of which can have its own message strategy.

Primary, Secondary, and Tertiary Audiences

One of the first things to do when developing health communication is to identify the **beneficiary**, the group of people most affected by the health problem. In some cases, this group is also the **primary audience**, defined as the group of people whose behavior you hope to influence through a communication intervention. Sometimes the beneficiaries are incapable of acting for themselves, for example, infants and young children or persons with a mental disability. In that case, the primary audience is made up of those whose actions directly affect the health outcome or who are making a decision. If you are encouraging vaccination of children for pertussis (whooping cough) or are providing guidance for emergency preparedness for those with disabilities, the caregivers are the primary audience whose behavioral change is sought; the beneficiaries are the children or the persons with mental disability.

In addition to your primary audience, you might also have to work with a **secondary audience** or **tertiary audience** to reach or influence the primary audience. These people can be allies to support a behavioral change, but sometimes they might themselves need to be convinced to change their opinions, or even actions, before the primary audience will be free to act on its own. Secondary audiences may include family members or friends who have influence on your primary audience. If you want to encourage someone to stop smoking, you will need the support of a spouse or partner if the smoker relies on their opinion. Similarly, if you want to encourage breastfeeding in first-time mothers, the baby's father or grandmothers are important influencers. Tertiary audiences may also be important. These groups often include **gatekeepers**—community leaders, healthcare professionals, and community advocates. They can support a behavioral change goal if they agree with it, or prevent its adoption if they disagree. For example, if you want to develop a health communication to emphasize the importance of human papillomavirus (HPV) vaccination for adolescent boys, you will need to persuade the parents (primary, because they make the health decisions) but also ensure that the responsible health professionals (tertiary) support the decision to vaccinate.

Audience Segmentation

Having defined your audience, the next step is to address differences that might exist within that audience, whether they are patients in a clinical setting or a wider audience in the population. **Audience segmentation** is a convenient strategy borrowed from commercial marketing to individualize messaging for different segments of the population. Although it would be easier to use one health communication approach to reach all those affected by the same health issue, a one-size-fits-all approach works no better in health communication than it does for clothing. Jay Conrad Levinson famously said, "Segmentation is saying something to somebody instead of saying nothing to everybody."[1] We will be more effective if we can reach and speak to a specific group of people who are likely to be interested in what we have to say. The Elaboration Likelihood Model posits that we can attract the interest of specific audience members by focusing on a topic in which they have already expressed interest or that they find meaningful. If we are going to be precise in our communication, we need to focus our efforts on a fairly small group of people—referred to as our *target market* or *target audience*. Thus, audience segmentation is a data-based method of identifying smaller target groups of people who share some relevant characteristics.

Early marketing professionals developed the concept of segmentation for marketing products, arguing that the key to marketing products was to identify subgroups of consumers by learning what their needs and desires were, and then developing products tailored to those needs. A marketer's mission is to know who the customers are, what those customers want and need, and where and how to reach them. Although we are not trying to get people to buy a certain brand of soda or potato chips in health communication, we are trying to "sell" a behavior, an attitude, or a belief about health. And we can use segmentation as a powerful tool to make the most of our resources. This strategy goes beyond just thinking about who is or is not participating in a health behavior; it expands to thinking about social influences, cognitive and attitudinal variables, and relevant demographics. People differ in their health knowledge, motivations and beliefs about health, behaviors, life experience, media use, and cultural values. So segmentation can be a useful way to understand these differences. One way to think about whether segmentation is needed in health communication is to ask yourself:

- Is it useful to separate users from nonusers because the messages may be different (e.g., people who do and do not smoke)?
- Are there separate groups that require different types of information or motivation to promote change (e.g., people who have tried to quit smoking before and really would like to quit or people who are not interested in quitting at all)? (Think about what you learned from the transtheoretical model and how this concept relates to the stages of change.)
- Are there groups that are likely to identify with different sources of information (e.g., new, young smokers vs. older smokers)? (Here, think about what you learned from the health belief model and how susceptible or severe these groups may think the consequences of smoking might be.)

The private sector subscribes to large marketing databases that divide the U.S. public into segments based on shopping, media choices, census tracts, and other data that are collected (increasingly without our knowledge) every time we use a credit card, place a phone call, go online, perform a search, or fill out a survey. In one common application, advertisers detect your online search for an item and then produce a timely pop-up ad for the same item in your newsfeed. Although we in health communication very seldom have the opportunity or resources to do such data-driven segmentation, we can use data that are available—and collect our own—to help us think about the specific needs of our audience and how messages could be constructed to address these different needs. In general, we use audience segmentation to:

- Group potential audiences by common experiences, attitudes, beliefs, or sociodemographic factors
- Gather greater insights from these segments
- Identify one or more segments as the intervention focus
- Craft messages that resonate best with this group
- Identify the best media channels for the segment

Segmentation in health communication can occur using a variety of strategies. If we consider the differences in the ability of audiences to receive and process information, we may be able to create communication that is targeted to these differences. For example, the Centers for Disease Control and Prevention (CDC) created what it called "energy balance audience segments" based on nutrition, physical activity, and weight control data obtained from the Porter Novelli Styles database, which included more than 20,000 responses from multiple waves of health and lifestyle surveys. The CDC used statistical analysis to generate the audience segments and then create specific audience profiles. These profiles could be used in a variety of ways, from one-on-one patient consultations to larger media campaigns aimed at increasing physical exercise or healthy eating.

In smaller scale programs, segmentation strategies are built from secondary resources (**secondary data**, such as those from health departments or local hospitals), complemented by local insights and research (**primary data**, such as local surveys, interviews, or observations). Health departments or community agencies may gather primary data and use those to segment an audience. For example, recall the earlier example of developing health communication to encourage HPV vaccination for adolescent boys. Consider some possible audiences for messages: parents of the boys, the boys themselves, healthcare providers providing the vaccine, and the general public. After choosing an audience, use secondary data

(e.g., who is likely to be vaccinated) and primary data (e.g., parent or provider surveys on barriers to vaccination for boys) to develop a segmentation scheme. **BOX 5-1** shows how this could be done, using parents as the key primary audience because they make healthcare decisions for their children. Segments could then be separated based on:

- *Demographic differences:* Age, gender, marital status, number of children, education level, occupation
- *Geographic differences:* Urban vs. rural vs. suburban; areas of high vs. low vaccination rates for other diseases
- *Sociocultural differences:* Language, cultural beliefs about vaccination, ethnicity, social class
- *Psychographic differences:* Attitudes about vaccination or health care
- *Stage of behavior change:* Knowledge of HPV, approval of vaccinations, intentions to vaccinate, self-efficacy in getting vaccine

This framework can be used to analyze all potential audiences and develop message strategies for each. It is also sometimes helpful to create **personas**, or "characters" based on data from each segment. Personas can clarify and bring to life the different needs of the larger audience and can become the foundation of your creative message and dissemination strategy. An illustration of teen personas from the CDC is shown in **FIGURE 5-1**.[2]

Segmentation can be beneficial to health communication planning because it can leverage audience segments that are easier to change. This may, in turn, increase social norms in the larger population. In the HPV vaccination example provided previously, if the parents most likely to vaccinate their sons can be persuaded to do so, HPV vaccination may become a social norm for all parents. This kind of leveraging is a powerful tool that uses scant resources effectively.

Targeting and Tailoring Messages

Once segmentation is used to define a population, two other tools are used to develop health communication messages: targeting and tailoring. **Targeting** means focusing on a segment of the population usually defined by common demographic or behavioral characteristics. Aiming communication interventions at a large general audience is like using a sawed-off shotgun to hit a bull's-eye; some buckshot will hit the target stand, some will hit the bull's-eye, and most will completely miss. To improve accuracy and conserve resources in health communication, we direct

BOX 5-1   Example of Segmentation: HPV Vaccination

HPV is the most common sexually transmitted disease, causing over 90% of all cases of cervical cancer in women, as well as the majority of anal and penile cancers in men.[a,b] The HPV vaccine has been tested on both boys and girls and is recommended to be given prior to the recipient becoming sexually active. The CDC recommends that all kids who are 11 or 12 years old get two shots of HPV vaccine 6 to 12 months apart. If older than 14, three shots are needed.[c] But uptake is not at desired levels. Approximately 60% of girls and 50% of boys aged 13–17 have received at least one dose of the vaccine,[d] but only 42% of girls and 37% of boys have received the required second dose.[d] Significant differences are seen by race, with Hispanics having the highest uptake, as well as those with lower family incomes and a history of flu vaccination. On the other hand, adolescents with private insurance and those who had college-educated parents were less likely to initiate the vaccine.[e]

A health communication intervention could use segmentation to think about how messages would be different for different groups.

Potential Audience	Possible Segmentation by			
Parents of Adolescents © Viktor88/Shutterstock.	**Sociodemographic Differences**	**Geographic Differences**	**Behavioral Differences**	**Psychographic Differences**
	Age of parents	Urban	Current use of flu vaccine	Beliefs in value of vaccine
	Income	Rural	Use of other preventive care services	Belief that HPV is sexually transmitted and not appropriate to vaccinate for in teens
	Private vs. public insurance	Suburban		General beliefs about vaccine safety

Modified from O'Sullivan GA, Yonkler JA, Morgan W, Merritt AP. *A Field Guide to Designing a Health Communication Strategy*. Baltimore, MD: Johns Hopkins Bloomberg School of Public Health/Center for Communication Programs; 2003.

[a] HPV-associated cancer statistics. Centers for Disease Control and Prevention website. https://www.cdc.gov/cancer/hpv/statistics/index.htm. Updated March 6, 2017. Accessed March 2, 2018.

[b] HPV vaccines: vaccinating your preteen or teen. Centers for Disease Control and Prevention website. https://www.cdc.gov/hpv/parents/vaccine.html. Updated August 24, 2017. Accessed March 2, 2018.

[c] HPV vaccine coverage maps—infographic. Centers for Disease Control and Prevention website. https://www.cdc.gov/hpv/infographics/vacc-coverage.html. Updated August 24, 2017. Accessed March 2, 2018.

[d] Reagan-Steiner S, Yankey D, Jeyarajah J, et al. National, regional, state, and selected local area vaccination coverage among adolescents 13-17 years—United States, 2015. *MMWR*. 2016;65(33):850-858.

[e] Holman DM, Benard V, Roland KB, Watson M, Liddon N, Stokley S. Barriers to human papillomavirus vaccination among US adolescents: a systematic review of the literature. *JAMA*. 2014;168(1):76- 82.

messages to smaller audience segments and target those messages to their needs. Aiming at the bull's-eye with a rifle, and coming relatively close, is better than shooting randomly or using a shotgun. The metaphor works for aiming health communication interventions at a specific group of people. Targeting is just a short-hand way of saying that you are using demographic, behavioral, cultural, or other factors in your communication strategy to reach specific audiences.

Tailoring, on the other hand, refers to communications that are fine-tuned for an individual person, based on individually collected information. These may be mass distributed, but they still reflect individual interests and do not make the assumption that "birds of a feather flock together," as targeting approaches tend to do.

Demographic Targeting

Demographic targeting is widely used in marketing. In the United States, there are radio, television, internet, and print media that reach out exclusively to children (of all ages) and to a spectrum of adults, from first-time parents to seniors. There are media segmented

Teens at-a-Glance

These composite profiles are for illustrative purposes only.

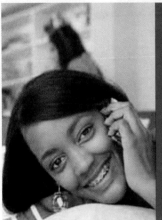

"I'm having a great time in high school, but I do worry about my future and what opportunities will be available to me. I want to be successful, healthy, and happy."

Katelyn Jackson (A Visible Teen*)
San Diego, California
Sophomore, Eastwood High School
Age: 14

❖ Is popular at school and is considered a trendsetter among her friends. Considers herself a fashion diva.

❖ Is a good student but worries about getting into her first choice of colleges.

❖ Is very conscious of her weight, tries to avoid sodas and fast food, and goes to the gym three days a week with one or both of her parents.

❖ Has her own cell phone and uses it to text her friends, access the Internet, and take and send photos to her friends.

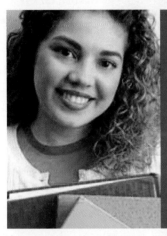

"I work very hard at school, and enjoy my friends and family. I'm called a "brainiac" because I spend a lot of time on my studies and extracurricular activities. I have high goals for myself and want to make my parents proud."

Alvarez (A Status Quo Teen)
Phoenix, Arizona
Senior, Palisades High School
Age: 17

❖ Comes from a very supportive family; both her mother and father graduated from college and are professionals.

❖ Makes high grades and takes advance placement classes in science and math; wants to go to an Ivy League college.

❖ Plays team sports and is physically active.

❖ Is considering a career in health care as either a pediatrician or a psychiatric social worker.

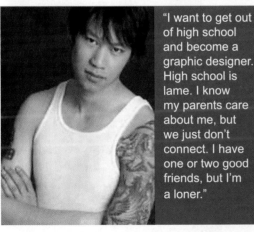

"I want to get out of high school and become a graphic designer. High school is lame. I know my parents care about me, but we just don't connect. I have one or two good friends, but I'm a loner."

Michael Cho (An Isolator Teen)
Worcester, Massachusetts
Junior, Calgary High School
Age: 17

❖ Wants to be in control of his life and often isolates himself from his peers and parents. Believes his parents don't understand him and has difficulty communicating with them about most things.

❖ Considers himself to be very creative; develops and posts his own video files online; dabbles in animation.

❖ Has challenges in core courses but excels in visual arts. Would like to become a digital graphic designer but is not sure how to make it happen.

❖ Can't wait to get out of high school.

FIGURE 5-1 Teen personas.

Reproduced from Audience insights: Teens 2. Strategic and proactive communication branch. https://www.cdc.gov/healthcommunication/pdf/audience/audienceinsight_teens.pdf

by gender identity, ethnic identity, and language. (e.g., think Telemundo). Increasingly, TV media aim at specific interests or hobbies (sports, gardening home improvement, gaming, etc.). We have been assaulted with targeting in mass media for so long that we are becoming oblivious. For the past 100 years of advertising, consumer product ads (e.g., laundry detergent, hand soap, food to be eaten at home, clothing) featured women and were directed at women, whereas big ticket items and spontaneous purchases (e.g., cars, televisions, sporting events, fast food) were targeted mostly to men. Although this is changing as gender norms and expectations evolve, advertisers still believe that certain products will be important to certain groups.

In health communication, demographic targeting takes place as a way to customize messages. So, for example, messages may change based on the race and ethnicity of the audience, the gender of those being targeted, or their beliefs. **FIGURES 5-2**, **5-3**, and **5-4**, from Act Against AIDS's *Doing It!* campaign, show how demographic targeting can occur. In this case, all adults were encouraged to get tested for human immunodeficiency virus (HIV) and to know their status. Using pictures and messages, the organization chose to target different adult segments with group-specific messages rather than use more general content.

Behavioral Targeting

There are times when demographic distinctions are less important than behavioral intention, or having an illness or condition. For example, women who hope to become pregnant will pay attention to just about anything with a baby in it; women who are not thinking

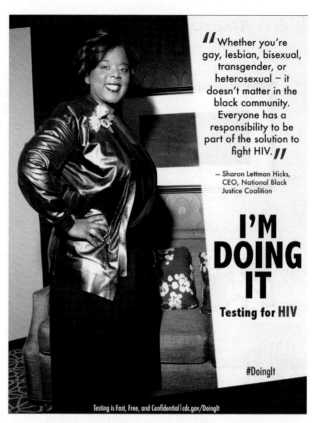

FIGURE 5-3 CDC "I'm Doing It" campaign targeting black women.

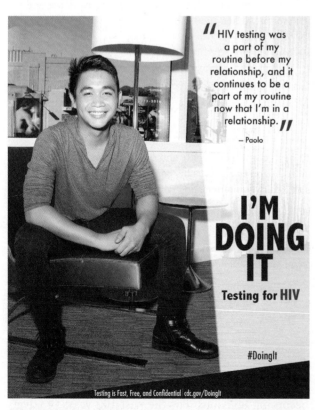

FIGURE 5-2 CDC "I'm Doing It" campaign targeting Latinos.

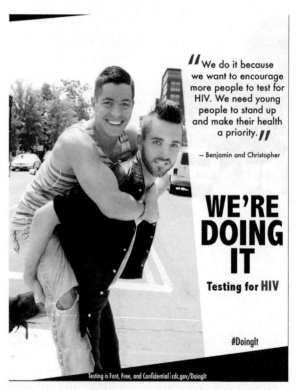

FIGURE 5-4 CDC "I'm Doing It" campaign targeting young gay men.

about having a baby will skip over the ads for prenatal vitamins and diapers. Men who have recently learned they have prostate cancer usually pay little attention to the ethnicity of the person on the cover of a brochure and prefer to see and hear from men of any background who have survived the disease.

Behavioral targeting can also be done within an ethnic population, targeting those who may think differently about the worth of the behavior. The Risk Communication Laboratory at Temple University developed a health communication intervention aimed at African American adults over the age of 50 who had limited literacy to encourage them to have a colonoscopy. They found that although this group *seemed* to be homogenous—they were the same race, the same age group, and all had limited literacy—they were very different in their behavioral intentions and beliefs about health and preventive medicine, making their intention to have a colonoscopy different. APPENDIX 5A outlines the way in which the developers were able to develop messages based on these differences.

In sum, targeting is a strategy to create materials that appeal to audience segments that share characteristics. The goal is that our intended audience will recognize themselves in these materials and respond positively.

Tailoring

Tailoring takes a more individualized approach to reaching groups. With tailoring, individualized communications are created by gathering personal data to determine the most appropriate strategy to meet that person's needs. We can collect this information by a variety of means, including quantitative methods such as surveys distributed via the mail, in person, an interactive website, or a smartphone, or using qualitative methods such as in-person interviews.

An example of how an interactive website can collect data to tailor communication is the CDC HIV risk assessment tool (FIGURE 5-5). Based on the answers a user gives, communication is customized according to HIV risk-relevant criteria. Displayed information is customized to a user-developed profile, including the terminology used for disorders, medications, procedures, and instructions.

Individual tailoring also often includes theory-based elements such as adoption readiness stage, self-efficacy, and outcome expectations. The University of Michigan Center for Health Communications Research has brought out its third version of a tailoring system to help health communicators plan for tailored interventions.[3] There are videos to explain

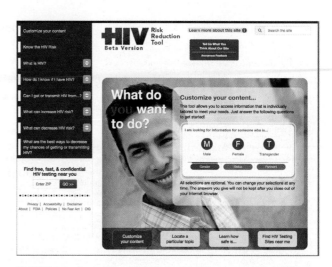

FIGURE 5-5 Customizable CDC HIV risk assessment tool.
Reproduced from HIV risk reduction tool. Centers for Disease Control and Prevention website. https://wwwn.cdc.gov/hivrisk/. Accessed May 10, 2018.

everything you need to know about tailoring health communication messages and materials at on their website. FIGURE 5-6 shows two tailored materials to illustrate the approach taken using the system. The tailoring variables, which you would get from each person targeted in the intervention, appear in the center column with the specific messages and images on either side. Visuals and text would then be modified based on individual answers so each person would have their own tailored communication based on their responses.

▶ McGuire's Hierarchy of Effects

For all the reasons discussed, creating health communication messages that are actually persuasive is difficult, regardless of the behavior or attitude of interest. So how do we create a message that grabs a person's attention, resonates with their own concepts, stimulates enough interest to be stored in memory, and favors the performance of a healthy behavior?

In the 1980s, William McGuire, a social psychologist who was interested in how people develop attitudes, took the **hierarchy of effects (HOE)** model from the fields of marketing and advertising and used it to develop a framework for health communication messaging.[4] The HOE model suggests several steps from perception to performance where messages succeed or fail. The audience must first tune in to the message and pay attention to it, including both understanding and thinking about it. The audience must also develop skills related to the health behavior addressed by the message. For instance, the audience—which could be an individual or a group—may learn the benefits of adhering to their

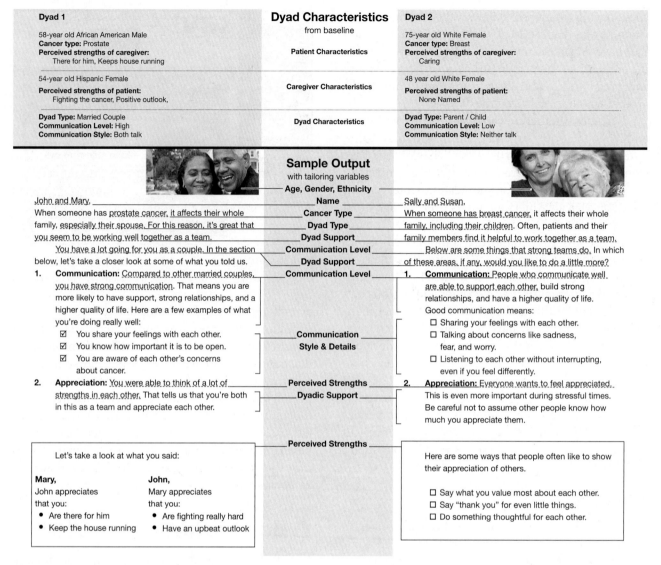

FIGURE 5-6 Tailoring example from Michigan.

Reproduced from University of Michigan Center for Health Communications Research.

blood pressure medication, where to get tested for HIV, or how to perform hands-only cardiopulmonary resuscitation. The audience must then agree with the position conveyed in the message, which may involve changing their previous attitude and replacing it with the new message. For the message to be successful, the audience must be able to access their memory, use it to develop the intention to act, and finally, use the relevant skills to perform a healthy behavior. This process is a lot to ask of anyone, a fact that underscores the need to design messages that take an audience through the entire process.

What variables are important for creating an effective communication message? In addition to the design of the message itself, some external characteristics are important, including attractiveness and credibility of the source. If the source does not seem to be credible, why should the audience

believe it? When designing a message, its style and organization are central to how the audience will respond to and understand it. Communication channel characteristics (especially directness) and characteristics of the audience members (e.g., culture, literacy, mood, education) are highly important. If the message is not crafted in a culturally relevant manner or is not at an appropriate literacy level for the intended audience, then the message will not be effective. This is not an exact science, however. What increases the success of reaching one step (e.g., attracting attention with fast-paced, flashy messages) may impede the success of reaching another step (flashy messages may grab attention but inhibit understanding), so we have to be very thoughtful when we construct and present communication messages. But McGuire has developed a set of guidelines that can help us get started.

12-Step Process

In McGuire's hierarchy, there are 12 steps for creating health communication messages.

1. The Message Must Get and Maintain the Attention of the Audience

If you do not capture and hold the audience's attention, then the rest of the steps will not matter. When people seek information, they usually want to get right to the bottom line—what is the key point or gist?—because most people do not want to expend much time or energy searching. When they find what they need, they are satisfied and search no further because the information was sufficient. Satisficing[5] (satisfy + suffice) is a term coined to describe this process. From a communication practice standpoint, it is important to provide information materials or one-on-one communication that conveys the gist of the main message(s) and that these main messages can be found easily and quickly.

Presentation is important. If creating written materials, make the message visually appealing with text and graphics, entertaining with word play and humor, and stimulating by involving emotions. Be sure to follow some key text rules, illustrated in **FIGURE 5-7**. To begin with, do not justify both margins of text. This causes uneven spacing between words and can confuse people with limited literacy. If you use columns of text, the best column width is 40–50 characters. This is short enough to allow the eyes to shift easily to the beginning of the next line, but long enough to maintain the flow of the text.

Get the graphics right. Photographs work best for showing "real-life" events, people, and emotions, but drawings work best for showing a procedure (e.g., drawing blood), depicting socially sensitive issues (e.g., drug addiction), and explaining an invisible or hard-to-see event (e.g., airborne transmission of the flu). Drawings should be simple and easy to understand, avoiding unnecessary details. Cartoons may be good to convey humor or set a casual tone, but use with caution—not all audiences understand them or take them seriously.

Other guidelines for using visuals in written messages include:

- Present only one message per visual.
- Provide captions so the visual can be understood without reading the text.
- Use visuals that emphasize or explain the text.
- Show the actions you want your audience to take.
- Make visuals easy to understand.

The best visuals are culturally relevant and sensitive to the concerns and needs of your audience. **FIGURE 5-8** illustrates some of these concepts.

2. The Strongest Points of the Message Should Be Given at the Beginning

Place the most important information at the beginning of the message; otherwise, the audience may lose interest before getting to the most important part. An example of this might be a message that states: "Always wash hands with soap and warm water for 20 seconds before and after handling food. Food and water can carry germs that may make you and your family sick." In this case, the most important information is how to wash your hands. This can be done if counseling a patient or in written materials that are provided either in a clinic or through media channels.

Human ability to process large amounts of information is limited.[6] So when people are exposed to a lot of information, or if it is complex or unfamiliar, they may tune it out or just remember the first or last item. (This is called a primacy or recency effect.) We often need to use less information (fewer words, fewer topics) in our messages and strive to highlight key points without overwhelming people. Except among persons highly involved in a particular health issue, providing more information will rarely help people better comprehend key messages.

3. The Message Should Be Clear

People should be able to identify the action you are asking them to take, the reason for taking that action, and the crucial evidence behind that reasoning. Use simple language, be direct, and do not overburden people with too much information. The best advice here is to speak or write as if you were talking to a friend. Do not use jargon or technical terms—say high blood pressure, not hypertension; fungus infection, not *coccidiodomycosis*. This is especially important when counseling patients in a clinical setting. If writing materials, use short lists and use bullets instead of commas. Remember that most humans acquire complex information slowly. To improve comprehension, slow the pace of content presentation and reduce the amount of content, including graphics and music. Do not cram too much in. It is also helpful to focus on what your audience needs to know and do, skipping details that are only "nice to know." For example, if you are writing a brochure on how to prevent Lyme disease, you do not need to tell the audience how and when it was discovered. Instead, tell them how to

Text Appearance Matters

The way your text looks greatly affects readability. Choosing the appropriate font style and size is important in creating health communication materials that are easy to read.

1. **Use font sizes between 12 and 14 points.**
   Anything less than 12 points can be too small to read for many audiences. Older people and people who have trouble reading or seeing may need larger print.

2. **For headings, use a font size at least 2 points larger than the main text size.**

   Examples of font sizes:
   This is 8 point.
   This is 10 point.
   This is 12 point.
   This is 14 point.
   This is 16 point.
   This is 18 point.

3. **Font Style**

   For the body of the text, use fonts with serifs, like the one used in this line. Serif fonts are usually easier to read than sans-serif fonts. This is because the serif makes the individual letters more distinctive and easier for our brains to recognize quickly. Serifs are the little "feet" on letters.

   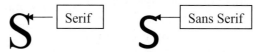

   Use sans serif fonts in headings and subheadings. Sans serif is more readable when your type must be small or when used on a website.

   Keep the following style tips in mind:

   > **Do not use ALL CAPS**

   - Do not use FANCY or script lettering.
   - Use both upper and lower case letters. Do not use ALL CAPS. ALL CAPS ARE HARD TO READ.
   - Use grammatically correct punctuation.
   - Use **bold type** to emphasize words or phrases.

   > **Limit use of light text on a dark background.**

   - Limit the use of *italics* or underlining. They are hard to read.
   - Use dark letters on a light background. Light text on a dark background is harder to read.

FIGURE 5-7 Rules for using text in health communication.

Reproduced from Centers for Disease Control and Prevention. *Simply Put: A Guide for Creating Easy-to-Understand Materials.* 3rd ed. Atlanta, GA: Centers for Disease Control and Prevention; 2009. https://www.cdc.gov/healthliteracy/pdf/Simply_Put.pdf.

prevent it. A good example of clear messaging is in **FIGURE 5-9**, a CDC communication on how to protect others from mosquito-borne illnesses if you are sick.

The hardest decision of all is whether you really need to use any or all of your hard-won data and statistics in a presentation or message. For whatever reason—low numeracy levels, cultural preference, or distrust or dislike of numbers—some people just are not interested in data-oriented messages. In those instances, data should not be used at all. However, if someone is highly involved in the health issue and if communicators have sufficient time to effectively

For example: If you are telling people to choose healthy snacks, such as fruit, Image A is effective because it shows them what to eat. It reinforces your message. Image B shows them what they should not eat, but on its own it gives them no visual link to what they should eat. Also, "X" is not universally known to mean "no".

For example: The mosquito depicted below is drawn several times larger than actual size to show what it looks like. Then it is shown next to a penny to demonstrate how big it really is.

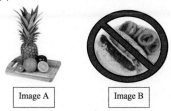

Image A   Image B

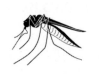

Enlarged to show detail   Shown to scale

FIGURE 5-8 How to use visuals in health communication.

Reproduced from Centers for Disease Control and Prevention. *Simply Put: A Guide for Creating Easy-to-Understand Materials.* 3rd ed. Atlanta, GA: Centers for Disease Control and Prevention; 2009. https://www.cdc.gov/healthliteracy/pdf/Simply_Put.pdf.

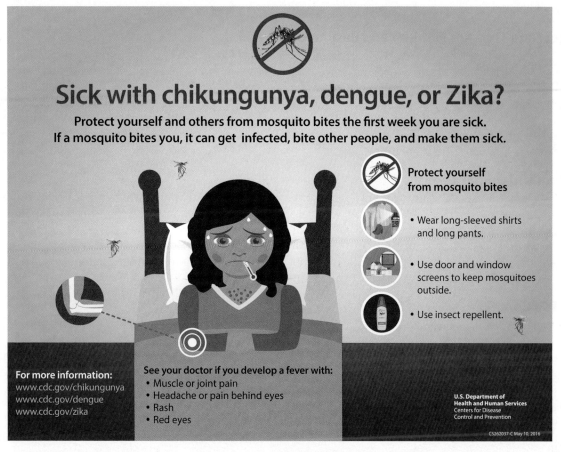

FIGURE 5-9 Example of clear communication: chikungunya, dengue, or Zika.

Reproduced from Sick with chikungunya, dengue, or Zika? Centers for Disease Control and Prevention website. http://www.cdc.gov/zika/pdfs/sick-with-chikv-denv-zika.pdf. Published May 10, 2016. Accessed March 24, 2018.

explain what data mean and how they are derived, then even individuals with low numeracy can increase their comprehension of data messages. Keep in mind that data messages usually resonate better with persons who[6]:

- Have lower levels of emotional involvement (e.g., fear, anger)
- Have higher levels of education
- Are less familiar with the topic or situation
- Have a position (advocacy) that is supported by the data

Especially when health communication is persuasive, we must make ethical choices about what data or other information to include or exclude. Much more is involved than crunching numbers for data tables and graphs.[7] Lay audiences usually see us as highly credible health information sources and communicators who have an important ethical responsibility to be honest and maintain their trust. If conclusions based on research findings are uncertain, it is better to say so rather than to communicate certainty that does not exist. For more on how to use data and statistics in communication, see **BOX 5-2**.

BOX 5-2 Using Data and Statistics in Health Communication

David E. Nelson

Minimize the Number of Data Items

Regardless of their level of numeracy, people have limited ability to process and understand complex information provided to them. This is referred to as cognitive burden or, when it comes to numbers, data overload. Unfortunately, we are often guilty of creating data overload for our audiences. We make the mistake of trying to show many numbers to help prove our points, failing to realize most audiences are not adept with numbers or scientific concepts.

Most people typically want us to communicate our main conclusion(s) and recommendations quickly so they can get the main point of the message. The "more is better" approach, when it comes to communicating health data, is an especially *ineffective* communication strategy and may even be counterproductive.[a] For lay audience persuasion the implication is clear: Be cautious and use data sparingly.[b] A general rule of thumb is to use only one or two numbers and to start with the more compelling number.

Select Data That Are Familiar and Easy to Understand

It is best to use numbers that audiences encounter more commonly. Frequencies (counts) using whole numbers such as 25 or 2000 are likely to be easily understood. Percentages are usually good choices, *except* for conveying personal health risk information (e.g., the probability of a smoker getting lung cancer).[c] However, fractional percentages, such as 0.8% or 0.002%, should be avoided because they are easily misunderstood. Indeed, using whole numbers without decimal points (e.g., 74% instead of 74.3%, or a relative risk of 3 rather than 3.2) is likely to facilitate understanding,[d] as does rounding of large numbers (e.g., 115,000 rather than 115,491). If proportions are used, such as 1 in *x*, use the lowest possible denominator (4 in 10 rather than 40 in 100).

Explain Unfamiliar Terms

We often mistakenly believe statistical or epidemiologic terms are understood by others. But statistical significance, probability, relative risk, and other concepts are not familiar to most people. Terms such as these need to be defined in plain language, and additional background material should be made available through websites or other means for those who may be interested in learning more. Care should always be taken to explain the meaning of numeric representations and to remind the audience of how to put data into context. Even the most commonly used public health statistics may be misunderstood without a supporting explanation.[a]

Provide Context

To understand what data mean, people need appropriate contextual information. It is a crucial role of health communicators to interpret health findings in full context and in full light of prior research. Any number without sufficient background information is meaningless unless it can be placed in its proper perspective. Simply reporting there were *Y* cases of influenza in New Mexico in February 2016 provides little meaning without further details about the number of influenza cases in past months or years so audiences can see whether the current number represents an increase, decrease, or no change over time.

Understanding probability data (i.e., statistical estimates of risk or benefit) is especially challenging for lay and even health professional audiences.[e] Sometimes a familiar analogy may help (e.g., Your chance of getting better with surgery is about 50%—like flipping a coin).

Relative risk estimates are good for helping to raise awareness about a health topic,[a] as demonstrated by common news media health stories proclaiming that, "New study shows food *A* cuts your risk of heart disease in half." But such information is often misleading when presented without the absolute risk numbers. "Doubling the risk" of cancer, for example, might mean that the absolute risk increased from 1 in 100,000 to 2 in 100,000—not a very big effect from an individual's standpoint. There is substantial evidence that presenting probability data as absolute risk estimates, especially in clinical settings, improves people's understanding.[e-g]

[a] Nelson DE, Hesse B, Croyle R. *Making Data Talk.* New York, NY: Oxford University Press; 2009.

[b] Zikmund-Fisher BJ, Fagerlin A, Ubel PA. A demonstration that "less can be more" in risk graphics. *Med Decis Making.* 2010;30:661-671.

[c] Fagerlin A, Zikmund-Fisher BJ, Ubel PA. Helping patients decide: ten steps to better risk communication. *J Nat Cancer Inst.* 2011;103:1436-1443.

[d] Witteman HO, Zikmund-Fisher BJ, Waters EA, Gavaruzzi T, Fagerlin A. Risk estimates from an online calculator are more believable and recalled better when expressed as integers. *J Med Internet Res.* 2011;13(3):e54. doi:10.2196/jmir.1656.

[e] Gigerenzer G. *Risk Savvy: How to Make Good Decisions.* New York, NY: Viking Penguin; 2014.

[f] Zipkin DA, Umscheid CA, Keating NL, et al. Evidence-based risk communication: a systematic review. *Ann Intern Med.* 2014;161:270-280.

[g] Akl EA, Oxman AD, Herrin J, et al. Using alternative statistical formats for presenting risks and risk reductions. *Cochrane Rev.* 2011;3:CD006776.

4. The Action You Are Asking the Audience to Take Must Be Reasonably Easy

If it's not reasonably easy, it is unlikely that they will follow through. Suggest easier behaviors that have fewer barriers, such as using condoms versus practicing abstinence. Or, instead of completely cutting pizza and other unhealthy foods from your diet, try to reduce the portion size. The Making Healthy Eating Easier campaign, developed by the Division of Community Health at the CDC, addresses this concept and uses easy-to-understand visuals (**FIGURE 5-10**).

For maximum impact and persuasion, health communication messages need to be properly framed. **Framing** a message gives it a context or even suggests a point of view or an interpretation with which it is to be understood. Whether consciously or unconsciously, we frame information to make it more interesting, more palatable, or even more frightening.

The frame itself has been demonstrated to have a direct impact on how someone hears, processes, and acts on information. So it is an important technique for persuasive health communication. For example, if we say that 1 in 20 people *die*, many people think the death rate is worse than if we said 19 out of 20 people *survive*. **Gain-framed appeals** state the advantages of taking an action (e.g., chance of survival), whereas **loss-framed appeals** state the disadvantages of not taking an action (e.g., chance of death).

Let's use the HPV vaccine example again: Gainforth and colleagues found that framing the HPV message in terms of the benefits of engaging in the behavior (gain frame) was more important to mothers of boys than the costs of failing to engage in the behavior (loss frame).[8] In contrast, an earlier study of college women found they were more motivated by lossframed messages if they identified themselves as sexually active. And the CDC Features website's September 2015 headline read, "Put 'HPV Cancer Prevention' on

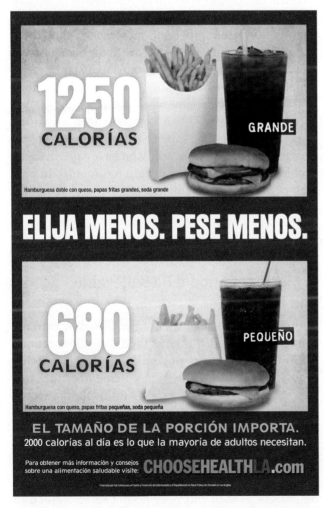
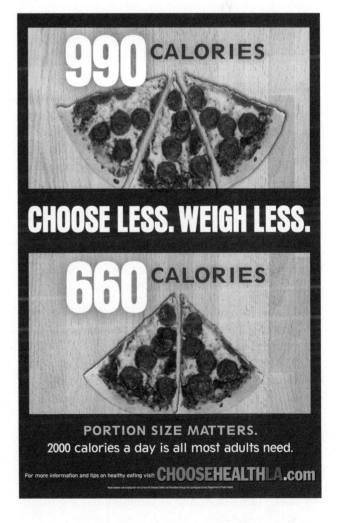

FIGURE 5-10 CDC campaign: Making Healthy Eating Easier.

Your Back-to-School Checklist,"[9] framing the HPV vaccine as (1) a routine immunization for school, and (2) cancer prevention.

In general, it is helpful to use gain frames rather than loss frames in your messaging—tell your audience what they *should* do instead of what they *should not* do. But there are reasons to use loss frames as well. There is consistent research showing that gain-framed messages are more effective at encouraging individual behavior change, such as smoking cessation, skin cancer prevention, or physical activity.[10] In these instances, use data to demonstrate the benefits of healthier behaviors, such as "regular use of birth control reduces your risk of an unplanned pregnancy by up to 99%." However, for disease detection (early identification of diabetes, screening for cancer), loss-framed messages are more effective[11,12] (e.g., "Persons who do not receive colorectal cancer screening tests on a regular basis are at more than double the risk of developing advanced colon cancer that has spread to others parts of the body").

5. The Messages Must Use Incentives Effectively

It is not enough to simply ask the person to do what you want. You need to explain why they should be interested in a change of behavior and what the incentive is. For example, being socially accepted, having physical attractiveness, avoiding embarrassment, not being isolated, and being trusted and respected are generally strong motivating factors for engaging in a behavior. However, in order to maximize these incentives, it is critical that you understand your audience ahead of time and build the incentives on their existing values. You can build these perceived incentives into your communication, increasing the persuasiveness. To maximize incentives:

- Use incentives that are either very negative or very positive. These tend to enhance the effectiveness of the message.
- Use emotional appeals to intensify motivation by highlighting severity. This may be especially true in a person or group who already sees themselves at risk.
- Discount the perceived benefits of an unhealthy practice (e.g., smoking does not really impress your peers).
- Use both positive and negative incentives.
- Make sure all incentives build on existing values of the audience.
- Make sure you ask your audience what incentives would motivate them before you use them.

6. Provide Good Evidence for Threats and Benefits

The key here is to show that the threats of the health issue or behavior and the benefits are real and likely. If the audience is already interested in the topic, you can use expert quotes, documentation, and statistics (using the guidelines discussed previously). If the audience is not interested in the topic, you instead would want to use dramatized case examples and personal testimonials to engage them in the topic.

7. The Messenger Needs to Be Perceived as a Credible Source of Information

The messenger should be helpful in attracting an audience's attention, personalizing abstract concepts, and modeling actions and consequences. They can also facilitate retention of the message because they are memorable. In the case of one-on-one communication with a patient or client, it may mean finding someone who the person can relate to or who seems most "like them." In the case of a communication campaign or community-based program, messengers should be chosen for how influential they are to the audience and may include celebrities, public officials, experts, "real" people, survivors/victims, or animated/costumed characters. In either clinical or public settings, often "people just like me"—that is, people who match the target audience profile—are the most credible spokespersons. These are real people who have experienced a problem and are willing to make a testimonial. In general, perceived power enhances messenger credibility, along with expertise, honesty, attractiveness, and similarity to the audience. Celebrities can be used to reach different audiences with appeals.

8. Messages Should Be Believable and Realistic

Remember that people are not persuaded by extreme claims or examples. Messages should provide accurate information that does not mislead, so avoid highly dramatic text, visuals, or video. Remember that two psychological principles strongly influence the acceptance or disbelief of health information: confirmation bias and selective exposure.[13,14] **Confirmation bias** means that we tend to interpret messages as confirming what we already believe. A corollary of this is that we tend to pay no attention to, or even tune out, messages with which we do not agree. **Selective exposure** means we like to obtain information from sources with which we agree. This means we generally have friends, choose media, and find information within groups who share similar beliefs and opinions and who tend to agree with us. Selective exposure is especially challenging because people have many available communication sources and can (and do) choose to be exposed only to those with whom they agree. This makes it difficult and expensive to produce a distinctive, scientifically sound health message that can attract the attention of someone who is not interested or does not agree with your thinking. Making your message as accessible as possible is key to holding attention.

9. Messages Need an Appropriate Tone for the Audience of Interest

In the case of a clinical encounter, the tone of the message needs to fit the circumstance—you would not want to crack a joke when you are talking to a patient about their cancer diagnosis. In the case of using media or other population-based communication, the tone of the message is how you use the aesthetic elements—imagery, lighting, and sound—to provide an atmosphere that reinforces the message appeal. Think of the music in *Jaws*, the documentary style of *The Office*, or the shaky camera in *The Blair Witch Project*; all these devices help to set a tone for what's to come. A serious tone is generally the safest, but be careful because it can be perceived as boring and unengaging. Avoid coming across as preaching to the audience. Being light and humorous is acceptable, but be careful what you say and how you say it. Humor generally requires more skill than might be suspected because people vary so widely in what they find funny. In addition, what the public finds funny changes very quickly. Finally, do not be offensive, preachy, or seem that you are being "mom." No one wants to be nagged!

As with all communication, it's important to pretest the messages and visuals before finalizing so you know if you have hit the right tone. A good example of this is the CDC emergency preparedness campaign, shown in **FIGURE 5-11**. Capitalizing on the popularity of zombies in television shows and movies, the campaign played with the idea of a "zombie apocalypse" and being prepared.

10. The Message Should Use an Appropriate Appeal

Rational appeals are usually successful with audiences that are already interested in the topic, whereas emotional appeals work for those not yet interested. A special note here: If you frighten your audience, make

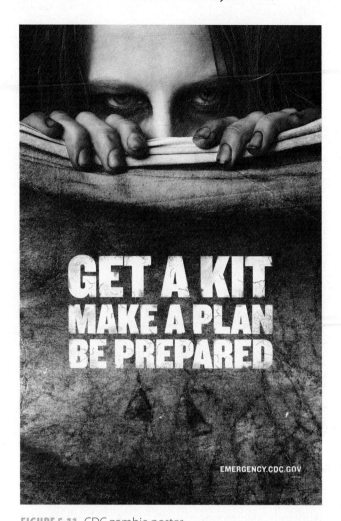

FIGURE 5-11 CDC zombie poster.

Reproduced from Zombie preparedness: poster. Centers for Disease Control and Prevention website. https://www.cdc.gov/phpr/zombie/posters.htm. Used with permission of Centers for Disease Control and Prevention

sure you also give them an easy way to alleviate the perceived threat. Give them realistic next steps. If you make people anxious and give them no way to reduce that anxiety, you may make the situation worse and they may increase undesired behavior rather than decrease it. This concept has been shown to be true in all types of health communication. In a meta-analysis of health communication studies, Witte and Allen found that "strong fear appeals and high-efficacy messages produce the greatest behavior change, whereas strong fear appeals with low-efficacy messages produce the highest levels of defensive response"; that is, they backfire.[15] Witte notes that if you scare people too much and do not show them how to overcome the obstacles preventing them from taking action, they freeze up and avoid the subject. A good example of this is abstinence-only counseling, school curriculum, and media campaigns that tell teens about all the horrible consequences of sexual activity, without providing information on safer sex strategies. Studies have shown that where these programs are prevalent, risk of teen sexual activity and rates of teen pregnancy are actually higher.[16]

11. The Message Should Not Harm or Be Offensive to the Audience

This is mainly a problem for negative messages that use fear appeals. It is important to recognize that some behaviors are not always a matter of personal choice and an individual's sole responsibility. The best strategy is to adopt a "do no harm" attitude. If you label behaviors as "bad," it blames the victim. They become much less likely to listen and incorporate the message into their behavior.

12. The Message or Campaign Should Use a Recognizable Identity

This one is not really applicable to interpersonal communication, but when developing a communication campaign, including the name, logo, and slogan, that identifies the messages as being from your organization will help the audience to remember the key messages because they will link individual messages with the rest of the campaign. It's best to make sure that this branding

is consistent and that elements convey what you are trying to get across. This is particularly important if the name of the organization is one that adds to the credibility and weight of the message. If the organization is not as essential to the message (e.g., the "pink ribbon" has superseded any one organization's role in communicating about breast cancer awareness; the "red dress" for women's heart disease is making similar headway in consumer recognition), then organizational branding is less important than establishing a consistent unifying brand for an entire campaign.

▶ Conclusion

We have presented some best practices for crafting relevant and meaningful health communication messages. By adopting and adapting the tested commercial marketing and advertising techniques of segmentation, framing, targeting, and tailoring, and by using McGuire's hierarchy to guide us, we can develop more effective health communication, whether we are counseling a client or patient or developing materials or media campaigns, to reach target audiences and improve health behavior.

Key Terms

Audience segmentation
Beneficiary
Confirmation bias
Framing
Gain-framed appeals
Gatekeepers

Hierarchy of effects (HOE)
Loss-framed appeals
Personas
Primary audience
Primary data
Secondary audience

Secondary data
Selective exposure
Tailoring
Targeting
Tertiary audience

Chapter Questions

1. Why is audience segmentation central to a social marketing approach in health promotion?
2. How can communications and interventions designed to scare their intended audience backfire? For what types of messages is the scare approach useful?
3. Describe the difference between tailoring and targeting messages. Based on these concepts, how are messages created?
4. Discuss the characteristics of an effective health communication message.
5. What is message framing? Give an example of a gain-framed appeal and a loss-framed appeal, and when you would use each.

References

1. Levinson JC. *Guerrilla Marketing: Easy and Inexpensive Strategies for Making Big Profits from Your Small Business.* 4th ed. Boston, MA: Houghton Mifflin; 2007.

2. Segmenting audiences to promote energy balance: resource guide for public health professionals. Centers for Disease Control and Prevention website. http://www.cdc.gov/nccdphp/dnpao/socialmarketing/pdf/audience_segmentation.pdf. Updated September 25, 2014. Accessed December 20, 2015.

3. Center for Health Communications Research. The Michigan Tailoring System website. http://chcr.umich.edu/mts. Published 2009. Accessed March 2, 2018.

4. McGuire WJ. Public communication as a strategy for inducing health promoting behavioural change. *Prev Med.* 1984;13:299-319.

5. Plous S. *The Psychology of Judgment and Decision Making.* New York, NY: McGraw-Hill; 1993.

6. Nelson DE, Hesse B, Croyle R. *Making Data Talk.* New York, NY: Oxford University Press; 2009.

7. Alonso W, Starr A, eds. *The Politics of Numbers.* New York, NY: Russell Sage Foundation; 1987.

8. Gainforth HL, Cao W, Latimer-Cheung AE. Message framing and parents' intentions to have their children vaccinated against HPV. *Public Health Nurs.* 2012;29(6):542-552.

9. Put vaccination on your back-to-school-list. Centers for Disease Control and Prevention website. http://www.cdc.gov/features/hpvvaccine/. Updated August 5, 2015. Accessed December 28, 2015.

10. Gallagher KM, Updegraff JA. Health message framing effects on attitudes, intentions, and behavior: a meta-analytic review. *Ann Behav Med.* 2012;43:101-116.

11. O'Keefe DJ, Jensen JD. The relative persuasiveness of gain-framed and loss-framed messages for encouraging disease detection behaviors: a meta-analytic review. *J Commun.* 2009;59:296-316.

12. Ferrer RA, Klein WMP, Zajac LE, Land SR, Ling BS. An affective booster moderates the effect of gain- and loss-framed messages on behavioral intentions for colorectal cancer screening. *J Behav Med.* 2012;35:452-461.

13. Heath C, Heath D. *Decisive: How to Make Better Choices in Life and Work.* New York, NY: Crown Business Random House; 2013.

14. Sparks GG. *Media Effects Research: A Basic Overview.* 5th ed. Independence, KY: Cengage Learning; 2015.

15. Witte K, Allen M. A meta-analysis of fear appeals: implications for effective public health campaigns. *Health Educ Behav.* 2000;27:591-615.

16. Kirby D. The impact of abstinence and comprehensive sex and STD/HIV education programs on adolescent sexual behavior. *Sex Res Social Policy.* 2008;5:18-27.

Appendix 5A

Demographic and Behavioral Targeting to Encourage Colonoscopy in Low-Literacy African Americans

Sarah Bauerle Bass and Thomas Gordon

Colorectal cancer (CRC) is the third leading cause of cancer death in the United States; however, survival rates are high if detected early through screening techniques such as colonoscopy.[1,2] African Americans, however, exhibit significantly lower rates of screening behavior and have significantly higher CRC mortality.[3] Targeted messaging has a long history as a health communication technique and has been used in encouraging CRC screening in minority populations with some success,[4-6] but not with people with low literacy, many of whom are older minorities.[7] Our goal was to create a targeted decision aid for this population to encourage understanding of the benefits of colonoscopy and to communicate CRC risk and colonoscopy need in older African American adults with low literacy.

To develop the messages, we first surveyed 102 low literacy African Americans between the ages of 50 and 74 years at a general internal medicine clinic in a large urban teaching hospital over an 8-week period. Literacy level was established using the eight-item standardized Rapid Estimate of Adult Literacy in Medicine–Revised,[8] and participants who scored a 6 or below were eligible for the survey. The questions on the survey fell into three categories: (1) personal attitudes and preferences regarding preventive screening and health maintenance (11 questions), (2) perceived barriers to having a colonoscopy (16 questions), and (c) perceptions of colonoscopy. Patient participants were asked to rate how much they agreed or disagreed with each of the statements on a 0–10 scale. To assess whether patient attitudes related to screening differed significantly enough to identify subgroups within the patient sample, a cluster analysis was conducted. The variables specified for clustering included 11 questions involving personal behaviors, attitudes, and preferences linked to health maintenance and preventive screening in general and colonoscopy specifically. This analysis found that there were three distinct cluster groupings, each of which was named to reflect their distinct characteristics: *Ready Screeners* (50%), *Fearful Avoiders* (30.4%), and *Cautious Screeners* (19.6%).

FIGURE 5A-1 presents the survey mean values across these three clusters. As illustrated, the Ready Screeners are characterized by a willingness to go to the doctor, an openness to having preventive testing to find medical problems early, and an overall sense that screening is "worth the effort." The Ready Screeners strongly agree that screening is a way to stay healthy and that if they had cancer they would want to know. They would comply if their doctor recommended screening, and they do not need to be pushed by family or friends to be screened. This group strongly believes that if they get cancer, it is "God's will." Overall, the Ready Screeners trust the medical establishment, are very positive about the benefits of screening, and display few barriers to having a colonoscopy. The majority (65%) had, in fact, had a colonoscopy. The main message strategy to motivate this group is to emphasize that doctors recommend colonoscopy and that it is worth the effort.

Approximately one-third of the sample (30.4%) was categorized as Fearful Avoiders. This group differed from the first in that they have a strong dislike of doctors and medical procedures. They not only profess a dislike of medicine, but also trust their bodies to tell them if there is a problem, making preventive

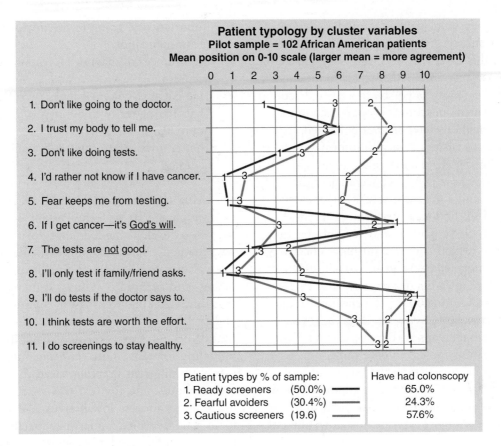

FIGURE 5A-1 Survey means across clusters.

Reproduced from Bass SB, Gordon TF, Ruzek SB, et al. Developing a computer touch-screen interactive colorectal screening decision aid for a low-literacy African American population: lessons learned. *Health Promot Pract.* 2013;14:589-598. Sage Publications.
http://journals.sagepub.com/doi/abs/10.1177/1524839912463394?journalCode=hppa.

screenings unnecessary. This self-trust appears to mask an overall fear of having medical tests and also a fear of receiving a cancer diagnosis—reflected in their agreement with the statement that "I would rather not know if I have cancer." Although they agreed that screening tests are "worth the effort" and should be done to stay healthy, especially if a doctor recommends them, few have acted accordingly—only 24.3% of this cluster had undergone a colonoscopy. Similar to the Ready Screeners, the Fearful Avoiders also believe that getting cancer is "God's will." Message strategies to motivate this group include emphasizing the importance of having a colonoscopy and its accuracy, that it is better to know you have cancer because screening can detect it early enough to be cured, and that family members would want you to be screened to be healthy.

The final cluster, Cautious Screeners, represented 19.6% of the sample. This patient type is similar to the Ready Screeners in many ways. They see screening tests as valuable and "worth the effort." They also strongly believe that screenings help a person "stay healthy." The main difference between this cluster and the Ready Screeners is that they are more likely to say they do not like going to the doctor—though less so than the Fearful Avoiders. The Cautious Screeners also do not feel overly influenced by a doctor's recommendation or by pressure from family or friends to be screened. This group is cautious in that they want to make their own decisions regarding health and, although they did not mind going to and talking with a physician, a physician's recommendation for screening is not their primary motivator to action. In addition, this is the only group that disagreed with the statement "Getting cancer is God's will," reflecting their independence of thought regarding illness and their health. More than half of the Cautious Screeners (57.6%) had already had a colonoscopy. The main message strategy recommendation for this group is to emphasize the importance of making a decision that could positively affect their health.

Once these target groups were established, we used a commercial marketing technique called *perceptual mapping* to discern message strategies. These methods yield three-dimensional computer models that represent how a survey group conceptualizes decision elements—in this case, the perceived risks and benefits of colonoscopy—and mathematical models messages designed to "move" a person to a desired action (intent to have a colonoscopy). Though used in marketing,[9] these methods have seen only limited application as a way to customize health information to a particular group. Perceptual mapping provides a valid representation of how people conceptualize the elements that constitute the most salient factors associated with their likelihood of performing the desired action, or with the cognitive and tangible barriers to the behavior, which allows us to more effectively develop highly targeted decision aids to address them and "move" them toward a desired decision. This can be done through demographic or behavioral targeting, or in this case, both.

Once perceptual maps are developed, vector analytic procedures are applied to determine a message strategy. To optimally position the target concept in the perceptual space, target vectors (dotted lines in FIGURE 5A-2) are used to start the mathematical vector resolution process. Figure 5A-2 depicts how different clusters thought about colonoscopy and what barriers or facilitators may exist in the decision-making process. The vectors identify optimum message associations for moving respondents (the aggregated "Self") within the model. These message strategies involve the dynamics of "pulling" concepts closer together by emphasizing their association, or "pushing" concepts farther apart by emphasizing their differences. The final form of the message (content, wording, imagery, and format) is then constructed to include and illustrate the concepts identified as optimal for addressing the respondent's concerns, knowledge, and perceptions of the risks/benefits. (For further details about our use of the perceptual mapping approach, see https://sites.temple.edu/turiskcommlab/ and references 10–13.)

A lack of resources prevented us from developing decision aids for the three groups, so we focused on a message strategy that would be applicable for all clusters. Specifically, we focused on the following messages, addressing the most significant barriers and facilitators of the three clusters to mathematically "move" the groups to being more willing to have a colonoscopy. They were as follows:

- Importance of going to the doctor and getting a recommendation
- Importance of having a colonoscopy and its accuracy
- That having a colonoscopy is "worth the effort"
- That it is better to know if you have cancer and not to fear it
- That family is important and would want you to be tested

Using these messages as the focus of the tutorial, we partnered with the Patient Education Institute, who develops the X-Plain tutorial series (http://www.patient-education.com), which is implemented in a variety of settings including hospitals, physician offices, and corporate wellness centers. We used the Institute's existing web-based colonoscopy tutorial and revised the tutorial to address the key messages found through our perceptual mapping and vector modeling analyses. Our resulting tutorial had significantly different graphics, used culturally appropriate photos, and the text was significantly altered not only to address low literacy needs, but also to focus on identified concepts. Specifically, instead of graphics we used photographs depicting African American patients, wrote text at a sixth-grade reading level, and added "testament" videos showing actual clinic patients from our study who had had a colonoscopy. These added features reinforced key messages, allowing users to see and hear people like them discuss the importance of having a colonoscopy. The text was also significantly altered by deleting much of the physiological–medical information about colon cancer and colonoscopy and focusing more on the psychosocial issues found to be important to our participants when making a decision about colonoscopy (see FIGURE 5A-3). This strategy proved to be highly effective. In a pilot randomized trial, participants who got the targeted decision aid rated the education more positively on all acceptability measures and were significantly more likely than controls to report that the education would be helpful to a patient who wanted information to make a decision. These participants also reported significantly more positive feelings about colonoscopy than controls and greater likelihood to be screened, and had significantly lower decisional conflict about getting a colonoscopy.

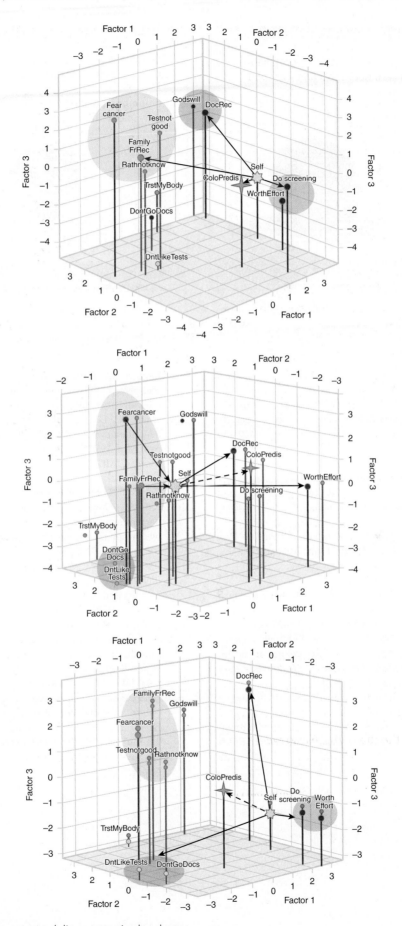

FIGURE 5A-2 Vector message modeling strategies by cluster.

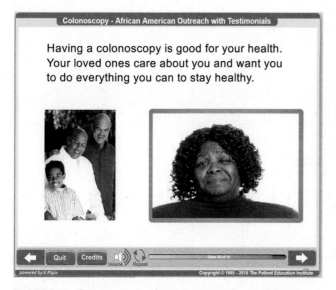
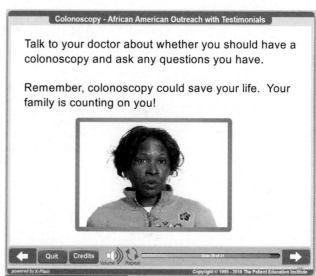

FIGURE 5A-3 Computer touchscreen tutorial screenshots.

Reproduced from Bass SB, Gordon TF, Ruzek SB, et al. Developing a computer touch-screen interactive colorectal screening decision aid for a low-literacy African American population: lessons learned. *Health Promot Pract.* 2013;14:589-598. Sage Publications. http://journals.sagepub.com/doi/abs/10.1177/1524839912463394?journalCode=hppa.

References

1. Cokkinides V, Bandi P, Seigel R, Ward EM, Thun MJ. Cancer facts & figures 2008. American Cancer Society website. http://www.cancer.org/acs/groups/content/@nho/documents/document/cped_2008.pdf.pdf. Accessed March 2, 2018.

2. Winawer S, Fletcher R, Rex D, et al. Colorectal cancer screening and surveillance: clinical guidelines and rationale—update based on new evidence. *Gastroenterology.* 2003;124:544-560.

3. Centers for Disease Control and Prevention. *Behavioral Risk Factor Surveillance System Survey Data.* Atlanta, GA: U.S. Department of Health and Human Services, Centers for Disease Control and Prevention; 2007.

4. Basch CE, Wolf RL, Brouse CH, et al. Telephone outreach to increase colorectal cancer screening in an urban minority population. *Am J Public Health.* 2006;96:2246-2253.

5. Morgan PD, Fogel J, Tyler ID, Jones JR. Culturally targeted educational intervention to increase colorectal health awareness among African Americans. *J Health Care Poor Underserved.* 2010;21(suppl 3):132-147.

6. Holt CL, Shipp M, Eloubeidi M, Fouad MN, Britt K, Norena M. Your body is the temple: impact of a spiritually based colorectal cancer educational intervention delivered through community health advisors. *Health Promotion Pract.* 2011;12:577-588.

7. Greiner KA, Born W, Nollen N, Ahluwalia JS. Knowledge and perceptions of colorectal cancer screening among urban African Americans. *J Gen Intern Med.* 2005;20:977-983.

8. Davis TC, Long SW, Jackson RH, et al. Rapid estimate of adult literacy in medicine: a shortened screening instrument. *Fam Med.* 1993;25:391-395.

9. Morgan MG, Fischoff B, Bostrom A, Atman CJ. *Risk Communication: A Mental Models Approach.* Cambridge, England: Cambridge University Press; 2002.

10. Bass SB, Gordon TF, Ruzek SB, Hausman AJ. Mapping perceptions related to acceptance of smallpox vaccination by hospital emergency room personnel. *Biosecurity Bioterrorism: Biodefense Strat Pract Sci.* 2008;6:179-190.

11. Bass SB, Wolak C, Greener J, et al. Using perceptual mapping methods to understand gender differences in perceived barriers and benefits of clinical trial participation in urban minority HIV+ patients. *AIDS Care.* 2016;28(4):528-636.

12. Bass SB, Gordon TF, Ruzek SB, et al. Developing a computer touch-screen interactive colorectal screening decision aid for a low-literacy African American population: lessons learned. *Health Promot Pract.* 2013;14(4):589-598.

13. Bass SB, Muniz J, Gordon TF, Maurer L, Patterson F. Understanding help-seeking intentions in male military cadets: an application of perceptual mapping. *BMC Public Health.* 2016;16:413. doi:10.1186/s12889-016-3092-z. http://bmcpublichealth.biomedcentral.com/articles/10.1186/s12889-016-3092-z. Accessed March 2, 2018.

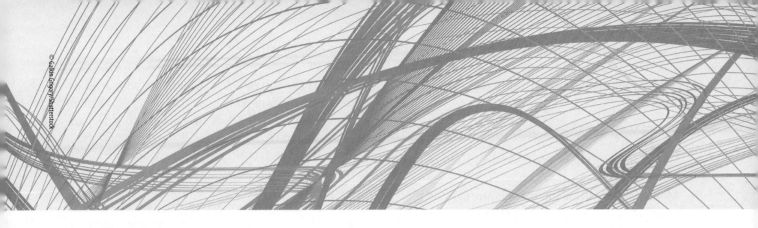

CHAPTER 6

Media and Communication Channel Selection and Planning: The Plot Thickens

Sarah Bauerle Bass, Claudia Parvanta, and Linda Fleisher

LEARNING OBJECTIVES

By the end of this chapter, the reader will be able to:

- Describe the strengths and weaknesses of different media channels used in health communication.
- Estimate levels of broadcast, print, and social media use in the United States.
- Use systematic and data-based approaches for selecting channels by audience, purpose, and reach.
- Develop a digital strategy.
- Discuss social inequities in media use.

▶ Introduction

As every generation evolves, the way we communicate with each other, and how we get and share information, changes. From cave paintings, drums, town criers, telegraphs, newspapers, radio, television, and now social media delivered through individual mobile devices (aka smartphones), the pace of communication technology change is breathtaking. A level of reach (how many people get a message) and tailoring to characteristics, once prohibitively expensive, can now be accomplished through social media

channels for almost nothing—and in the blink of an eye. In addition, mainstream media, such as network and cable TV, radio, and even print magazines, still draw tremendous audiences and have credibility unmatched by their social media counterparts. Augmented reality—where computers can put you in a "real world"—is knocking on the opportunity door. But "old fashioned" forms of communication—think brochures—are still a viable option. What's a health communicator to do?

These days we have multiple media options at our disposal to attract specific audiences, not only in different geographic locations or at specific times of day (the traditional media market approach), but also at specific:

- Phases of life, from childhood through our senior years
- Stages of a condition (good or bad), an illness, or a disease
- Moments in a behavior change journey, such as awareness, contemplation, preparation, action, and maintenance

How are different communication channels used to reach specific audiences defined by these various and changing criteria? We will help you build an effective communication strategy to accomplish your goals—be they to engage, inform, or persuade—with one or more audiences.

▶ The Big Media Picture

The Pew Research Center reports that 89% of Americans use the internet. The 11% that do not are mainly individuals over the age 65 (34% of the 11%), earn less than $30,000 annually (19%), have less than a high school or only a high school education (51%), and reside in rural locations (22%).[1] Nearly all Americans use TV and radio. The general trend in the United States is to replace broadcast programs aired at set times (TV, radio) and print media with digital versions that can be accessed on demand through personal devices; however, this varies by demographics and time of day. According to a Nielsen's 2016 data for average platform use throughout a weekday, the average adult spends 4 hours and 9 minutes watching live TV, 1 hour and 52 minutes listening to an AM/FM radio, 1 hour and 43 minutes using an app or the web on a smartphone, 32 minutes using an app or the web on a tablet, 57 minutes on the internet on a computer, 30 minutes watching time-shifted TV (DVR), 14 minutes on a multimedia device, 13 minutes on a gaming console, and 7 minutes using a Blu-Ray device.[2]

As can be seen from the Nielsen data, broadcast media still provide the most powerful channels to reach large numbers quickly. Think about how many people *watch* a 15-second Super Bowl ad. (Whether anyone recalls the ad the next day is another matter.) But broadcast media are not yet able to customize or reach specific audience segments interactively, an important advantage of digital and interactive media channels. Together, broadcast and interactive media provide an array of outlets for health communication. The relative merits depend on audience factors, as well as how much time, personnel, and money you have at your disposal. Many health communication

campaigns attempt to reach an audience with a variety of media in hopes of reaching as many people as many times as possible. The Los Angeles County Department of Public Health did this through a multimedia campaign (print, transit, social media, television, and radio) called *Sugar Pack* that addressed added sugar in drinks (APPENDIX 6A). The lesson from Appendix 6A is that multiple communication channels can be used to get multiple messages across to multiple audiences.

▶ Communication Channels

A health communicator has a myriad of communication channels to choose from when deciding how best to reach an audience. But not every channel is right to reach them, depending on media use preferences and the characteristics of the channel. So let us examine the pros and cons of different channels.

Traditional Media Channels

Traditional media channels—TV, radio, magazines, transit ads—have been around so long that we sometimes do not even think about them because they are such a part of our daily lives. But they remain important options to think about when deciding on how to get our message across.

Television

Data from the Neilsen Company show 116.4 million homes with TV in the United States and 296.8 million people older than 2 years living in these homes during the 2015–2016 TV season.[3] Overall, Americans spend nearly 30 hours a week watching TV, although the amount of time spent varies greatly by demographic group. In 2015, those classifying themselves as Asian American had the least amount of TV viewing with an average of 16 hours a week; those self-identifying as aged 65+ averaged a weekly 48 hours of TV viewing.[4] The good news for health communicators is that half of all people living in a community will watch their local news on the TV, and many watch smaller cable networks that have "niche" viewing, like Cartoon Network or ESPN. These media buys (purchases of time on paid media) are much less expensive than national network programming. The main downside to television is the need for high-quality content, which translates into professional media production and acting talent. Other cons include the passive nature of TV (although interactive TV is coming) and the difficulty of finding content in the clutter of competing advertisements and programs.

Because of the high cost of television advertising, health communication campaigns often rely on **public service announcements (PSAs)**. Broadcast stations are obligated to provide free air time as a public service, but it is the station's prerogative to select the time slots. Many stations use their unsold advertising time, often in the early morning hours, to run PSAs, meaning few people will see them. Production quality is a major factor in the airing of the PSA. Some cable stations (e.g., MTV and BET) will incorporate well-made PSAs into time slots that appeal broadly to their audiences. So, although you relinquish control over the broadcast schedule for a PSA, some stations and markets will give you better air times for your target audience.

The **Advertising Council** (http://adcouncil .org) has built its reputation on matching nonprofits and government agencies with top communication companies to produce high-quality campaigns across multiple platforms. Its TV spots are legendary: Buzzed Driving is Drunk Driving, Friends Don't Let Friends Drive Drunk, Smokey the Bear, and others you have seen throughout your lifetime. The Ad Council takes on about 50 issues a year; the primary sponsor underwrites production costs, but talent and quite a bit of air time are donated. A recent campaign on increasing awareness of autism is illustrated in **FIGURE 6-1**.

Radio

Radio remains the most popularly consumed media channel, with 93% of surveyed Americans tuning in at least once a week.[5] Listening format varies greatly by market (geographic location), making radio one of the most customizable mass media available. Since 2014, the category of country music, with a 15.2% listenership, has surpassed "news, talk, information," which has a 10.6% share. All other music forms—for example, Top 40, adult contemporary, rock, classics, urban—fall into single-digit percentages of listeners; however, even single digits represent *millions* of people tuning in every day.

The main cons of radio are that people are often in locations where they cannot write down pertinent information (e.g., in their cars), so the messages you design should be both catchy and memorable. It is also generally less expensive to buy air time compared to TV, and you may be able to barter to have some paid and some free PSAs run. Again, professional expertise in copy and voiceover are important to attract station managers to run your radio PSAs. The more professional it sounds, the more likely it is to be run.

For both television and radio, entertainment education strategies are effective ways to engage a loyal audience and create cross-channel opportunities for interaction. Try to work with specific local stations

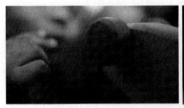 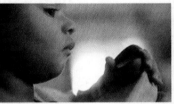 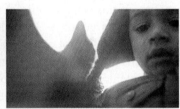

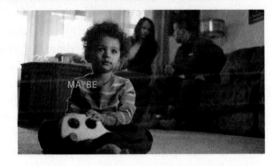 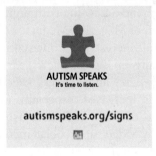

This ad shows clips of a little boy playing repetitively with a truck's wheels as his parents try to explain his behavior, saying maybe it's because of this, maybe it's because of that. Then on screen it says "Maybe is all you need to find out more about autism". An announcer tells viewers to learn the early signs of autism at AutismSpeaks.org.

FIGURE 6-1 Ad Council TV spot.
Reprinted courtesy of Ad Council.

BOX 6-1   Transcript of 30-Second Radio Ad on High Blood Pressure from the Ad Council

Psst. It's me, your heart. High blood pressure is serious, and if you think I'm just going to keep ticking away, you're wrong. I can quit whenever I want, but I like my job. Just treat me better. Maybe we can do some exercise on occasion? After all, we're in this together.

Don't let your heart quit on you. High blood pressure can lead to a stroke, heart attack, or death. Get yours to a healthy range before it's too late. Find out how at heart.org/bloodpressure. A message from the American Heart Association, the American Stroke Association, and the Ad Council.

Reprinted courtesy of Ad Council.

and hosts to involve them in an issue directly. **BOX 6-1** shows the copy for a 30-second radio ad produced by the Ad Council to promote awareness of high blood pressure risk.

Print/Magazines

A Pew Research Center study reported that newspaper readership has been steadily declining since 2000. By 2014, fewer than 20% of 18- to 24-year-olds and fewer than 60% of those 65 and older were reading a daily newspaper.[6] If this were the end of the story, we could kiss newspapers goodbye. But, although only 56% read the print version of a newspaper, the rest use other platforms, including internet and mobile, to read the same content. This means newspaper content is still read, making it a continued important place for health communication.

Magazines have also found a new life with digital audiences. The Association of Magazine Media found that readership of general-interest print magazines also has fallen substantially in the past few years,[7] including the *National Enquirer* and *Reader's Digest*. But digital readership has increased, especially for magazines that attract and measure audiences using print, digital, web, mobile, video, and social media platforms.[7] Like their print counterparts, online magazines present highly targeted, curated content and have faithful viewerships.

Billboards and Transit Ads

These types of communication are in many ways some of the oldest. Think about how people got information before there were highways. Posters would be placed in public squares or on buildings. Now, billboards are a ubiquitous form of communication; it is estimated

that there are between 560,000 and 780,000 billboards just on federal roads in the United States. Combining local and state roads, there are likely over 2 million highway billboards in the United States today.[8] Digital billboards are also becoming more common because of lower production price, ability to display multiple ads, and wide range of visual and graphic options. Because people are only seeing billboards quickly as they drive by, billboards should never be used to present complicated health information. But short messages—wear sunscreen, put your baby to sleep on their back—can be presented on billboards and, especially in certain areas where people may drive by the same billboard every day, these messages can be effective.

Similarly, transit ads are used to reach many people over an extended period. In regions with a bus system, an advertisement on a bus is like a moving billboard that travels 14 hours a day. It is estimated that a single ad on the side of a bus will be seen 240,000 to 350,000 times in a week.[9] Other options in larger urban centers include subway ads, posters in bus stands, and taxi advertising. Like billboards, transit ads should be focused on the needs of the community that will see the messages, and message content must be simple and memorable to be effective.

Digital and Social Media

Social Media Usage

Increasingly, health communication is engaging and interacting with specific audiences through social media because it can create "buzz" and give a heightened sense of authenticity to messages.[10] Remember the "ice bucket challenge," which raised awareness and funds for ALS (amyotrophic lateral sclerosis, sometimes called Lou Gehrig disease)? This challenge raised $115 million for the ALS Association, helped 15,000 patients, funded more than 150 research projects, and helped identify three new genes that will be used to develop new therapies.[11] The use of social media allowed this challenge to go viral and resulted in a significant increase in fundraising, as well as awareness of ALS. As this example illustrates, the adoption of social media reflects a widespread sense that these tools are necessary to reach demographic groups that are abandoning traditional technologies (e.g., television) and getting less of their information from expert sources.

FIGURE 6-2 shows an infographic of the leading social media platforms in use in 2015. Nearly two-thirds of U.S. adults (65%) reported using social networking sites, with 90% of young adults (18–29 years

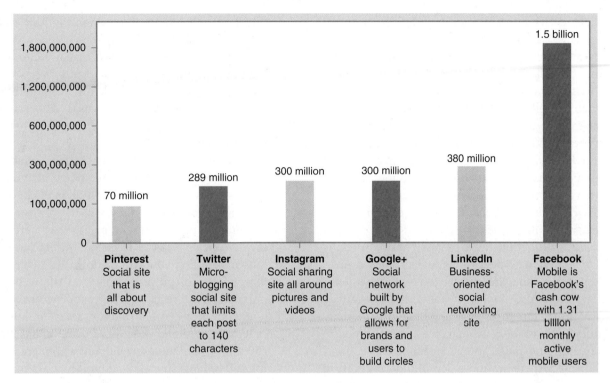

FIGURE 6-2 Marketing industry report of social media platform use, 2015.

Data from Leverage Media. http://www.leveragemedia.com.

old) using them, and 35% of those over 65. There were small or no differences by gender (68% women, 62% men) or ethnicity (65% white, 65% Hispanic, 56% African American). However, residents in rural areas (58%) were significantly less likely to use social media sites than their urban (64%) or suburban (68%) counterparts.[12]

It is no surprise that teens and young adults use social media frequently and preferentially. In a 2015 Pew survey of teens (13–17 years old), the authors reported that "...92% of those surveyed go online daily—including 24% who say they are online almost constantly." **TABLE 6-1** shows the percent of social media use in adults and the percent increase over the past year. By race/ethnicity, similar rates are seen, with African Americans spending the most time of social media (just over 6 hours a week) and Asian Americans the least (5 hours, 25 minutes a week).[13]

Social Networking Sites

There are many online sites and services that allow users to create personal profiles, post content, and invite friends, colleagues, or strangers to interact with this content. Sites tend to attract different followers, and the popularity of sites and their features often change. Major sites in use at this writing include the following:

TABLE 6-1 Percentage of Total Media Time Spent on Social Media by Age, 2016

Age	Average Overall Time Spent on All Media Weekly	Percent of All Media Time Spent on Social Media	Percent Increase from Previous Year
18+	25 hours, 7 minutes	22%	36%
18–34	26+ hours	24%	21%
35–49	31+ hours	22%	29%
50+	20+ hours	20%	64%

Data from The Neilsen Company. *2016 Nielsen Social Media Report: Social Studies: A Look at the Social Landscape.* http://www.nielsen.com/content/dam/corporate/us /en/reports-downloads/2017-reports/2016-nielsen-social-media-report.pdf. Published 2016. Accessed June 15, 2018.

■   *Facebook* leads social networking with the most users and functions. As of the end of 2017, Facebook had 2.13 billion monthly active users (defined as someone who has logged in to Facebook during the last 30 days) and 1.4 billion daily active users.[14] Facebook is also a major international phenomenon—84% of Facebook's daily active users are outside of the United States and Canada.[14]

- *Twitter* is a real-time information network that enables millions of users to send and read messages of up to 280 characters or less called tweets. Tweets can be posted to Twitter via text message, mobile websites, or a variety of mobile and web applications. Of the site's 313 million monthly active users, 82% access Twitter via mobile devices. Like Facebook, a majority of users (70%) are from outside the United States.[15]
- *LinkedIn* functions as a professional networking site. Individuals post individual profiles equivalent to a résumé and receive job announcements. Recruiters use LinkedIn for initial candidate screening. Organizations use LinkedIn to share information about conferences, post links to research and publications, and hold discussions. Currently there are more 546 million users from over 200 countries. Of these, 40 million are students and recent college graduates.[16]
- *Google+* is a social media platform that uses "circles" that create categories for your connections and "hangouts" that allow for video chats with up to 10 people. An instant upload feature automatically sends pictures and videos from a cellphone to a private photo album. Although Google+ has over 2 billion profiles, a 2015 review showed that only about 9% have posted public content, most of which are comments related to YouTube.[17]
- *YouTube* is a major site for sharing user-created videos. The videos and associated comments serve as a forum for users to connect with others having a common interest. Expected to generate almost $4 billion in gross revenue in 2018,[18] YouTube currently has 6 billion hours of video viewership per month. One billion videos are viewed on mobile phones each day. It is estimated that almost one-third of internet users have used YouTube.[19]
- *Pinterest* serves as an online bulletin board where individuals collect and "pin" media from other online sources. Users create thematic boards that are searchable by the public. Women outnumber men 4 to 1 on the site (175 million total users), which trends toward commercial products and resources. Over 9 million users connect their Pinterest account to their Facebook account.[20]
- *Instagram* is an online mobile photo and video-sharing service that lets users share privately or publicly, often by connecting to other social networking sites like Facebook, Twitter, Tumblr, and Flickr. Of more than 800 million monthly users, 500 million are active daily users.[21]
- *Tumblr* is a microblogging platform used for sharing photos, videos, quotes, and text. It has more than 550 million users and 396 million blogs. Most users are millennials, aged 18–35 years. Almost 80% of users access the service through their mobile devices.[22]
- *Flickr* is an image- and video-hosting social network where users can find free, attributable images.[23] Owned by Yahoo, 90 million Flickr users share a million photos daily.
- *Reddit* is an entertainment, social news networking, and news website. Registered users can submit content and vote (up or down) to determine the position of posted content on the webpage, much like Pinterest's bulletin board system. Content entries are organized by areas of interest called "subreddits." Reddit currently has over 250 million unique users, 60% of whom are male. It has 8 billion page views a month and 5 million comments are made a day. There are over 850,000 subreddits.[24]

Each of these sites can be used as a health communication channel, and each has its own positives and negatives. We will use Twitter as an example of how to use a social media site. **BOX 6-2** illustrates the basics of using Twitter.

As noted, Twitter allows for sharing of tweet information and also for making a collection of tweets that has a unique URL so they can be used and shared as a unit. Suggestions for using Twitter appear almost daily. Some advice is very simple, such as keeping tweets short (62 characters instead of 280), adding pictures or videos, tweeting after lunch (because everyone else is rushing to do it in the morning), and using hashtag (#) links to specific topics wisely. In addition to basic messaging, the Centers for Disease Control and Prevention (CDC)[25] recommends using other Twitter-based activities, such as:

- *Twitter chats:* Scheduled events that allow organizations or programs to communicate with their followers. Chats include free-flowing discussions, question and answer sessions, and the dissemination of information to a large audience through sharing or retweeting of content.
- *Twitterview:* A type of interview in which the interviewer and the interviewee are limited to short-form responses of 280 characters per message.
- *Twitter Town Hall:* A scheduled forum that allows followers to submit questions on a specific topic. Responses can be delivered through live tweets, video, or live stream.

BOX 6-2 Twitter Basics

There are a number of ways to use Twitter that maximize your reach and establishes your credibility to users. Some of the most common things to do include:

1. Retweet, reply to tweets, and react to tweets. If you are new to Twitter and do not have many followers yet, one way to increase your visibility is to retweet or reply to other tweets. This is especially important if the organization or Twitter handle you are retweeting or replying to has a lot of followers because if you are interacting with their tweets, they may interact with yours. And if they interact and follow you, some of their followers may too. It also establishes you as someone who is keeping up with what is going on.

2. Mention others and use @ signs and hashtags (#). Mention other Twitter users by their username (i.e., @username), or use established hashtags in your tweets. This is another way to build your audience. People/organizations and all their followers will see a mention, making it more likely that they interact with your tweets. Try posting a message about a person or organization doing work in your community or is well known for their expertise in a health area. Using hashtags is another important way to gain visibility, especially if the hashtags are well-known phrases or ways that people may search for information. Look at what hashtags other people/organizations are using and use those, too, because if a user clicks or taps on the hashtagged word, they will see all the tweets that have included that hashtag. Again this is a great way to bring traffic to you and build your following.

3. Use some of the advanced features on Twitter. Once you have mastered how to tweet, retweet, reply, or react, think about some of the other things you can do on Twitter, like using lists, direct messages, and likes. Also, use images, gifs, or videos in your tweets. These are eye catching and increase the chances that someone will pause and read at your tweet. You can also connect your other social media pages to Twitter to make sure you are using consistent content across platforms.

The bottom line with Twitter, and really any social media platform, is that to gain followers and get people to see and interact with your postings, you have to regularly engage with the platform and post items that people think are important and memorable. You can get more information if you go to the Twitter Help Center at https://help.twitter.com/en/twitter-guide.

- *Live tweeting:* Tweets from an event to highlight key points of a presentation, audience engagement and comments, and play-by-play moments, often used to allow conferences' nonattendees to follow the events.

So, what's the downside to using any social media? Two words: direct engagement. Direct engagement allows for two-way social and emotional communication with specific groups formed around a condition, a persona, or an intervention, but it is also a double-edged sword. Constant review of content is required to prevent inaccurate or distorted information and to stay updated as things change. Maintaining a timely presence and oversight can be daunting. However, under the right circumstances and when used appropriately and efficiently, digital media can become a powerful resource. The 3forMe campaign in Philadelphia used social media in a health context to urge human papillomavirus (HPV) vaccination in teenagers. The campaign also used Facebook ads and a connected website to increase awareness of the benefits of vaccination (see **BOX 6-3**, **FIGURES 6-3** through **6-6**, and **TABLE 6-2**).

When digital media are just a small piece of a larger communication channel puzzle, or the target audience does not use digital media regularly, other channels must be sought.

Cell Phone Texting and mHealth

Estimates from a Pew internet study[26] indicate 83% of U.S. adults and 84% of those living in U.S. urban areas[27] own a mobile phone. Mobile phones have, in fact, become an integral part of our daily lives. We use them not only for talking, texting, and email, but also for social media, banking, shopping, and searching for information. Almost half of mobile phone owners have a smartphone, with African Americans and Latinos reporting smartphone ownership (47% and 49%, respectively) at higher rates than whites (42%).[26,27] They are, in fact, these groups' main way to access the internet. This indicates that using mobile devices to address health is a viable way to reach many audiences. Phones are usually turned on, which allows for interactive communication and on-demand access to resources.[28] Because of the near-saturation use of mobile phones, they are becoming an important channel for health communication, primarily through text messaging or mHealth applications. These channels can also enhance patient–provider communication outside the clinical setting.

Text messaging (or short message service) is the social media used most often in health communication interventions. These interventions have addressed many health issues, from diabetes self-management to

BOX 6-3 Reaching Adolescents for HPV Immunization Using Facebook

Salini Mohanty, Emily Gibeau, Ayla Tolosa-Kline, and Caroline Johnson

Human papillomavirus (HPV) is the most common sexually transmitted infection in the United States. HPV infection can cause cancers including cervical, vaginal, and vulvar cancer in women and penile cancer in men.[a] Additionally, HPV infection can cause anal cancer, oropharyngeal cancer (cancer of the back of the throat), and genital warts in both men and women.[a] The Advisory Committee on Immunization Practices (ACIP) recommends that all adolescents receive the three-dose HPV vaccine series at age 11 or 12 years.[a] The goal is to have adolescents receive all three doses of the HPV vaccine before they may be exposed to the virus through sexual contact. Unfortunately, in Philadelphia, the fifth largest city in the United States, HPV vaccine uptake has lagged behind the desired goal of 80% for three-dose series completion.[b,c]

To improve HPV vaccine initiation and series completion among adolescents, the Philadelphia Department of Public Health (PDPH) launched an HPV vaccine education campaign through Facebook called *3forMe*. With the assistance of graphic designers, web designers, and focus groups, the 3forMe campaign was created to engage adolescents with specific messages about the risk of HPV infection, the benefits of HPV immunization, and announcements for vaccination through Facebook. The social media platform Facebook was chosen for the 3forMe campaign for multiple reasons including previous success of a health communication campaign by the PDPH and high usage of this platform among adolescents. Take Control, a Facebook campaign created by the PDPH, had previously been successful in engaging adolescents to order condoms by mail. Also, the majority of adolescents (81%) use at least one type of social media platform, and 77% specifically report using Facebook, which makes it an appropriate social media platform to reach and engage adolescents.[d]

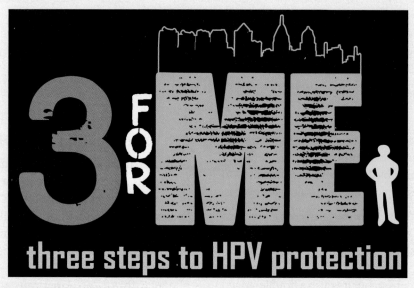

FIGURE 6-3 Logo for 3forMe campaign.
Reproduced from Philadelphia Department of Public Health. 3forMe website. http://www.3formephilly.org/.

The aims of this project were to: (1) provide education about and promote access to HPV vaccination for adolescents through Facebook; (2) provide HPV immunization at adolescent events (basketball tournaments, health fairs) throughout Philadelphia, which would be advertised through the 3forMe Facebook page; and (3) provide HPV immunization to adolescents who schedule appointments to visit a PDPH clinic in response to the 3forMe Facebook campaign. In addition to the Facebook page, we created a website (Figure 6-4), which included the opportunity for adolescents to sign up for immunization appointments.

Over the course of 1 year, six Facebook advertising campaigns, costing $2500–$3000 each, were developed to direct adolescents to the 3forMe Facebook page and website. Adolescents with a Facebook account who self-identified as 13–18 years of age and living in Philadelphia were prioritized to receive advertisements (Figures 6-5 and 6-6). Advertisements, which ran for two-week periods, were displayed on the right side of the Facebook login page and varied by themes, images, and text, each linking to HPV immunization and selected for relevance to an adolescent audience.

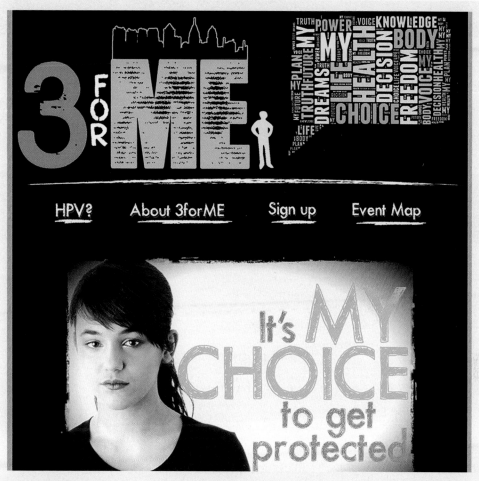

FIGURE 6-4 3forMe website homepage.

Reproduced from Philadelphia Department of Public Health. 3forMe website. http://www.3formephilly.org/.

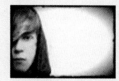

3forME

"I used a condom. I still got genital warts. If I'd known I would've gotten the HPV shot."

You like 3forME.

FIGURE 6-5 Facebook ad for 3forMe, My Life.

Reproduced from Philadelphia Department of Public Health. 3forMe website. http://www.3formephilly.org/.

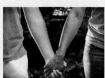

3forME

Protect yourself, Protect others. Sign up to get the FREE HPV vaccine & bring a friend.

You like 3forME.

FIGURE 6-6 Facebook ad for 3forMe, Have You Told Someone You Love.

Reproduced from Philadelphia Department of Public Health. 3forMe website. http://www.3formephilly.org/.

Facebook Insights provides access to real-time analytics related to Facebook activity (Table 6-2). These analytic tools allowed our team to gain a better understanding of how adolescents were interacting with our page and which messages were most successful in engaging adolescents.[e] Our team measured three main outcomes for the marketing campaigns: (1) *reach*, which is the number of individuals who saw any activity related to our page including posts, ads, and comments; (2) *engagement*, which is the number of individuals who clicked, liked, commented on, or shared 3forMe page posts; and (3) *likes*, which are the number of individuals who became fans of our page.[f]

(continues)

Between July 2012 and July 2013, the 3forMe Facebook page ran six sets of advertising campaigns, which on average reached 155,110 adolescents and engaged 2106 of them per campaign. In total, all campaigns accrued more than 3400 unique fans. Each campaign had varying success rates based on key metrics. During advertising campaigns, there were sizable increases in all metrics compared to nonadvertising campaign periods. Increased campaign reach and engagement did not necessarily translate to an increase in the number of likes for the Facebook page. For example, the disease risk campaign had the highest reach and engagement; however, this did not translate to an increase in the number of adolescents liking the Facebook page.

TABLE 6-2 3forMe Metrics for Facebook Campaign

Campaign	Dates	Theme	Reach	Likes
1	7/12–7/26/2012	Ownership	167,489	606
2	8/29–9/12-2012	Back-to-school	177,896	231
3	12/6–12/20/2012	Disease risk	204,663	422
4	5/6–5/20/2013	Disease risk and peer support	150,842	426
5	6/17–6/30/2013	Summer protection and peer support	147,878	670
6	7/17–7/31/2013	Philly-centric	81,896	1065

The Philadelphia-centric theme was most successful in gaining likes for the 3forMe page, although it had the lowest reach. Advertising campaigns that focused on a sense of community, protecting oneself during the summer months, and independence to make decisions about immunization were more successful in gaining likes than campaigns that focused on routine care, risk reduction, and prevention of disease transmission. Adolescents readily engaged with posting comments or questions to the 3forMe Facebook page. Campaigns that attracted the most likes also attracted the most comments. Most adolescents provided endorsements of HPV vaccine; some asked questions, usually about vaccine side effects or potential discomfort. On occasion, a participant would post inaccurate information about the vaccine, which would immediately be addressed by staff. Although adolescents were encouraged to sign up for HPV immunization appointments at the PDPH through the Facebook page and website, few adolescents ($n = 152$) chose to do so.

The 3ForMe campaign was developed to speak directly to adolescents about HPV infection and the benefits of HPV immunization. Messaging on the Facebook page primarily focused on adolescent empowerment, responsibility, and prevention. Based on Facebook metrics, the campaign was well received and far-reaching. However, the greatest limitation of our study was its inability to determine if adolescent engagement through social marketing translated into changes in HPV vaccine-seeking behavior. Although some HPV immunizations were given as a direct result of the campaign, it is unknown whether the campaign ultimately affected HPV immunization rates on a larger scale.

Communication permeates every aspect of public health. *Healthy People 2020* has made a priority of combining health communication strategies and health information technologies to improve health and service delivery to the public.[c] The exponential growth of social media since 2004 makes it an attractive tool for health communication, especially Facebook—arguably the most mature of the top social networks. With more than 1 billion registered users, Facebook can support health promotion campaigns that are targeted, measurable, near real-time, and inexpensive. The reach and speed of social networking sites make them very appealing for pushing information to the public. Other studies have also reported success in health promotion messaging, although it has been difficult to assess whether social media engagement translates into action or behavior change.[f,g]

Social networking sites are intended to engage users in dialogue, with both the host and other participants. We found that adolescents were very open to expressing their opinions on the 3forMe Facebook page. When using social media such as Facebook for health education and promotion, it is essential that the site be monitored daily, so that questions and misinformation can be addressed promptly. Additional research is needed to assess the impact of social marketing campaigns on adolescent health behavior and outcomes.

[a] Genital HPV infection - fact sheet. Centers for Disease Control and Prevention website. https://www.cdc.gov/std/hpv/stdfact-hpv.htm. Published December 28, 2016. Accessed March 5, 2018.

[b] Centers for Disease Control and Prevention. National and state vaccination coverage among adolescents aged 13-17 years—United States, 2012. *MMWR*. 2013;62(34):685.

[c] Healthy People 2020. U.S. Department of Health and Human Services, Office of Disease Prevention and Health Promotion website. http://www.healthypeople.gov. Accessed March 5, 2018.

[d] Social media fact sheet. Pew Research Center website. http://www.pewinternet.org/fact-sheet/social-media/. Accessed March 21, 2018.

[e] Borthakur D, Gray J, Sarma JS, et al. Apache Hadoop goes realtime at Facebook. *Proceedings of the 2011 ACM SIGMOD International Conference on Management of Data*. Athens, Greece: Association for Computing Machinery; 2011:1071-1080.

[f] Friedman AL, Brookmeyer KA, Kachur RE, et al. An assessment of the GYT: Get Yourself Tested Campaign: an integrated approach to sexually transmitted disease prevention communication. *Sex Trans Dis*. 2014;41(3):151-157.

[g] Guse K, Levine D, Martins S, et al. Interventions using new digital media to improve adolescent sexual health: a systematic review. *J Adolesc Health*. 2012;51(6):535-543.

physical activity, weight loss, and medication adherence.[28] Most have shown significant benefits to participants and positive changes in health behavior. Factors that increase successful use of test messaging include weekly messages, bi-directionality (meaning the participant can text back), personalization (using their name and other details), and tailoring to clinical needs (e.g., health status).

Health communication has started to use mobile messaging to share messages. In 2015, the Pew Research Center included the use of messaging apps in its survey and found that 36% of smartphone owners reported using apps such as WhatsApp, Kik, or iMessage, and 17% used apps that automatically delete sent messages, such as Snapchat or Wickr. Nearly half of 18- to 29-year-olds used these free messaging apps when connected to WiFi to avoid data charges on their mobile phone plan.[1] **APPENDIX 6B** provides an example of how Text4baby, the largest mHealth initiative in the United States, addressed the Zika threat by targeting pregnant women.

mHealth, or mobile health, can use texting as a component, but is more broadly defined as using mobile communications—such as tablets or smartphones—for health services and information.[29] These devices can create, store, retrieve, and transmit data in real time between users and the communicator or institution. Mobile device communication allows for easy accessibility and personalized, tailored messages, and also provides the ability to connect users with each other. A doctor can communicate with patients about their health; a health communicator can provide prevention information or encouragement.

There are many applications for mHealth communication. Within a patient population, healthcare providers can send and receive messages about health behavior, send reminders about medications, or connect patients with other patients to provide social support, all outside the boundaries of a physical healthcare setting. An example of this is the FOCUS mobile phone intervention, designed to prevent relapse in people with schizophrenia after release from the hospital. Users can respond to clinical assessment measures, communicate with a case manager, and select on-demand modules for medication adherence, mood regulation, sleep, social functions, and coping with hallucinations. The system prompts patients to do self-assessments three times a day and provides opportunities to talk or meet with case managers as needed.[30]

Another strategy is to use mHealth to target a specific group to encourage healthy behaviors not connected to a healthcare provider or facility. The Text 2 Survive project, run by the Illinois Department of Public Health, uses text messaging to provide minority youth with accurate information about HIV/AIDS. The user also can access lists of nearby (based on zip code) clinics for HIV testing and places to get free condoms. Incentives are used to encourage use of the app and the listed venues.[31]

Most mHealth interventions have been used to target self-defined networks of users and the places frequented by others in their networks. One could imagine using these media to form networks of health consumers, based on disease, condition, behavior, or goals. Then it would be possible to address the network audiences and build social or economic capital to promote health and healthy behaviors. For example, applications such as Whrrl and Yelp, which currently are used to locate stores and restaurants, could be used to encourage patronization of healthier food establishments, parks, gyms, clinical services, or any other health resource within a defined community of targeted consumers, patients, or caregivers.[32]

mHealth and texting in health communication are not without their challenges, however. Conducting these types of health communication interventions can be complex and underscore the need for close collaboration with technology experts, reliance on existing technology infrastructure, and input from end users. It is critical that in-depth planning and subsequent testing with the intended audience occur before these technologies are used as a new application. For many, particularly those with more limited incomes, smartphones are the sole access to the Internet. This has implications for the development and delivery of content. Important factors are the size of the screen, the amount of information that can be easily absorbed looking at a phone screen, and how "sticky" the information is—how long it will stay with the person after they see/read/experience it.

Websites and/or Blogs

A website, a collection of electronic pages at a single address, can be entirely under your control. Likewise, anyone can have a blog, which is a chronological collection of content you post with the expectation that others will comment on what you have said. Websites may contain blogs, or blogs may link to websites. These sites keep your content together for easy access and retrieval by your intended audiences and create/maintain your identity, brand, and credibility.

Most smartphone and computer users will explore online when they have questions about their health, and most use browsers and search engines (e.g., Google, Bing, Yahoo, or Safari) to find information on the web. There are two ways to get users to view your messages. **Inbound marketing** is the process of designing your site to be so visible, accessible, and interesting that users will want to visit your site to find what they are looking for. **Outbound marketing** encourages users to visit a site by sending interruptive media (tweets, pop-up ads, email blasts) to their device. In either case, when a viewer gets to your website, you want them to stay a while, look at your content, and take some action. Think of yourself as a host welcoming guests. You want to do everything possible to make them comfortable and attend to their needs. In brief, your content needs to be useful, findable, aesthetically pleasing, and especially because this is health communication, it needs to be accurate.

HubSpot's[33] survey of marketing benchmarks from more than 7000 businesses showed relationships between webpage features—number of website pages, landing pages, blog posts—and the volume of traffic for these pages. Here are a few highlights:

- Websites with 51–100 pages generate 48% more traffic than those with 1–50 pages. And those with more than 1000 pages see five times the traffic as those with fewer than 51 pages.
- The more landing pages the more leads. A **landing page** is how you get to a website. For most websites, the landing page is their home page, but there are reasons to have multiple landing pages (not necessarily connected to the main website) to attract different kinds of audiences and audiences from other platforms. Most websites use **click through** landing pages with the goal of persuading the user to move onto another destination page in the site.[34]
- There appears to be a linear relationship between the number of monthly blog posts and inbound traffic, with no sharp break in the trend. Webpages with 15 or more posts per month will see five times more traffic than those with none.

What is the downside? Websites and blogs must be updated constantly with new information to avoid appearing out-of-date. Expert website design is needed to maximize usability and access to information. Constant diligence and attention are needed to control content, especially from users. Targeting information to a specific audience is difficult; websites use a more general communication strategy.

Virtual Worlds and Gaming

Shegog and colleagues state that 97% of U.S. teens play computer, web, console, or mobile games. Of these, 31% of teen gamers play daily and another 21% play three to five days per week.[35] Gaming provides a highly customizable format for reaching adolescents through young adults with health-related content. Within the realm of gaming, virtual worlds provide an immersive experience that enables the user to enact decisions and experience consequences, albeit on a fantasy or dramatic plane. An example of how gaming can affect health behavior is Pokémon Go. In July 2016, in its first week, it became the most downloaded app in history; in the first two weeks it was downloaded 30 million times from 30 different countries.[36] It incorporates virtual, physical, and social dimensions as part of the game, which involves collecting virtual characters on your cell phone by walking to catch the Pokémon that have been placed in real public locations, such as parks, streets, buildings, and public spaces.[37] Interestingly, use of the app appears to have increased the daily physical activity of those using it.[38] Without being a "health app" per se, its effects on physical activity are clear, in that you cannot play the game unless you are walking or moving out in the environment. As with most trends, however, it went out of style quickly. Pokémon Go was a big hit—and then it was not. The trick is trying to develop content that has staying power and will continue to engage users. In **APPENDIX 6C**, descriptions and examples of using virtual worlds and gaming with health content are provided.

Gaming is an exciting application of technology that is just beginning to be explored in health communication. It can provide extensive player involvement and a unique channel for delivering health behavior communication in an engaging and entertaining format. However, the challenges of complicated coding and design components and long development time can be daunting. In addition, gamers expect certain capabilities and genres during games—fantasy, storytelling, interactivity—and health behavior games need to fit this mold. One part of gaming is eliciting emotion, which is strongly linked to memory or retention, and might also enhance or inhibit behavior change.[39] Stories are designed to evoke this emotion, and games need to incorporate this into a health behavior frame. This requires sophisticated, persuasive communication that goes beyond the typical health appeals used in other communication channels.

Old-Fashioned, "Low-Tech" Health Communication

Pamphlets

Although media—old and new—are more "glitzy" and exciting, more "old-fashioned" forms of communication should not be overlooked. The standard health pamphlet is a communication medium that goes back at least 200 years, when publications concerning health and treatments for a variety of physical and mental issues were available (see **FIGURES 6-7** and **6-8**). Although many of these were created to sell remedies or elixirs to "cure" everything from an upset stomach to cancer, the health pamphlet or brochure has continued to be an important and economical way to reach a large population with health information. Nowadays, health-related brochures are produced commercially for a variety of different health issues and are a staple at health departments, clinical settings, and social service agencies. Just think about your most recent visit to the doctor's office and you know that the brochure is alive and well. In general, brochures are cheap and easy to produce, especially with the availability of publishing software such as Adobe InDesign. Brochure content can be updated easily and can be targeted or tailored

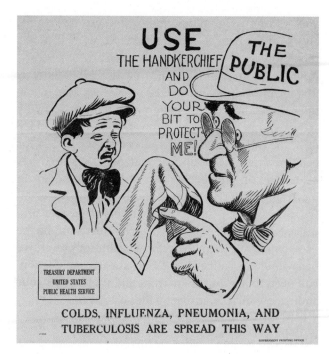

FIGURE 6-7 Turn-of-the-20th-century brochure on spreading germs.

Reproduced from Treasury Department, United States Public Health Service. U.S. Government Printing Office.

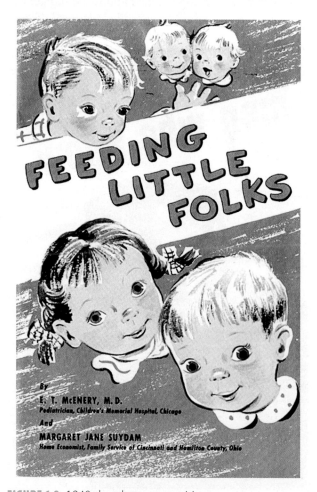

FIGURE 6-8 1940s brochure on nutrition.

Reproduced from Center for the History of Medicine at Countway Library, Harvard University. https://cms.www.countway .harvard.edu/wp/wp-content/uploads/2015/12/0003752_dref.jpg.

with a variety of graphics, photos, and text. Brochures also have the benefit of being portable; users can take them home and read them at their leisure.

One downside of using a pamphlet/brochure is that it can easily be overlooked or even avoided by the intended audience, simply because there are so many others competing for attention in the doctor's office or in the mail. And although they are used widely for health communication, little systematic research has been done on the effectiveness of brochure design in increasing comprehension or affecting health behavior. Information about the causes and consequences of a disease, for example, should be well understood by the user to motivate them to perform healthy or preventive behaviors.[40] As with all types of health communication, you need to do your homework and understand your audience, which can drive up the cost of production.

Posters

Posters have been used for advertising since the late 19th century and are an effective tool for influencing health behavior. **FIGURE 6-9** shows a poster used in World War II warning soldiers about the dangers of sexually transmitted diseases (called venereal disease back then). Similar campaigns have used posters to display information about nutrition, HIV prevention, and just about any other health issue you can name.

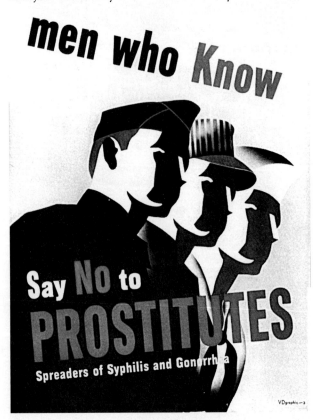

FIGURE 6-9 Say no to prostitution, World War II poster.

The benefits of posters for increasing awareness about a health issue are the variety of locations in which they can be hung and their low expense. As with pamphlets/brochures, available software allows for easy layout of posters, and printing can be done relatively cheaply. However, extensive testing of messages and graphics should be done with a subset of the intended audience to ensure the posters are providing effective messages without unintended interpretations or consequences. The content must be factual, brief, and, as far as possible, matched to audience characteristics. Posters are not the place for a lot of information. Instead, they should set a mood or raise awareness about a health issue.

Health Education

For this discussion we take health education to mean health communication exclusive of patient–provider interactions. This is often school- or community-based; a health educator talks with the target community about a health issue, perhaps using visual aids like posters, handouts, or displays. Although the most prevalent is certainly classroom teaching, an increasingly popular approach to health education is **edutainment** (*edu*cation + enter*tainment*), using stories, entertainment, and theater for health and social education. Many edutainment strategies use media (think *Sesame Street* for kids or a prime-time television series like *NCIS* that features a health issue). Community-based edutainment can take the form of street theater, puppet shows, or role-playing activities.[41] Photo novellas (graphic novels, or comic books for adults) can be used to address health issues using narrative, emotional appeal, and low literacy accessibility as features. Edutainment is particularly useful when audience comprehension is a major issue. It has been used internationally in a variety of settings to present health information in an entertaining way. **APPENDIX 6D** outlines an edutainment project called *East Los High* aimed to address health and social issues in Latina/o youth.

Another growing area of health education is the use of **lay health advisors**, respected members of a community who have been trained to talk about a health issue with their peers. Lay health educators strengthen already existing community network ties[42] and contribute a unique understanding of what is needed to improve health outcomes.[43] For example, in Latino communities lay advisors called *promotoras* have been used successfully to affect health behavior. The *Salud es Vida* program used a promotora-led Spanish language educational group session on cervical cancer screening to reach immigrant Latina women from farms in Southeast Georgia. Besides the education session, a toolkit was provided to the promotoras that included brochures, a flipchart, a short-animated video, and in-class activities to use in the sessions. Subsequently, there was a significant increase in cervical cancer screening in women who attended these sessions,[44] suggesting that engagement of community members with their peers in health education has a positive impact on health behavior.

▶ Communication Channel Selection

When planning a communication channel strategy, the paramount objectives are to engage, inform, and persuade. Some communication channels and formats are best for information, whereas others are more suited to persuasion. The challenge is to select the best communication channels for our message mix and determining the best use of these channels to get the most efficient and powerful communication. The ultimate decision in selecting communication channels should be based on who your target audience is already listening to, viewing, or reading. The following provides some guidance on how to select communication channels for specific audiences.

Criteria for Selecting Channels of Communication

There are four main criteria to use when selecting communication channels for health communication:

1. Which communication channels does your target audience use and have access to?
2. Which communication channels does your target audience say they like?
3. Which communication channels are most effective for communicating the content and images to the audience?
4. Where is your audience in its stage of behavior adoption (e.g., ready to act vs. just contemplating), and what communication channels might be most effective in moving them?

First, you need to match the communication to the message content. Is the channel a credible source of information, motivation, or persuasion for your target audience? For example, if you are trying to get people to stop smoking, would a *meme* (an expression coined by Rickard Dawkins in 1976 for something

that spreads virally through a culture, now especially through social media) distributed on Facebook be enough? You would need to think about the communication format and whether it lends itself to the content of the message. Richer communication media, such as face-to-face communication and some emerging technologies, tend to be more effective for conveying ambiguous messages because they allow for discussion and immediate feedback, transmission of both verbal and visual information, and greater personalization. Important richness factors include the following[45]:

- *Interactivity/feedback:* The ability of communicators to interact directly and rapidly with each other
- *Language variety:* The ability to support common (natural, informal, conversational) language as distinct from more formal, specialized, or abstract languages (e.g., medical, legal, or mathematical)
- *Tailoring:* The ability to modify the message based on the needs of the recipient in real time
- *Affect:* The ability to transmit feeling and emotion

Is the concept you want to communicate more visual or auditory? Is it better to use both? Are written words even needed? These questions help you think about which channel is most appropriate. Next, consider the frequency and reach of the communication channel. **Frequency** is the number of times you can get your message to your audience. **Reach** is how many people you actually reach with your message. Depending on your target audience, you may need more frequency to raise awareness of an issue or more reach to contact a large population. Sometimes you need both.

Another thing to think about is the production needs and costs. Some communication channels are costlier than others and need more expertise and personnel. Recall the earlier discussion of gaming and virtual reality. These types of interventions often have a long development time and require detailed knowledge of computer coding, computer graphics, and more. Other communication channels take no time to push information out, such as a tweet, a text message, or a Facebook post. It is worthwhile to assess the complexity of your message to see if more complicated channels are needed and if you have the additional budget, personnel, and expertise that may be required.

Sometimes the best approach is to create a *channel mix*, using a variety of communication channels to increase the likelihood that your target audience will see and hear your message. Success depends on an adequate and efficient mix of channels; the goal is to mix channels so that balance gives you a more effective strategy than trying to achieve it all with one channel. Many of the communication channels discussed in this chapter are used extensively for entertainment as well as information, particularly television, radio, and the internet.

Person, Place, and Time: Mediated Touchpoints in a Customer Journey

The first and last consideration in choosing a communication channel strategy is the individual who will receive your message. The **customer journey** is an individual's experiences that begin with *becoming aware* of an offering—be it an idea, product, or service—and continues through *actions taken*. The journey may end with adoption of the idea or purchase of the product, or it might include post-purchase or adoption advocacy. In our case, our "customer" is the patient/client/person we are hoping to reach with a health message that we want them to adopt or use to change behavior. The opportunities for a health communicator to engage with these customers during their journeys are referred to as **touch points**. Touch points can be tangible structures or services normally associated with branding, including buildings, signage, staff clothing, packaging, and products, but they also include *every* communication interaction. Whether it's a live phone call, a billboard, a TV ad, or a tweet, you choose a media channel because of its potential to deliver the right kind of touch at the right point (place and time) for the intended recipient.

So how do we understand the customer journey? What do they want—information, encouragement, validation, a sense of community, a reward? What else? A map of their media use can be complex, particularly when there are several audiences. It still boils down to answering the basic who, what, where, when, why, and how questions for each audience and behavior change goal.

▶ A Final Word: How Media Use and Health Disparities Are Related

It is important to end with a caution to ensure we think about health communication in a broad context. Although it is easy to get caught up with the most exciting technology of the time, remember that the promise of health communication rests on the ability to reach broad and diverse audiences. Communicating via mobile technology and web-based health websites is often less expensive than using traditional channels but requires the audience to have access to internet infrastructure. Studies indicate that those with higher rates of health disparity—the poor, the elderly, ethnic minorities, those with low health literacy, immigrants, those who did not graduate high school—are also those who fall into the "digital divide," without access to hard-wired broadband. These groups are also often the audiences we are trying to reach with health-protective messages. An intervention based only on emails and websites may actually *increase* health disparities by providing health communication that is inaccessible to the group with greater need.

Few technology-based interventions are designed with the appropriate contextual, cultural, and linguistic approaches to facilitate the equitable utility and impact of health communication across populations. It is our responsibility to develop health communication interventions and communication channel strategies within an ecological context[46] and to ensure that our messages are understandable and accessible by more than one segment of our intended audience.[47]

Mobile phones are a good example. As discussed earlier, the overwhelming majority of Americans have wireless phones, and almost two-thirds own a smartphone, with similar penetration among racial/ethnic and income groups. For those with low household incomes and levels of education, smartphones may be the only access point for online resources and services. The Pew Internet Survey[48] found that some 13% of Americans with an annual household income of less than $30,000 per year are smartphone-dependent for online access. By comparison, just 1% of Americans from households earning more than $75,000 per year rely only on their smartphones for online access. Similar findings across race/ethnicity show that 12% of African Americans and 13% of Latinos are smartphone-dependent, compared with only 4% of whites. Although they might be able to use their smartphones to get online, access can be interrupted by financial stresses and technical constraints. In this study, 30% of smartphone-dependent Americans report they "frequently" reach the limit of their data plan, and over half say that this happens occasionally. These emergent communication technologies hold great promise, but health communicators must develop strategies to counteract the relative lack of internet access in the digital divide where their target populations often reside.

Access to modern communication channels is only one barrier to successful receipt of a communication message. Almost half of adults in the United States have basic or below health literacy skills. Coupled with a record 61.8 million U.S. residents (native-born, legal immigrants, and undocumented immigrants) speaking a language other than English at home—an increase of 2.2 million from 2010[49]—the need for culturally and linguistically relevant health communication is staggering. We have the opportunity to increase health equity through broad dissemination of health information and interventions to populations suffering health inequities, especially through mobile devices. Our challenge is to design culturally relevant and accessible mHealth communications, which will require community engagement and community-based partnerships to be successful.[50]

▶ Conclusion

There are a dizzying number of communication channels available for distributing health information. The last decade has seen the rise of social media as a powerful tool to reach and interact with not only a selected audience, but also individuals. New opportunities for communicating and persuading with health information have been developed and will continue to appear. But it is important to not "throw out the baby with the bathwater"; some of the standard, more traditional forms of health communication—brochures, health education, television—are still very effective with certain audiences. The trick is to understand the communication barriers and opportunities for each audience. The challenge is to keep up with the new communication methods, add them to the established ones, and choose the best mix for each target audience.

Key Terms

Advertising Council
Click through
Customer journey
Edutainment
Frequency

Inbound marketing
Landing page
Lay health advisors
mHealth
Outbound marketing

Public service announcements (PSAs)
Reach
Text messaging
Touch point

Chapter Questions

1. What does the phrase "not all social media are digital, not all digital communications are social" mean? How does this relate to how public health organizations use digital media?
2. Describe, with examples from the chapter, two ways health communicators can integrate new methods with established communication channels.
3. Discuss the biggest downfall to using any type of social media for health communication.
4. Describe what mHealth is and how it can be used. What are the benefits of using mHealth?
5. How do health communicators select the channel of communication for their messages? What factors must be considered?

References

1. Anderson M, Perrin A, Jiang J. 11% of Americans don't use the internet. Who are they? http://www.pewresearch.org/fact-tank/2018/03/05/some-americans-dont-use-the-internet-who-are-they/. Published March 5, 2018. Accessed March 21, 2018.
2. The Nielsen Company. *The Nielsen Total Audience Report: Q2 2016.* http://www.nielsen.com/content/dam/corporate/us/en/reports-downloads/2016-reports/total-audience-report-q2-2016.pdf. Published 2016. Accessed June 15, 2018.
3. Nielsen estimates 116.4 million TV homes in the U.S. for the 2015-16 TV season. Nielsen Company website. http://www.nielsen.com/us/en/insights/news/2015/nielsen-estimates-116-4-million-tv-homes-in-the-us-for-the-2015-16-tv-season.html. Published August 28, 2015. Accessed March 6, 2018.
4. The total audience report Q2 2015. Nielsen Company website. http://www.nielsen.com/content/dam/corporate/us/en/reports-downloads/2015-reports/total-audience-report-q22015.pdf. Published 2015. Accessed March 6, 2018.
5. All things considered: comparable metrics offer a solid line of sight for the industry. Nielsen Company website. http://www.nielsen.com/us/en/insights/news/2015/all-things-considered-comparable-metrics-offer-a-solid-line-of-sight-for-the-industry.html. Published June 23, 2015. Accessed March 6, 2018.
6. Newspapers: daily readership by age. Pew Research Center Media and News Indicators Database. http://www.journalism.org/fact-sheet/newspapers/. Published June 1, 2017. Accessed March 21, 2018.
7. Magazine Media Factbook 2016/17. MPA: The Association of Magazine Media website. http://www.magazine.org/sites/default/files/MPA-FACTbook201617-ff.pdf. Published 2016. Accessed March 21, 2018.
8. Billboard fact sheet. Scenic America website. http://www.scenic.org/storage/PDFs/scenic%20america%20

billboard%20fact%20sheet.pdf. Published 2014. Accessed March 6, 2018.

9. Transit Advertising website. http://transitadvertisinginc .com. Accessed August 16, 2016.

10. Schein R, Kumanan W, Keelan J. Literature review on effectiveness of the use of social media: a report for Peel Public Health. http://www.peelregion.ca/health/resources /pdf/socialmedia.pdf. Accessed March 6, 2018.

11. Progress since the ice bucket challenge. ALS Association website. http://www.alsa.org/fight-als/edau/ibc-progress -infographic.html. Accessed August 2, 2016.

12. Perrin A. Social networking usage: 2005-2015. Pew Research Center website. http://www.pewinternet.org/2015/10/08/2015 /Social-Networking-Usage-2005-2015. Published October 8, 2015. Accessed March 6, 2018.

13. The Neilsen Company. *2016 Nielsen Social Media Report: Social Studies: A Look at the Social Landscape.* http:// www.nielsen.com/content/dam/corporate/us/en/reports -downloads/2017-reports/2016-nielsen-social-media-report .pdf. Published 2016. Accessed June 15, 2018.

14. Company info. Facebook website. http://newsroom.fb.com /company-info/. Published 2016. Accessed August 2, 2016.

15. Company. Twitter website. https://about.twitter.com /company. Published 2016. Accessed August 8, 2016.

16. About us. LinkedIn website. https://press.linkedin.com/about -linkedin. Published 2016. Accessed August 2, 2016.

17. Enge E. Hard numbers for public posting activity on Google Plus. Stone Temple website. https://www.stonetemple.com /real-numbers-for-the-activity-on-google-plus/. Published April 14, 2015. Accessed March 6, 2018.

18. Net advertising revenues of YouTube in the United States from 2015-2018. Statista website. https://statista.com /statistics/289660/youtube-us-net-advertising-revenues/. Accessed March 21, 2018.

19. Statistics. YouTube website. https://www.youtube.com/yt /press/statistics.html. Published 2016. Accessed August 8, 2016.

20. Pinterest by the numbers: stats, demographics & fun facts. Omnicore website. http://www.omnicoreagency.com /pinterest-statistics/. Published October 26, 2015. Accessed August 17, 2016.

21. Smith C. By the numbers: 180+ interesting Instagram statistics (June 2016). DMR website. http://expandedramblings.com /index.php/important-instagram-stats/. Updated July 14, 2016. Accessed August 17, 2016.

22. Smith C. By the numbers: 95 amazing Tumblr statistics & facts. DMR website. http://expandedramblings.com /index.php/tumblr-user-stats-fact/. Published July 14, 2016. Accessed August 17, 2016.

23. Smith C. By the numbers: 14 interesting flickr stats. DMR website. http://expandedramblings.com/index.php/flickr -stats/. Published July 14, 2016. Accessed August 17, 2016.

24. Reddit statistics and facts. DMR Business Statistics website. https://expandedramblings.com/index.php/reddit-stats/. Accessed March 21, 2018.

25. The Health Communication Social Media Toolkit. The Centers for Disease Control and Prevention. CDC website. https://www.cdc.gov/healthcommunication/toolstemplates /socialmediatoolkit_bm.pdf. Accessed March 21, 2018.

26. Smith A. Trends in cell phone usage and ownership. Pew Research Center website. http://www.pewinternet .org/2011/04/28/trends-in-cell-phone-usage-and-ownership/. Published April 28, 2011. Accessed March 6, 2018.

27. Smith A. Americans and text messaging. Pew Research Center website. http://www.pewinternet.org/2011/09/19 /americans-and-text-messaging/. Published September 19, 2011. Accessed March 6, 2018.

28. Hall AK, Cole-Lewis H, Bernhardt JM. Mobile text messaging for health: a systematic review of reviews. *Annu Rev Public Health.* 2015;36:393-415.

29. Vital Wave Consulting. *mHealth for Development: The Opportunity of Mobile Technology for Healthcare in the Developing World.* Washington, DC: UN Foundation/ Vodafone Foundation Partnership. http://www.globalproblems -globalsolutions-files.org/unf_website/assets/publications /technology/mhealth/mHealth_for_Development_full.pdf. Published 2009. Accessed March 6, 2018.

30. Ben-Zeev D, Scherer EA, Gottlieb JD, et al. mHealth for schizophrenia: patient engagement with mobile phone intervention following hospital discharge. *JMIR Ment Health.* 2016;3(3):e34. doi:10.2196/mental.6348.

31. Innovation profile: texting service enhances minority youth access to HIV/AIDS information and testing. Agency for Healthcare Research and Quality website. http://www .innovations.ahrq.gov. Published 2010. Accessed March 2011.

32. Gibbons MC, Fleisher L, Slamon R, Bass SB, Kandadai V, Beck R. Exploring the potential of Web 2.0 to address health disparities. *J Health Commun.* 2011;16(suppl 1):77-89. doi:10 .1080/10810730.2011.596916.

33. Marketing benchmarks from 7,000+ businesses. Hubspot website. http://cdn1.hubspot.com/hub/53/Marketing- Benchmarks-from-7000-businesses-UPDATE.pdf. Published 2015. Accessed December 9, 2015.

34. What is a landing page? Unbounce website. http:// unbounce.com/landing-page-articles/what-is-a-landing -page/. Published 2015. Accessed March 6, 2018.

35. Shegog R, Peskin MF, Markham CM, et al. 'It's your game- tech': toward sexual health in the digital age. *Creat Educ.* 2014;5(15):1428-1447. doi:10.4236/ce.2014.515161.

36. Grubb J. Sensor tower: Pokémon Go has already passed 30M downloads and $35M in revenue. Venture Beat website. http://venturebeat.com/2016/07/19/sensor-tower -pokemon-go-has-already-passed-30m-downloads-and -35m-in-revenue/. Published July 19, 2016. Accessed March 6, 2018.

37. Clark AM, Clark MTG. Pokémon Go and research: quali- tative, mixed methods research, and the supercomplexity of interventions. *Int J Qual Methods.* 2016;15(1):1-3. doi:10.1177/1609406916667765.

38. Strange A. It's true, 'Pokémon Go' is becoming a fitness craze. Mashable website. http://mashable.com/2016/07/12 /pokemon-go-fitness/#ZJ235gzkZ8q4. Published July 12, 2016. Accessed March 6, 2018.

39. Thomas R. The influence of emotional valence on age differences in early processing and memory. *Psychol Aging.* 2006;21(4):821-825. doi:10.1037/0882-7974.21.4.821.

40. Rogers RW. Cognitive and physiological processes in fear appeals and attitude change: a revised theory of protection motivation. In: Cacioppo JT, Petty RE, eds. *Social Psychophysiology: A Sourcebook.* New York, NY: Guilford; 1983:153-176.

41. Piotrow PT, de Fossard E. Entertainment-education as a public health intervention. In: Singhal A, Cody MJ, Rogers EM, Sabido M, eds. *Entertainment-Education and Social Change: History, Research, and Practice.* New York, NY: Routledge; 2004:39-60.

42. Institute of Medicine. *Unequal Treatment: Confronting Racial and Ethnic Disparities in Health Care.* Washington, DC: Institute of Medicine; 2003.

43. Witmer A. Community health workers: integral members of the health care work force. *Am J Public Health.* 1995;85:1055-1058.

44. Luque JS, Tarasenko YN, Reyes-Garcia C, et al. Salud es vida: a cervical cancer screening intervention for rural Latina immigrant women. [published online ahead of print January 12, 2016]. *J Cancer Educ.* doi:10.1007 /s13187-015-0978-x.

45. Health Communication Capacity Collaborative (HC3). *A Theory-Based Framework for Media Selection in Demand Generation Programs.* Baltimore, MD: Johns Hopkins Bloomberg School of Public Health Center for Communication Programs; 2014.

46. Green L, Kreuter M. *Health Promotion Planning: An Educational and Ecological Approach.* 4th ed. Boston, MA: McGraw-Hill; 2004.

47. Bernhardt JM, Fleisher L, Green BL. Opportunities and challenges to using technology to address health disparities. *Future Oncol.* 2014;10(4):519-524.

48. Smith A. U.S. smartphone use in 2015. Pew Research Center website. http://www.pewinternet.org/2015/04/01 /us-smartphone-use-in-2015/. Published April 1, 2015. Accessed March 6, 2018.

49. Camarota SA, Zeigler K. One in five U.S. residents speaks foreign language at home, record 61.8 million. Center for Immigration Studies website. http://cis.org//sites/cis .org/files/camarota-language.pdf. Published October 2014. Accessed March 6, 2018.

50. Fleisher L, Bass SB, Gonzales E, et al. Best practices in culturally appropriate health education approaches. In: Kinsey P, Louden DM, eds. *Ethnicity, Health, and Well-Being—An African American Perspective.* Lincoln University, PA: Lincoln University Press; 2013.

Appendix 6A

Los Angeles County's Sugar Pack Health Marketing Campaign

Noel Barragan and Tony Kuo

The Los Angeles County Department of Public Health (DPH) is tasked with protecting and promoting the health and well-being of the county's nearly 10 million residents. Preventing and controlling chronic conditions such as obesity, high blood pressure, and diabetes are among its top priorities. Overweight/obesity is linked to a myriad of diseases, including hypertension, stroke, type 2 diabetes, sleep apnea, some cancers, and depression, to name a few.[1] In Los Angeles, nearly 60% of adults are overweight or obese, approximately 9.3% have been diagnosed with diabetes, and 26.4% have been diagnosed with hypertension. Additionally, nearly a quarter of children in grades 5, 7, and 9 are obese.[2,3] These rates do not affect all populations equally; they are disproportionately higher among the most vulnerable populations (i.e., those who are low income). For instance, in Los Angeles's most affluent communities, the prevalence of childhood obesity is less than 5% as compared to more than 30% in the county's most impoverished communities.[4]

As part of its ongoing effort to address the significant burden of overweight/obesity in Los Angeles, DPH launched a health marketing campaign aimed at educating the public about the sugar content in sugar-sweetened beverages (SSBs). Funded by the Centers for Disease Control and Prevention, the campaign encourages people to reduce their consumption of these beverages. SSBs are liquids that are sweetened with various forms of sugar (e.g., regular sodas, sports drinks, or energy drinks) and usually have little or no nutritional value.[5] Excess SSB consumption has been linked to increased weight gain and is the top source of added calories in the U.S. diet.[6,7]

DPH launched the Sugar Pack health marketing campaign in October 2011. The campaign was largely informed by the New York City Department of Health and Mental Hygiene's Pouring on the Pounds campaign, which visually connected SSBs to packs of sugar and body fat, and included bold slogans such as "You are drinking yourself fat."[8] Final campaign visuals and messaging were vetted by focus groups comprising residents of Los Angeles County cities with high rates of obesity. Informed by the focus groups' understanding of the association between SSB consumption and health and their response to the proposed campaign (TABLE 6A-1), the campaign's feature message depicted a 20-ounce regular soda with the slogan "You wouldn't eat 22 packs of sugar. Why are you drinking them?" (FIGURE 6A-1). Parallel messages were also developed for a 20-ounce sports drink ("You wouldn't eat 12 packs of sugar. Why are you drinking them?") and a 16-ounce energy drink ("You wouldn't eat 17 packs of sugar. Why are you drinking them?").

The campaign was launched under the department's umbrella branding *Choose Health LA* at a press event attended by local television, print, and radio media outlets. This initial stage of the campaign consisted of a social media and online presence (e.g., website, Facebook page, sendable e-cards), and print education materials (i.e., posters, educational fliers) distributed to local schools and other DPH partners. The press event led to a number of English, Spanish, and Asian language news articles and spots on local radio.

Several months after the initial launch, additional funding became available to support outdoor media buys and the development of a video that could be shared through online channels (FIGURE 6A-2).

To optimize reach on a limited budget and target messaging to the most vulnerable populations, media buys on billboards and the local Metro served as the primary paid vehicle for campaign distribution. Based on focus group results, the visuals exclusively featured the soda image. The local Metro ridership was chosen as the target audience because of its

TABLE 6A-1 Selected Findings from Focus Group Testing of the Sugar Pack Campaign Messages and Creative Concepts Prior to Launch

Knowledge, attitudes, and beliefs about SSBs	"I don't think soda is good for anybody period. But we do drink it, yes we do."
	"I think they are healthy in moderation, not every day to drink it. If you are out there burning the calories, working it off."
	"When I was younger, when I was sick, I was always told to drink [name brand sports drink]. It doesn't weight you down … [name brand sports drink] is like water, but good water for you."
	"They say that dark soft drinks are more harmful. But you think that [name brand sports drink] is not that bad, is not so harmful…."
	"I grew up drinking it. My father did not take it away from me. I turned out all right."
	"If you want to have soda or lemonade, you are not going to get diabetes or become overweight from that one drink."
	"It's not the worst thing, just don't overload it."
Opinions and reactions to the Sugar Pack campaign messages and creative concepts*	"Seriously, 23 packs* of sugar? That's crazy."
	"You see how much is on the label. But when you have a visual, you see more of a clear picture of how much you are really intaking."
	"I was astonished. It was like we had a bandage over our eyes. It was really shocking. We know they are harmful, but we are always tempted to drink even though you know."
	"You have coffee and you put two little envelopes. … But if you have a soda, and then you realize that it has 23* packs of sugar. That is too much. Imagine for a child."
	"I actually feel differently about soda already [after] seeing that. I kind of don't want to go outside and drink the soda I have in my car. … I know I am going to drink soda, that is not going to stop, but thinking about chugging sugar. It kind of grosses me out."
	"I'm actually ashamed. I never did make an issue of keeping sodas away from [my kids]."
	"It is shameful to know that you are bringing this and making it okay for them to drink it, and especially if you are setting the example, they are going to grow up thinking my mom did it so it is ok for me to do it."
	"Obviously you would just not give your kid 23* packs of sugar. But seeing how much is in there. I know there is sugar in soda. I just did not think about how much."
	"I have been shown commercials like this for years about soda … and it never stopped me from drinking soda and it didn't stop me from giving it to my kids."

*The number of sugar packs was updated from 23 to 22 to reflect shrinking consumer packaging in the size of a standard sugar pack. Campaign messages are based on 1/10-ounce or 3-gram sugar packs.

large size and its demographics (e.g., lower income).[9] Beginning in February 2012, a total of 2399 placements were displayed for 8 weeks. Anecdotally, DPH staff noted that many of the advertisements were not removed or replaced promptly at the conclusion of the negotiated time period. This allowed the campaign to be displayed longer than planned. Placements included billboards, bus taillight displays, bus interior cards, bus shelters, exterior rail, interior rail cars, and posters. In total, more than 350 million impressions

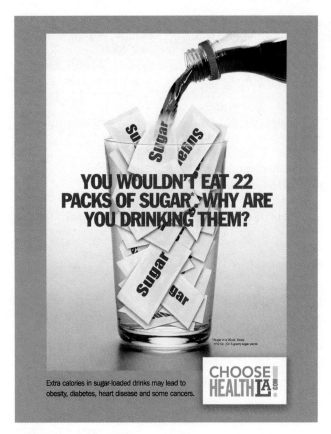

FIGURE 6A-1 Sugar Pack campaign: 20-oz soda.
Image courtesy of Los Angeles County Department of Public Health's Choose Health LA initiative, 2011.

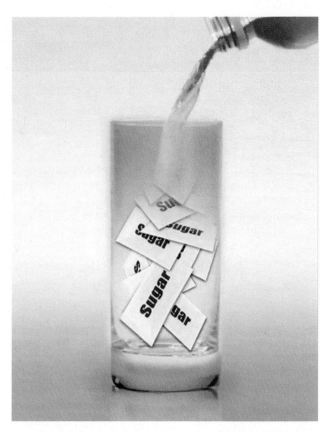

FIGURE 6A-2 Sugar Pack campaign: sports drink video.
Image courtesy of Los Angeles County Department of Public Health's Choose Health LA initiative, 2012.

were generated. In addition to being shared online, the Sugar Pack video was played on transit televisions over a 12-week period, starting in January and ending in April 2012.

The initial positive reception of the campaign and additional grant funding opportunities led to the health marketing campaign being relaunched several months later in July 2012. In this second round, both the soda and sports drink visuals and messages were used. This round lasted approximately 5 weeks. There were a total of 2374 placements, which generated more than 155 million impressions. As with the initial round of paid placements, advertisements were not removed/replaced immediately at the conclusion of the 5-week period.

The Sugar Pack campaign's implementation and dissemination has been shaped over time by the availability of funding support and opportunities. By utilizing a combination of media platforms, DPH optimized

the campaign's reach and impact. For example, use of online tools, in addition to more traditional media outlets, has allowed the campaign to maintain a web presence years after funding support ended. Online videos can still be viewed more than 6 years after the campaign's initial launch (https://www.youtube.com/watch?v=wKhi8uaoDeo and https://www.youtube.com/watch?v=2wlkr34JkWE). The strategic placements of ads on city transit platforms allowed for dissemination among not only thousands of bus and train/subway riders, but also drivers caught in Los Angeles's infamous traffic. The use of clear and concise messaging was a critical component to maximizing the impact of this relatively small budgeted campaign in an already flooded media market. Visuals and lessons learned from this health marketing campaign informed similar efforts in other jurisdictions across the United States.

References

1. Adult obesity causes & consequences. Centers for Disease Control and Prevention website. https://www.cdc.gov /obesity/adult/causes.html. Published August 15, 2016. Accessed March 5, 2018.

2. Los Angeles County Department of Public Health, Office of Health Assessment and Epidemiology. *Key Indicators of Health by Service Planning Area.* Los Angeles, CA: Los Angeles County Department of Public Health; 2017. http://publichealth.lacounty.gov/ha/docs/2015LACHS /KeyIndicator/PH-KIH_2017-sec%20UPDATED.pdf.

3. Los Angeles County Department of Public Health. *Parks and Public Health in Los Angeles County: A Cities and Communities Report.* Los Angeles, CA: Los Angeles County Department of Public Health; 2016. http://publichealth. lacounty.gov/chronic/docs/Parks%20Report%202016 -rev_051816.pdf.

4. County of Los Angeles Public Health. *Parks and Public Health in Los Angeles County: A Cities and Communities Report.* http://publichealth.lacounty.gov/chronic/docs/Parks%20

Report%202016-rev_051816.pdf. Published May 2016. Accessed March 5, 2018.

5. U.S. Department of Health and Human Services and U.S. Department of Agriculture. *Dietary Guidelines for Americans 2015–2020.* 8th ed. https://health.gov/dietaryguidelines/2015 /resources/2015-2020_Dietary_Guidelines.pdf. Published December 2015. Accessed March 5, 2018.

6. Malik VS, Pan A, Willett WC, Hu FB. Sugar-sweetened beverages and weight gain in children and adults: a systematic review and meta-analysis. *Am J Clin Nutr.* 2013;98(4): 1084-1102. doi:10.3945/ajcn.113.058362.

7. Welsh JA, Sharma AJ, Grellinger L, Vos MB. Consumption of added sugars is decreasing in the United States. *Am J Clin Nutr.* 2011;94(3):726-734. doi:10.3945/ajcn.111.018366.

8. Obesity. City of New York website. http://www1.nyc.gov /site/doh/health/health-topics/obesity.page. Published 2016. Accessed March 5, 2018.

9. Barragan NC, Noller AJ, Robles B, et al. The "sugar pack" health marketing campaign in Los Angeles County, 2011-2012. *Health Promot Pract.* 2014;15(2):208-216. doi:10.1177/1524839913507280.

Appendix 6B

Text4baby as a Surveillance/Information Dissemination Tool During Zika Outbreak

Jodie Fishman

▶ Zika in the United States in 2016

In early 2016, concerns about Zika skyrocketed as the virus reached pandemic levels. Linked to microcephaly in babies whose mothers had Zika while pregnant, the virus poses specific and dangerous threats to pregnant women. In early 2016, the Centers for Disease Control and Prevention (CDC) issued travel warnings for pregnant women traveling to areas infected with Zika and confirmed sexual transmission of the disease on U.S. soil. Continued warnings that local transmission would likely occur in the continental United States were realized in early August, as south Florida saw local outbreaks, first in the Wynwood neighborhood of downtown Miami and then in Miami Beach. As this outbreak continues, government agencies and others involved continue to set guidelines and release new information. To date (as of March 7, 2018) 5673 cases of Zika have been reported in the United States (excluding territories), 229 of which were locally acquired mosquito-borne cases.[1]

▶ Enter Text4baby

Text4baby (**FIGURE 6B-1**), the largest mobile health initiative in the nation, has used the power of cell phone technology to share important health and safety information with expectant women and moms with infants under age one since its launch in 2010. The service can also be used by dads, partners, family members, or friends who want to follow a woman's journey through pregnancy and baby's first year. Participants receive free, customized health information, safety tips, interactive surveys, and appointment

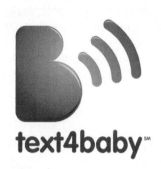

FIGURE 6B-1 Text4baby logo.
Reproduced from Text4baby website. https://www.text4baby.org.

reminders through at least three text messages per week and a free app—timed to the user's due date or baby's birthdate—all at no charge to the user. Through these educational messages, Text4baby aims to educate, and ultimately to improve maternal and child health outcomes.

The Messages

Text4baby's messaging topics include breastfeeding, smoking cessation, nutrition and physical activity, mental health, oral health, safe sleep, car seat safety, immunizations, developmental milestones, and many more. Dozens of federal agencies and national, state, and local organizations provide input into the content development.

Text4baby also sends urgent messages on recalls, changes in guidelines relevant to pregnant women and new moms, and information about outbreaks and safety during events like natural disasters. Examples include the Tylenol recall in 2010, Similac formula recall in 2010, updated car seat safety guidelines in 2011, pertussis outbreak in 2012, and information on food safety during power outages to users in affected states after Hurricane Sandy in 2012.

When a user signs up for Text4baby, the only data she (or he) provides at registration are the baby's due date/birth date and their zip code. Therefore, the Text4baby team has the ability to send messages by geographic location, down to the zip code level. Several sets of interactive messages give users the opportunity to respond to questions on specific topics and to receive follow-up information based on their responses. Interactive messaging sets the focus on health insurance coverage status for mom and baby, flu vaccination, appointment reminders, and more.

Reach and Demographics

Ninety-two percent of American women own a cell phone, and 66% own smartphones. Over 80% of cell phone owners send or receive text messages. People of color are more likely to text than their white counterparts, and low-income Americans text more than high-income Americans.[2] In September 2016, Text4baby had reached 1.1 million users across the country. Although most users are pregnant women and new moms with babies under age one, Text4baby also targets dads, partners, and other loved ones of pregnant women or new moms who want to follow the pregnancy/new mom journey.

Data collected upon sign-up are limited, but surveys of participants have helped paint a picture of Text4baby users[3]:

- Average age: 27
- 52% reported incomes under $16,000
- 52% are first-time mothers
- 28% are African American
- 44% are currently married
- 82% finished high school
- 53% are on Medicaid

Partnerships

Text4baby is jointly operated by ZERO TO THREE and Voxiva, Inc. Thanks to a partnership with the CTIA Wireless Foundation, all messages are free to the end user, and if a user has a limited texting plan, Text4baby messages do not count toward their monthly totals. A number of mobile carriers support Text4baby, making the service available in all 50 states and U.S. territories.

The program, a true public–private partnership, is made possible through a broad range of organizations including government agencies, corporations, academic institutions, professional associations, and nonprofit organizations. Additionally, Text4baby relies on more than 1400 outreach partners across the country to help enroll users and keep them engaged. These partners include providers, nonprofits, state and local health departments, Medicaid and Women, Infants and Children agencies, health plans, and more.

Data and Evaluations

Text4baby research and evaluations—conducted internally and externally—show that:

- *The program is reaching its target audience.* Participants enroll early in their pregnancy, tend to live in zip codes with high poverty levels, and come from low-income households.[3,4]
- *Text4baby is well-received.* According to an evaluation conducted by the U.S. Department of Health and Human Services, Health Resources and Services Administration, 99% of participants would recommend the program to a friend or family member, and 90% read the messages and found them useful.[5]
- *Text4baby impacts knowledge and behavior.* Text4baby moms are nearly three times more likely to believe they are prepared to be new mothers,[6] and compared to nonusers, they better understand the importance of prenatal care and prenatal vitamins, the risk of alcohol use, safe sleep practices, the best time to deliver in a healthy pregnancy, and the meaning of full-term.[5,7] Text4baby mothers who did not plan to be vaccinated for flu because of cost and received a text on how to access free and low-cost influenza vaccines were nearly two times more likely to report vaccination, and those who did plan to be vaccinated who received a reminder were two times more likely to report vaccination.[8]

▶ Text4baby's Zika Response

Given the ability to quickly reach women across the country with important health information—and to reach pregnant women or those thinking of becoming pregnant again soon—Text4baby is uniquely well positioned to share crucial information on Zika.

Activities

Starting in February 2016, Text4baby began sending one message per month to users nationally, with slightly different messages for pregnant women and new moms. Some messages included a link to a survey to collect data on user attitudes and practices related to Zika. When a user receives a message outside of the three per week timed to her due date or baby's birthdate, there is often a small spike in user cancellations. (One of the most frequently reported reasons for user cancellation is that they receive too many messages.) Sending one message per month on Zika has helped walk the fine line between getting users the information they need and keeping them enrolled.

Working with the CDC's Zika Response Team, the Text4baby team also started sending targeted messages to users in areas with active Zika transmission, including the U.S. Virgin Islands and Puerto Rico. That partnership also included sharing Text4baby promotional materials for inclusion in Zika prevention kits in those areas.

Text4baby began sharing information on Zika through other channels as well, including social media and *TEAM Text4baby*, an email newsletter targeted at graduates of the program (those whose babies have reached age 1)—knowing that many recent graduates tend to get pregnant again relatively quickly.

Using the program's public–private partnership base, staff members convened a federal partner meeting with a focus on Zika in May 2016. Text4baby acted as host, convening federal agencies to share current Zika messaging, resources, and best practices on Zika communication. Lastly, Text4baby created a state customization service to help states and localities reach women in their location with more specific text messages and other tailored messaging.

Selected Zika Messages

Messages to pregnant Text4baby users included information on travel warnings, preventing mosquito bites, preventing Zika through protected sex, cases in the United States, resources, and more (see FIGURE 6B-2). Messages to new moms differed slightly, and included information on delaying trying to conceive if they or their partner had traveled to an area with Zika, and protecting their baby/children and themselves from Zika (see FIGURE 6B-3). Messages to users in areas with active transmission focused on connecting users to local resources and providing them with information specific to where they live—including where to go for free Zika testing and free prevention kits.

Surveys

To inform Text4baby's Zika strategy and messaging—and inform Text4baby's partners' efforts as well—Text4baby surveyed users in March 2016 and July 2016 to assess level of concerns regarding Zika, users' sources of information, and informational needs. The

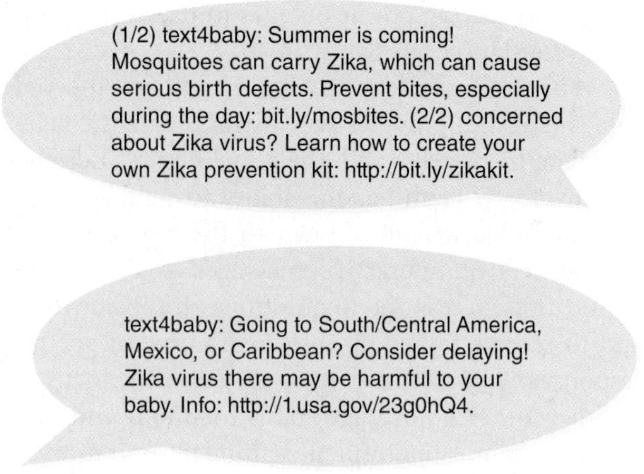

FIGURE 6B-2 Sample text messages: national.
Reproduced from Text4baby website. https://www.text4baby.org.

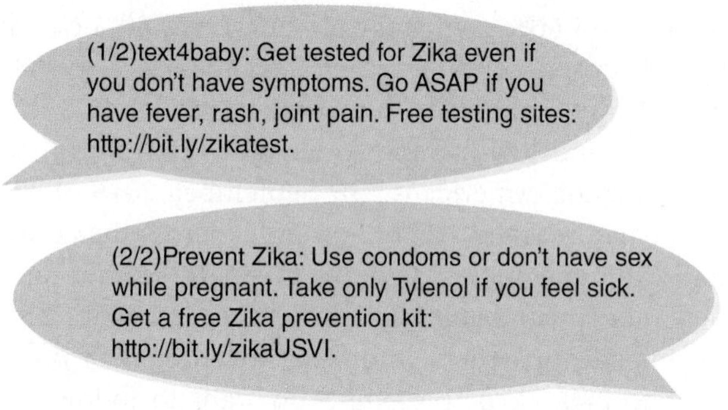

FIGURE 6B-3 Sample text messages: U.S. Virgin Islands.
Reproduced from Text4baby website. https://www.text4baby.org.

March survey went to just pregnant users ($n = 470$), and the July survey went to both pregnant and new mom users ($n = 1627$). The July survey repeated questions asked in March to gauge any shift in answers as summer/mosquito season arrived, as well as included new questions about users' knowledge of how to protect themselves from Zika and their current means of protection. Response rates were typical for survey links without an incentive sent via text message to Text4baby users and hovered around 2% for both respondents who received Text4baby messages in English and those who received them in Spanish (hereafter referred to as English-language and Spanish-language respondents). Though response rates were relatively low, Text4baby was able to collect hundreds to thousands of responses within 1–2 days of sending each text. Depending on the group, between 4% and 7% of respondents reported taking both the March and July surveys.

Just weeks after Text4baby's July survey, the first cases of local transmission in the United States occurred in South Florida—and other national Zika polls starting popping up. A CNN poll showed that just 23% of Americans were worried about Zika (including those who were only somewhat worried)[9];

a *Washington Post* poll showed that 35% were at least somewhat worried, with only 12% reporting being very worried.[10] Those results—failing to poll two extremely important groups in response to Zika—did not match Text4baby's. Text4baby's July Zika survey showed that 90% of all respondents strongly agreed or agreed that they were concerned about Zika (see **FIGURE 6B-4**). However, the percentage of pregnant English-and Spanish-language respondents who reported strongly agreeing (versus agreeing) that they were concerned about Zika decreased from March to July.

Alarmingly, only 1 in 3 respondents strongly agreed or agreed that they knew how to protect themselves from getting Zika (see **FIGURE 6B-5**). Other results showed the top measures pregnant respondents were taking to protect themselves (see **FIGURE 6B-6**)—the number-one measure among English-language respondents was avoiding travel to areas with Zika (71%), and the number one measure among Spanish language respondents was using insect repellant (72%).

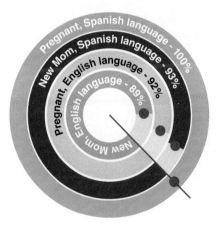

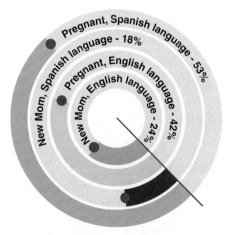

The number-one reported source for Zika information among both English- and Spanish-language pregnant respondents in both March and July was newspaper/TV/radio. Less than 1 in 3 pregnant respondents reported getting information on Zika from her healthcare provider (see **FIGURE 6B-7**).

Overall, Spanish-language respondents (both pregnant and new moms) were less likely to report avoiding travel to areas with Zika, more likely to report not doing anything to prevent Zika, being more concerned about Zika and future pregnancies (new moms), and wanting information from Text4baby on Zika more frequently.

Conclusions and Opportunities

Based on these survey results, Text4baby began looking into sending different messages to Spanish-language users and altering the frequency of messaging to that audience. The team is able to gauge cancellation rates separately for Spanish-language and English-language users, thereby allowing Text4baby staff to determine if more frequent and/or tailored messaging changes cancellation rates by language of user.

The Text4baby team also shared survey results with partners who work with providers, including the American Congress of Obstetricians and Gynecologists, the National Association of Pediatric Nurse Practitioners, and the Association of Women's Health, Obstetric and Neonatal Nurses. By sharing results with these organizations and others, Text4baby aimed to work together to increase dialogues about Zika among providers and pregnant women.

Survey results also highlighted the need to reinforce the differences between pregnant women and the general population, as well as the opportunity to use Text4baby as a surveillance tool. Within 2 days of sending each survey via text message, Text4baby had collected hundreds of responses, creating the ability to quickly share information on the needs of pregnant women nationally as well as by state. This information can help Zika coordinators across the country continue to identify needs in their areas and get the appropriate information out to those in need across the country.

As of September 2016, Text4baby continued to send monthly, national text messages, as well as more specific messages to users in areas with active Zika—and began tweaking messages to gauge what resonated most with users. This included using a more personal tone with a direct message from a Text4baby staff member who was also pregnant. Next steps include enhancing utilization of other means of communication, including social media and email; coming up

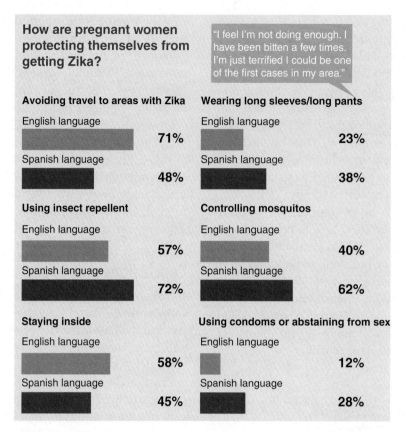

FIGURE 6B-6 Survey responses: how pregnant women are protecting themselves.
Reproduced from Text4baby website. https://www.text4baby.org.

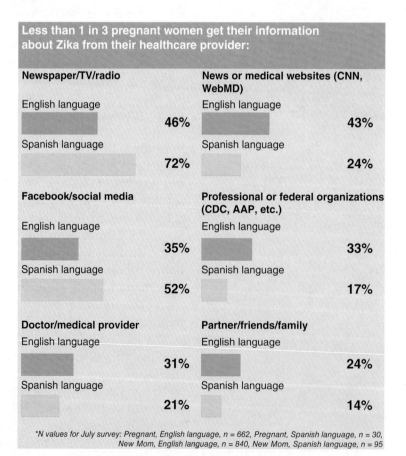

FIGURE 6B-7 Survey responses: information from healthcare provider.
Reproduced from Text4baby website. https://www.text4baby.org.

with new ways to meet Spanish-language users' needs related to Zika; and continuing to survey users as needed.

Using a mobile health program like Text4baby during a national outbreak can be an effective way to reach target audiences quickly, on the device that Americans always carry with them. Text4baby and others who reach a specific target audience must look for new ways to enhance communication with their users in times of outbreaks or other similar situations. Programs such as Text4baby can also be used as a surveillance and information gathering tool not only during public health crises, but also for other health behaviors and outcomes. Health information by text message remains a useful tool for quickly disseminating crucial health information to large numbers of people.

References

1. Zika cases in the United States. https://www.cdc.gov/zika/reporting/case-counts.html. Centers for Disease Control and Prevention website. Published March 8, 2018. Accessed March 21, 2018.

2. Anderson M. Technology device ownership: 2015. Pew Research Center website. http://www.pewinternet.org/2015/10/29/technology-device-ownership-2015. Published October 2015. Accessed March 5, 2018.

3. Martinez, KM, Uekusa S. 2013 national survey of Text4baby participants. California State University, San Marcos website. https://www.csusm.edu/anthropology/docsandfiles/text4baby.pdf. Published January 29, 2015.

4. Understanding the impact of Text4baby. Text4baby website. https://partners.text4baby.org/templates/beez_20/images/HMHB/final%20impact%20factsheet.pdf. Published June 17, 2015. Accessed March 5, 2018.

5. U.S. Department of Health and Human Services, Health Resources and Services Administration. *Promoting Maternal and Child Health Through Health Text Messaging: An Evaluation of the Text4baby Program—Final Report.* Rockville, MD: U.S. Department of Health and Human Services; 2015.

6. Evans WD, Wallace JL, Snider J. Pilot evaluation of the Text4baby mobile health program. *BMC Public Health.* 2012;12:1.

7. Evans WD, Wallace Bihm J, Szekely D, et al. Initial outcomes from a 4-week follow-up study of the Text4baby program in the military women's population: randomized controlled trial. *J Med Internet Res.* 2014;16(5):e131.

8. Text4baby as a surveillance tool for influenza vaccination. National Adult and Influena Immunization Summit website. https://www.izsummitpartners.org/content/uploads/2016/08/Text4baby-as-a-Surveillance-Tool-for-Influenze-Vaccination-08-09-2016.pdf. Accessed March 21, 2018.

9. Agiesta J. Few fear Zika following first mosquito-borne cases in US. CNN website. http://www.cnn.com/2016/08/03/politics/zika-olympics-us-mosquito/. Published August 3, 2016. Accessed March 5, 2018.

10. Guskin E, Clement S. Americans are still not worried about Zika, poll finds. *Washington Post* website. https://www.washingtonpost.com/news/to-your-health/wp/2016/08/09/americans-are-still-not-worried-about-zika-poll-finds/. Published August 9, 2016. Accessed March 5, 2018.

Appendix 6C

The Use of Virtual Worlds in Health Promotion

Joan E. Cowdery and Sun Joo (Grace) Ahn

▶ Virtual Reality Technology

Virtual reality technology can refer to a variety of applications but typically consists of some type of immersive 3-D experience for the user. Virtual reality environments are created by digital devices that simulate multiple layers of sensory information so that users are able to see, hear, and feel as if they are in the real world[1] and have the perception of existing in an alternate space. Depending on the purpose of the application, these spaces can mimic the real world or be highly fantasized, as is the case in many gaming environments. Early virtual reality applications, such as flight simulators, have expanded into many areas of health care including surgery simulations and trainings.

Although the initial application of virtual reality technology and the development of virtual worlds took place in the gaming realm, more recent applications have included social networking, education and training, and health care. One of the defining characteristics of virtual worlds is that they generate simultaneously shared spaces.[2] In addition to fostering real-time social interaction, virtual worlds allow users to have a physical presence in these shared spaces. Users in virtual worlds exist and interact in these computer-simulated environments where participants create what is commonly known as an avatar, a digitally constructed form of virtual representation that marks a user's entity.[3]

▶ Publicly Available Spaces

Unlike previous gaming applications that required additional equipment, current virtual technologies are readily available to anyone with a computer and an internet connection. There are a plethora of publicly available spaces where one can interact with others

for a variety of reasons for little to no cost. Many are game-specific and targeted toward specific age groups; for example, Virtual Worlds for Teens (http://virtualworldsforteens.com) and Twinity (http://www.twinity.com). The list of online virtual worlds continues to grow, so any attempt to provide a current list would be instantly outdated. One of the oldest, largest, and most active virtual worlds is Linden Lab's Second Life (http://www.secondlife.com). Current estimates indicate approximately 1 million regular monthly users with 70,000 concurrent users. In Second Life, residents can shop, attend business meetings, take classes, participate in trainings, swim, ski, watch a live concert, and do just about anything that one could do in real life. The geography of Second Life is organized as islands. One of the most popular and frequently visited is Health Info Island (http://http://secondlife.com/destination/28). Created and funded by a grant from the National Library of Medicine, HealthInfo Island has grown from a resource for health information to include over 120 support groups for patients and caregivers, as well as mental health simulations and an area for individuals with disabilities called Virtual Ability Island (http:// http://secondlife.com/destination/1160).

An increasing number of real-world health-related institutions and organizations have begun to promote the use of virtual worlds and have created virtual world presences. For example, the National Institutes of Health has suggested the use of virtual reality technology for research and education on diabetes and obesity because of the potential to engage patients in interventions that focus on healthy eating and physical activity.[4] Given that interactive technologies have been used to facilitate the delivery of health information and interaction among patients, caregivers, and health professionals, the application for health behavior change interventions seems plausible.

Use of Virtual World Technology in Health Communication

Virtually Experiencing the Consequences of Negative Health Behaviors

Virtual worlds offer novel media characteristics that allow researchers and healthcare practitioners to implement new strategies in approaching health behavior change that may have been difficult or impossible with traditional tools and media platforms. One such characteristic is the virtual acceleration of time,[5] wherein users are able to transcend the temporal boundaries of the physical world by experiencing digitally depicted events of the past or future in the virtual worlds. For instance, with the help of simulated sensory information via digital devices, users may be able to virtually experience the negative future consequences of present problematic health behaviors, allowing users to construe the health risks as personally relevant[6] and temporally imminent.[5] The increased sense of relevance and urgency through the virtual experience encourages individuals to reduce problematic health behaviors.

The virtual acceleration of time would be particularly useful for healthcare issues because one of the greatest challenges of communicating health risks is the large temporal gap that exists between present health behaviors and future negative health consequences. This gap explains why individuals tend to have a more rosy view of distant futures.[7] It may be that individuals are unaware of how imminent the health risk may be; for example, smoking a cigarette is unlikely to lead to immediate illnesses or fatality. The length of time it takes for negative health outcomes to manifest renders the causal relationship between the present cause (smoking) and future outcomes (e.g., lung cancer) abstract and difficult to grasp. Relatedly, earlier research demonstrates that when health messages are able to present the risk (i.e., a negative health consequence) to be temporally proximal, they are effectively able to elicit behavioral modification.

Virtual Selves

Another novel characteristic of virtual worlds is a byproduct of the plasticity of avatar creation. With the development of advanced digital technology, users may now easily create photorealistic avatars that share realistic physical feature similarities with the self. For example, imagine a health pamphlet that features a virtual entity that looks photorealistically like you, rather than a typical, but unfamiliar person; you would be more likely to pay attention and feel that the message is personally relevant.[8] Moreover, once the photorealistic virtual self is created, computer software is easily able to manipulate its appearance—the virtual self may be aged to make you look like you are in your 60s, or its physique may be altered so that it looks like the virtual self has gained weight—and these virtual selves may be plugged in to create health messages that allow individuals to realize that the health risk may influence everyone, including themselves.

In one such study, the effect of virtual experiences that incorporate virtual acceleration in time and photorealistic virtual selves on health attitudes and behaviors in the physical world were explored in the context of soft drink consumption.[5] Participants either saw a pamphlet, which was either tailored to the self or untailored, or were exposed to both the pamphlet and a virtual depiction of it. The six-page full-color pamphlet provided specific information on the health risks of soft drinks, with an emphasis on weight gain and obesity. In the virtual experience, participants wore a head-mounted display—goggles that provides three-dimensional perception through stereoscopic views of the virtual world—and observed either a virtual self or an unfamiliar, generic virtual human (i.e., virtual other).

During the two-minute virtual experience, participants saw the virtual self or virtual other imbibe a soft drink and continue to gain weight. Two years in the physical world were depicted in two minutes in the virtual world. Self-reported soft drink consumption intentions were assessed immediately following experimental treatments, and actual soft drink consumption was measured one week following experimental treatments (**FIGURE 6C-1**).

Results indicated that immediately following experimental treatments, the effect of tailoring significantly affected intentions to consume soft drinks in the future. Messages, regardless of whether they were presented in a pamphlet or in virtual worlds, led to shorter perceived distance between the self and the health risk, and in turn, higher involvement. The increased involvement ultimately led to lower intentions to consume soft drinks than untailored messages. Interestingly, however, the effect of tailoring seemed to dissipate over time. One week following experimental treatments, only the effect of medium was significant. The participants who were given the pamphlet coupled with the virtual experience perceived shorter

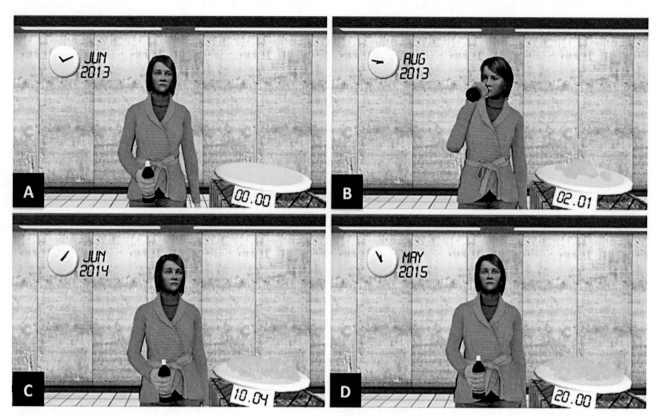

FIGURE 6C-1 Virtual reality soda consumption.
Created by Sun Joo (Grace) Ahn. Used with permission.

temporal distance between their present health behaviors and future health outcomes, which led to greater perceived imminence of the risks related to soft drink consumption. The increased risk then resulted in significantly lower soft drink consumption than with participants who only saw the pamphlet. This experiment provided strong preliminary evidence for the potential of incorporating virtual experiences as a part of multicomponent and multimedia health promotion campaigns.

In another study, Ahn and colleagues demonstrated that not all virtual representations used to promote health behaviors need to take on human forms.[9] A virtual pet system was developed, guided by the framework of social cognitive theory,[10] to systematically promote physical activity in children through goal setting, vicarious experiences, and positive reinforcement. A kiosk was built to present the virtual pet system, using a laptop and a flat-screen television stationed on top of a rolling cart. A Microsoft Kinect for Windows device with motion-detecting capabilities was mounted on top of the television (**FIGURE 6C-2**). In the study, children's physical activity was measured with an activity monitor and synchronized with a unique pet so that they would interact with their personalized pet for the duration of the intervention. The integration of the activity monitor with the virtual pet system allowed

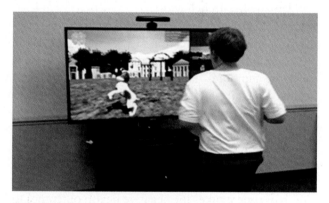

FIGURE 6C-2 Virtual kiosk with pet avatar.
Created by Sun Joo (Grace) Ahn. Used with permission.

children to use this system with minimal or no technical expertise; they simply had to plug the activity monitor into the computer, and the system would automatically synchronize the activity data with the child's unique virtual pet and update the system as necessary.

The interaction cycle was a repetition of goal setting, evaluation, and reinforcement processes. Upon first engaging with the virtual pet, children were asked to personalize their pets (e.g., selecting the collar color, selecting the tag color, naming the pet, etc.). The virtual pet then asked children to establish self-set physical activity goals, which were designed to promote physical activity self-efficacy by way of mastery experiences; that is, by setting and meeting goals for behavior change and recognizing one's ability to overcome challenges along the way, individuals gain confidence in their capacity to engage in that particular behavior. Similarly, the goal-setting feature in the virtual pet was designed to allow children to repeatedly engage in the experience of setting and meeting physical activity goals to promote mastery experiences.

Once the goal was set, children engaged in physical activity away from the kiosk, wearing the physical activity monitor. When children felt that they had met their physical activity goal, they returned to the kiosk and plugged the activity monitor into the computer. The computer then automatically synchronized the unique identifier chip embedded in the activity monitor to that child's unique virtual pet and brought the pet up on the screen while also evaluating the physical activity recorded on the activity monitor. If the child was unable to meet the goal, the virtual pet verbally informed the child that they had failed to meet the physical activity goal and encouraged the child to go back to engaging in physical activity. If the child did meet the goal, the virtual pet invited them to teach it a trick using verbal and gesture commands detected by the Kinect for Windows device. For instance, the child could verbally command, "Fetch!" and see a virtual ball appear on the screen. They could then make a throwing motion toward the Kinect, and the ball would fly into the virtual world, following the trajectory of the child's physical arm. The virtual pet would then chase after the ball and bring it back. Because the underlying assumption was that the virtual pet would be engaging in physical activity in the virtual world while children stayed physically active in the physical world, the tricks began with simpler ones (e.g., sit, stay) and eventually more sophisticated ones as children met more goals and the virtual pet became more fit (e.g., fetch, moonwalk). Once the child taught their virtual pet one trick, the pet asked them to set a new physical activity goal, and the cycle would repeat.

When compared with children in the control group who were given an identical computer system with the same functionalities but without the virtual dog, children who interacted with the virtual dog engaged in approximately 1.09 more hours of physical activity daily. Self-report survey data revealed that

interacting with the virtual dog led children to feel confident about their abilities to set and meet physical activity goals, which in turn, heightened their beliefs that physical activity is good for them.[10]

▶ Strategies, Challenges, and Implications for Future Use

Although virtual technologies offer a multitude of health promotion opportunities, they are not without challenges. Although widely available and accessible, these virtual worlds can be transient, as can the resources and programs contained within them. It is therefore incumbent upon health communication planners to be diligent in knowing what currently exists and in updating materials frequently.

Future areas of research inquiry should include the examination of how people create and interact with online personas and how such interaction might translate to real-world behavior change. The creation and use of avatars presents a unique dynamic for exploration regarding the receptivity to health messages. Understanding how participants process health information relevant to the needs of their real-world selves versus the perceived needs of their in-world avatars is crucial. Future research should also include the examination of how our experiences in virtual worlds change with long-term participation.

Finally, virtual systems are becoming more accessible and affordable through gaming platforms and consumer-grade devices. In the near future, it may be possible to send tailored health promotion messages directly to individuals' homes to existing infrastructures of virtual worlds. Sophisticated head-mounted displays are now available for a few hundred dollars and are easily incorporated into everyday computing systems as a plug-and-play device. Moreover, a number of large companies, including Samsung, Facebook, Apple, and Sony, are vying to create the most sophisticated yet affordable head-mounted display for consumers, signaling a virtual revolution in the near future. Similar to the progression of the internet and the mobile revolutions, the virtual revolution is likely to transform traditional patterns of health communication and health promotion campaigns.

References

1. Blascovich J, Bailenson JN. *Infinite Reality—Avatars, Eternal Life, New Worlds, and the Dawn of the Virtual Revolution.* New York, NY: William Morrow; 2011.
2. Ondrejka C. Education unleashed: participatory culture, education, and innovation in Second Life. In: Salen K, ed. *The*

Ecology of Games: Connecting Youth, Games, and Learning. Cambridge, MA: MIT Press; 2008:229-251.
3. Ahn SJ, Fox J, Bailenson JN. Avatars. In: Bainbridge WS, ed. *Leadership in Science and Technology: A Reference Handbook.* Thousand Oaks, CA: Sage; 2011:695-702.
4. Ershow AG, Peterson CM, Riley WT, Rizzo A, Wansink B. Virtual reality technologies for research and education

in obesity and diabetes: research needs and opportunities. *J Diabetes Sci Technol.* 2011;5(2):212-224.

5. Ahn SJ. Incorporating immersive virtual environments in health promotion campaigns: a construal-level theory approach. *Health Commun.* 2015;30(6):545-556.

6. Ahn SJ, Fox J, Hahm JM. Using virtual doppelgängers to increase personal relevance of health risk communication. *Lecture Notes Comp Sci.* 2014;8637:1-12.

7. Trope Y, Liberman N, Wakslak C. Construal levels and psychological distance: effects on representation, prediction, evaluation, and behavior. *J Consum Psychol.* 2007;17:83-95.

8. Ahn SJ, Bailenson JN. Self-endorsing versus other-endorsing in virtual environments: the effect on brand attitude and purchase intention. *J Advertis.* 2011;40(2):93-106.

9. Ahn SJ, Johnsen K, Robertson T, et al. Using virtual pets to promote physical activity in children: an application of the youth physical activity promotion model. *J Health Commun.* 2015;20(7):807-815.

10. Bandura A. *Social Learning Theory.* Englewood Cliffs, NJ: Prentice Hall; 1976.

Appendix 6D

Health Promotion and Social Change Through Storytelling Across Communication Platforms

Hua Wang and Arvind Singhal

▶ The Power of Stories in Health Communication

From time immemorial, stories have played a vital role in entertaining, educating, and engaging human beings. Passed from one generation to another, stories allow human societies to preserve culture, build identity, and instill moral values. In the past several decades, storytelling has proliferated widely—beyond the oral tradition and the printed word—to ride the popularity of mass media channels (such as radio and television) and the modern digital platforms (such as web-streaming services, YouTube, and the like). Accordingly, in the vast expanse of literature on storytelling in the modern mass and social media, an area of scholarship and practice in the field of communication called "entertainment-education" (also known as edutainment) has emerged and gained in prominence.

This edutainment strategy purposely uses a narrative and storytelling-centered approach to promote alternatives to tackle various health problems, for example, promoting exercise and cancer screenings; reducing teenage pregnancy and sexually transmitted diseases; and preventing the spread of cholera, malaria, and Zika. Such narrative efforts work by helping increase the audience's knowledge about critical issues, fostering favorable attitudes, changing overt behaviors, and transforming social norms.[1-3]

Between the 1970s and the early 2000s, edutainment programs were predominantly in the form of radio and television dramatic serials, and were broadcast in countries of Latin America, Asia, and Africa to tackle issues of reproductive health, family planning, HIV/AIDS, and domestic violence.[1,2] Using fictional melodramatic narratives, they educated audiences about contraceptive methods, modeled positive sexual attitudes and behaviors, and improved the reproductive health of millions in developing countries. Over the years, communication platforms used for such efforts have diversified to include live theater, music videos, cartoon/comic books, digital games, and so on.[3,4] However, in more media-saturated environments such as North America and Europe, edutainment initiatives face stiff competition from other commercial entertainment media outlets. In order to earn high audience ratings, sexual and health content on commercial entertainment channels is usually highly explicit, often inaccurate, and devoid of discussion about risks and associated consequences. To overcome these challenges, institutions like Hollywood Health & Society in the United States and the Center for Media and Health in the Netherlands offer consultation to creative writers and producers to accurately portray critical health information in the popular media.[4]

▶ Theories of Narrative Engagement and Persuasion

Edutainment programs are grounded in theories of narrative engagement and persuasion that explain the factors and processes that facilitate changes in the audience's knowledge, attitudes, and behaviors. In contrast to political campaigns, embedding educational messages in entertainment narratives represents a genre of implicit persuasion.[5] Certain elements of narrative-based entertainment help suspend audience disbelief and reduce their resistance to persuasion.[6] They are also grounded in social cognitive theory, an agentic framework of psychosocial change with a dual path of influence: direct exposure to media models and indirect social learning through interpersonal discussions.[7] The transportation-imagery model posits that narratives can be highly immersive, prompting the audience to pay attention, generate mental imagery of a prospective potentiality, and transport them into a world of different time and space.[8,9] In addition, narratives resonate particularly well with the audience when they perceive the stories to be realistic and can identify with the characters based on existing similarities or desirable attributes.[9-11] Further, theories of culture-centric health promotion emphasize that narratives built with familiar cultural markers are especially effective when targeting minority populations.[12]

Recent meta-analyses have demonstrated the advantages of using narratives in health interventions: Narratives have a sizably significant impact on combined changes in attitudes, intention, and behavior, even if they have a relatively small effect size in individual outcomes. Narratives are powerful interventional tools for eliciting affective audience response, and evidence suggests that those delivered through audio and video are more effective than print.[12,13] Moreover, empirical studies show supporting evidence of narrative-based interventions for racial/ethnic minority groups to reduce disparities.[14,15]

▶ Benefits of Storytelling Across Platforms

Telling stories across different communication platforms (also known as transmedia storytelling) is an innovative media programming trend. Instead of telling the story on a single medium, narrative elements are creatively coordinated across different media platforms to build a story world, engage a broader spectrum of audience, and provide them an enriching experience beyond pure entertainment. *The Matrix* is an excellent example where key bits of the overarching storyline were conveyed through the trilogy movies, a series of animated shorts, two comic book story collections, and video game tie-ins.[16] This approach has also been commercially successful with many entertainment franchises such as *Star Wars* and *Pokémon*. Entertainment media producers are increasingly collaborating with nongovernmental organizations (NGOs) and public health professionals to create prosocial programming.

Storytelling across platforms can offer the audience different points of entry into the narrative world, because some people may prefer movies whereas others enjoy games. Each element stands as an independent medium and narrative experience, yet also contributes to the larger picture through the puzzles and clues that encourage people to extend their participation across multiple platforms over time. Therefore, unity and variety are two critical characteristics that enable this approach of storytelling to engage people from all walks of life via their own choice of media and art forms.[17] It is particularly useful for reaching young audiences, who are savvy entertainment consumers and can easily navigate across multiple platforms. They have grown up with similar cross-platform experiences of commercial entertainment as part of their everyday life, so this approach holds promise as a health promotion and education interventional tool.

▶ Cross-Platform Storytelling with a Purpose

East Los High is arguably the first entertainment program intentionally designed to leverage storytelling across platforms to address health and social issues among Latina/o youth in the United States.[18] *East Los High*, a Hulu original series that debuted in June 2013, is a story set in a fictional high school in East Los Angeles, a predominantly Latino area in Los Angeles County with high rates of poverty, low educational attainment, low household income, and an urgent need to promote safe sex and reduce teen pregnancies. Among the main characters are Jacob, a graduating senior and popular football jock; Jessie, an intelligent, attractive junior who secretly admires Jacob, and is a newbie on the school's Bomb Squad dance team; Maya, Jessie's cousin, a troubled runaway, who takes refuge in Jessie's home and would soon become Jacob's heartthrob; Ceci, a lead dancer of the Bomb Squad, who is sexually active, becomes pregnant, and finds her life turned upside-down; and Vanessa, captain of the Bomb Squad, who trades sex for favors and discovers she is HIV positive. The plot simmers further when Jessie, a member of the "virgin club," is forced to disclose her secret as things get hot between her and Jacob; Maya, scarred by a past rape, rebuilds her life through work in a restaurant owned by Jacob's father; Ceci, deserted by her boyfriend after pregnancy, considers abortion but decides to keep her child; Vanessa, jealous and vengeful, orchestrates Jessie's seduction and repents as she copes with HIV.

Not only did these characters subvert the gardener, maid, and gangster stereotypes of Latino/a characters portrayed in the media, Hulu also made an exception that allowed the producers to promote the show's website (eastloshigh.com) at the end of each episode, where viewers were nudged to explore additional content through nine other digital platforms. Viewers, for instance, could access Ceci's vlogs. After being abandoned by her boyfriend, the pregnant Ceci is taken in by a women's shelter where she learns about services available for pregnant teens, including options to give birth and raise the child, give up the child for adoption, or terminate the pregnancy. Viewers could access six of Ceci's vlogs linked to different episodes as the major storyline unfolded in the online drama. In the vlogs, the audience could see Ceci talking about her feelings of being a pregnant teen, the physiological changes in her body, and the socioeconomic and cultural challenges she faced. From there, viewers could visit the *East Los High* resources page, use widgets to find local health clinics, and click on external links for additional information. These additional narrative components were also promoted on popular social networking sites. In four seasons, *East Los High* covered topics such as sexual and reproductive health, domestic violence, lesbian, gay, bisexual, transgender, queer (LGBTQ) identity, and undocumented immigrants, while earning five Emmy nominations (including outstanding new approaches drama series) and numerous accolades such as the Cannes Lions Award.

In addition to the Hulu drama series, *East Los High* provided viewers content through extended scenes, the *Siren* newspaper, Ask Paulie, Ceci's vlogs, Maya's recipes, dance tutorials, La Voz with Xavi, comic strips, and StayTeen public service announcements. It also had a comprehensive resources page with embedded health service widgets.

▶ Program Evaluation Methods

The multifaceted nature of cross-platform storytelling for health promotion requires the use of different research methods to better capture and evaluate the impact of the audience's experience. Our research team adopted analytics tracking to assess audience reach, which monitored web traffic to the *East Los High* website and to NGO partners' websites and widgets; a viewer survey to assess narrative engagement and intended outcomes; and a lab experiment with *East Los High* nonviewers to compare the effect of cross-platform storytelling with other forms of narrative presentation.[17]

Anonymous and unobtrusive tracking data were collected through Google Analytics from May 2013 to January 2014 to capture audience reach during the preprogram publicity and premier of Season 1 and after it ended. Number of visitors, pageviews, average

duration, and geographic location were recorded. Geographic information system software generated spatial-temporal dynamic visualizations of the geographic diffusion of web traffic over time. Two NGO partners (Planned Parenthood and StayTeen.org) independently monitored and shared statistics of their website traffic and health service widgets on the show's website.

An online survey was embedded on the *East Los High* website and promoted on social media with custom incentives. Between August and September 2013, 202 viewers who watched at least 20 of the 24 *East Los High* episodes completed the survey, including 110 Latina females who were 23 years old or younger—the program's primary target audience (**TABLE 6D-1**). Some 55% of those watched the entire series more than once, and 87% consumed the additional content rolled out on the *East Los High* website. They answered closed- and open-ended questions about their impressions of the program; their engagement with its narrative elements; their interpersonal discussions about the show; and their knowledge, attitudes, and behavioral intentions related to sexual and reproductive health. Measures of audience experience were derived from established scales of transportation, identification, and narrative engagement (**TABLE 6D-2**); health-related outcome measures were adapted from the 2013 Centers for Disease Control and Prevention's Youth Risk Behavior Survey.

A two (nondramatic vs. dramatic narratives) by three (text vs. multimedia vs. cross-platform) partial factorial design was used in a lab experiment from June to August 2014 at the University of Texas at El Paso to test the effect of different storytelling formats on *East Los High*'s target audience. It included 136 Latinas age 18–28 with sufficient English proficiency who had not seen *East Los High* or similar programs such as *Degrassi* and *16 & Pregnant*. They were randomly assigned to one of the following five conditions.

- Condition 1 ($n = 30$) was a true control group without any intervention.
- Condition 2 ($n = 21$) was a nondramatic text version of *East Los High* presented as a newspaper story.
- Condition 3 ($n = 21$) was a dramatic text version, presented as an *East Los High* script.
- Condition 4 ($n = 32$) was an online drama, presented as an abbreviated version of the *East Los High* Hulu original series.
- Condition 5 ($n = 32$) was a cross-platform version, presented as an online drama along with selected elements extended across different communication platforms.

TABLE 6D-1 Characteristics of *East Los High* Viewer Survey Participants, United States, 2013

Characteristics	Yes Responses (%)	
	Total Sample (*n* = 202)	Primary Target* (*n* = 110)
Sex		
Female	91	100
Ethnicity		
Hispanic/Latino	78	100
Age		
12–17	25	35
18–23	50	66
24–30	15	0
31–60	10	0
Education		
Elementary school	1	2
Middle school	10	11
High school	64	72
Bachelor's degree	20	12
Master's and beyon	5	0
Household Annual Income		
< $20,000	39	43
$20,000–$49,999	35	43
$50,000–$79,999	19	7
≥ $80,000	7	0
Pregnant Teen Connection		
Self	9	5
Mother	21	22
Aunt	15	19
Sister	14	12
Cousin	41	48
Niece	4	2
Friend	68	76
Acquaintance	35	34

*The primary target audience of *East Los High* was Latina teenage girls and young women because they are critical to the issues of safe sex and teen pregnancy and are also avid consumers of dramas and online video streaming.

Reproduced from Wang H, Singhal A. *East Los High*: transmedia edutainment to promote the sexual and reproductive health of young Latina/o Americans. *Am J Public Health*. June 2016;106(6): 1002-1010. Reprinted with permission of the publisher, The American Public Health Association.

TABLE 6D-2 *East Los High* Audience Narrative Engagement, United States, 2013

Item	Total Mean (SD)	Target Mean (SD)
Audience Program Rating[a]		
1. Storyline appeal	4.68 (0.79)	4.61 (0.83)
2. Enjoyment of Hulu drama series	4.88 (0.45)	4.93 (0.26)
3. Enjoyment of transmedia extensions	4.56 (0.86)	4.58 (0.83)
4. Production quality	4.74 (0.53)	4.73 (0.55)
5. Wanting more	4.96 (0.23)	4.97 (0.17)
Audience Narrative Engagement[b]		
1. Attention focus	1.34 (0.50)	1.35 (0.49)
2. Narrative understanding	1.37 (0.56)	1.31 (0.49)
3. Narrative presence	1.51 (0.67)	1.49 (0.68)
4. Perceived realism	1.35 (0.51)	1.30 (0.48)
5. Cognitive processing	1.42 (0.62)	1.42 (0.62)
6. Emotional engagement	1.44 (0.62)	1.46 (0.67)
Audience Character Identification[c]		
1. Feel like you know...		
▪ Jacob	1.43 (0.70)	1.40 (0.70)
▪ Jessie	1.57 (0.82)	1.48 (0.77)
▪ Maya	1.45 (0.81)	1.53 (0.88)
▪ Ceci	1.72 (0.94)	1.70 (1.04)
▪ Vanessa	1.91 (1.05)	1.91 (1.12)
▪ Abe (Ceci's abusive boyfriend)	3.14 (1.34)	3.19 (1.42)
▪ Freddie (Vanessa trades sex for favor)	3.24 (1.33)	3.13 (1.31)
▪ Ramon (Maya's rapist)	3.09 (1.30)	2.98 (1.25)
2. You like...		
▪ Jacob	1.31 (0.70)	1.22 (0.62)
▪ Jessie	2.28 (1.40)	2.21 (1.44)

(continues)

TABLE 6D-2 *East Los High* Audience Narrative Engagement, United States, 2013 *(continued)*

Item	Total Mean (SD)	Target Mean (SD)
■ Maya	1.51 (0.99)	1.52 (1.00)
■ Ceci	1.55 (0.76)	1.51 (0.72)
■ Vanessa	2.73 (1.50)	2.62 (1.50)
■ Abe (Ceci's abusive boyfriend)	3.72 (1.43)	3.55 (1.51)
■ Freddie (Vanessa trades sex for favor)	3.40 (1.46)	3.25 (1.47)
■ Ramon (Maya's rapist)	3.76 (1.40)	3.63 (1.45)

[a] 1=poor; 5=excellent.

[b] Items are based on Green and Brock (2000) and Russelle and Bilandzic (2009). 1=strongly agree; 5=strongly disagree.

[c] Items are based on Moyer-Gusé E. Toward a theory of entertainment persuasion: explaining the persuasive effects of entertainment-education messages. *Commun Theory.* 2008;18:407-425; Murphy ST, Frank LB, Chatterjee JS, et al. Comparing the relative efficacy of narrative vs nonnarrative health messages in reducing health disparities using a randomized trial. *Am J Public Health.* 2015;105(10):2117-2123.

Reproduced from Wang H, Singhal A. *East Los High*: transmedia edutainment to promote the sexual and reproductive health of young Latina/o Americans. *Am J Public Health.* June 2016;106(6): 1002-1010. Reprinted with permission of the publisher, The American Public Health Association.

The content was carefully selected according to the program's objectives, and the messages were identical across all conditions. **FIGURE 6D-1** shows that repeated measures of narrative engagement, knowledge (correct condom use, birth control pills, emergency contraception), attitudes (sex education, women's rights to choose, HIV/STD testing, importance of sex communication), and behavior (protection during last sex intercourse, sex communication) occurred at baseline, posttest, and 2-week follow-up.

▶ Lessons Learned from *East Los High*

Viewership and web traffic to the *East Los High* website suggested that the audience responded to the show with great enthusiasm. In addition to the millions of viewers who watched *East Los High* on Hulu, hundreds of thousands visited the *East Los High* website to access full episodes, extended content across platforms, and additional resources. Tens of thousands of visits occurred even after Season 1 ended. The trend over 9 months indicated that viewers were spending more time on the *East Los High* website, and almost half returned for multiple visits, showing the potential of transmedia

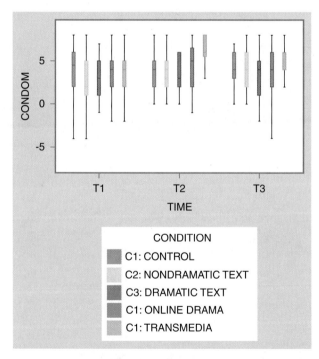

FIGURE 6D-1 Clustered boxplots of knowledge about correct condom use over time by condition, El Paso, Texas, 2014.

Note: CONDOM is the sum of 8 items about correct condom use, with each correct answer coded as 1 and each incorrect answer coded as -1. The boxplots show the distributions of CONDOM knowledge scores for the 3 different time periods across all 5 conditions. Each box represents the interquartile range; the whiskers at the top and bottom of the box indicate the upper and lower quartile; and the middle line in each box represents the median. Descriptive U3 effect size statistics60 indicated that at T2, 94% of participants in C5 had higher scores than those in C4, and 97% of participants in C5 had higher scores than those in C3, C2, and C1; at T3, 69% of participants in C5 had higher scores than those in C2, and 91% of participants in C5 had higher scores than those in C4, C3, and C1.

Reproduced from Wang H, Singhal A. *East Los High:* transmedia edutainment to promote the sexual and reproductive health of young Latina/o Americans. *Am J Public Health.* June 2016;106(6):1002-1010. Reprinted with permission of the publisher, The American Public Health Association.

edutainment for creating a sustainable platform for large-scale, longer-term audience engagement. Moreover, the *East Los High* website served as a portal that drove viewers to additional health and social services via embedded widgets and referral to NGO partners' websites. These tight connections between the intervention exposures and an infrastructure for follow-up actions (e.g., personalized health information seeking) can greatly enhance the enabling environment for behavior change. Further, *East Los High* was widely popular across the United States and around the world, reaching geographic areas with the highest Latino populations, teen pregnancy rates, and poverty rates. This suggests that culturally sensitive interventions can help address, and even reduce, disparities in minority groups.

The viewer survey offered a snapshot from 202 *East Los High* fans, who were predominantly young Latina females with low socioeconomic status, and hence at risk for teen pregnancy. Their high ratings of the program and their fervent desire for more such programs suggest that the transmedia edutainment approach was effectively implemented in the program. Viewers consistently demonstrated high levels of narrative engagement, carefully attended to the show, understood the nuances of characters and their stories, felt immersed in the story world, related content to their real-life experiences, actively reflected on the plotlines, and were emotionally engaged. Further, among the target audience group of Latina females, *East Los High* spurred interpersonal discussions. They talked to their friends, siblings, parents, and relatives about the show face-to-face and also via social media, text messages and phone calls. They reported a high level of awareness of various health services for testing and assistance to pregnant teens, but somewhat lower levels of actual testing behavior or knowledge about where to seek help. After watching *East Los High*, they indicated learning new information (correct condom use, birth control pills, and emergency contraception), displayed higher levels of behavioral intentions (using and recommending testing and pregnancy services), and appreciation for the comprehensive resources on the *East Los High* website. Overall, the survey results suggested that *East Los High* resonated well with its target audience—they perceived the program to be compelling, educational, and transformative. Their enthusiasm suggests that narrative-based transmedia edutainment interventions like *East Los High*

can cultivate a fan base for deeper learning, lasting engagement, and broader social change.

The lab experiment added evidence of the *East Los High* effects on 136 nonviewers who fit the characteristics of its target audience and were randomly assigned to one of the five conditions: C1/control group, C2/nondramatic text, C3/dramatic text, C4/online drama, and C5/cross-platform. Although the messages embedded in the stimuli were identical, the results varied. There were encouraging positive trends over time and tendencies showing advantages of cross-platform storytelling; however, most were not statistically significant, which warrants future investigation. However, one revealing result was regarding the knowledge of correct condom use, where transmedia yielded significantly better outcomes than other conditions over time. This may have benefited from the extended scene of Maya's conversation with a health counselor about condom use that was one of the selected transmedia extensions in C5. This suggests that even though the message of promoting condom use for safe sex and preventing sexually transmitted infections and unplanned pregnancies is the same across all experimental conditions, using transmedia to highlight critical and accurate information as incorporated in the dialogue with a main character can give the intervention a turbocharged boost. Among the nonviewers, 30% reported searching for information and discussing *East Los High* after their participation in the experiment, although few watched full episodes or started following *East Los High* on social media. It suggested that the self-selection among *East Los High* fans can make a difference in how they interact with the content, and future interventions should be mindful about the match between the edutainment themes and presentation styles with the characteristics, motivations, interests, and media habits of potential target audience.

In conclusion, entertainment-education programs, especially those that employ transmedia storytelling across multiple platforms, offer an adaptive and versatile approach to reaching target audiences as well as providing a broad reach, deep engagement, and more positive and sustainable outcomes. *East Los High* is exemplary in that it is rewriting what is programmatically possible in the media landscape in the 21st century.[17]

The text in this appendix is largely based on the original research article Wang H, Singhal A. *East Los High*: transmedia edutainment to promote the sexual and reproductive health of young Latina/o Americans. *Am J Public Health*. June 2016;106(6):1002-1010.

References

1. Singhal A, Rogers EM. *Entertainment-Education: A Communication Strategy for Social Change.* New York, NY: Routledge; 1999.

2. Singhal A, Cody MJ, Rogers EM, Sabido M, eds. *Entertainment-Education and Social Change: History, Research, and Practice.* New York, NY: Routledge; 2004.

3. Wang H, Singhal A. Entertainment-education through digital games. In: Ritterfeld R, Cody MJ, Vorderer P, eds. *Serious Games: Mechanism and Effects.* New York, NY: Routledge; 2009:271-292.

4. Singhal A, Wang H, Rogers EM. The entertainment-education communication strategy in communication campaigns. In: Rice RE, Atkins C, eds. *Public Communication Campaigns.* 4th ed. Beverly Hills, CA: Sage; 2013:321-334.

5. Slater MD, Rouner D. Entertainment-education and elaboration likelihood: understanding the processing of narrative persuasion. *Commun Theory.* 2002;12:173-191.

6. Moyer-Gusé E. Toward a theory of entertainment persuasion: explaining the persuasive effects of entertainment-education messages. *Commun Theory.* 2008;18:407-425.

7. Bandura A. Social cognitive theory for personal and social change by enabling media. In: Singhal A, Cody MJ, Rogers EM, Sabido M, eds. *Entertainment-Education and Social Change: History, Research, and Practice.* Mahwah, NJ: Erlbaum; 2004:75-96.

8. Green MC, Brock TC. The role of transportation in the persuasiveness of public narratives. *J Pers Soc Psychol.* 2000;79:701-721.

9. Murphy ST, Frank LB, Moran MB, Patnoe-Woodley P. Involved, transported, or emotional? Exploring the determinants of change in knowledge, attitudes, and behavior in entertainment-education. *J Commun.* 2011;61:407-431.

10. Busselle R, Bilandzic H. Measuring narrative engagement. *Media Psychol.* 2009;12:321-347.

11. Shen F, Sheer VC, Li R. Impact of narratives on persuasion in health communication: a meta-analysis. *J Advertising.* 2015;44(2):105-113.

12. Lee H, Fawcett J, DeMarco R. Storytelling/narrative theory to address health communication with minority population. *Appl Nurs Res.* 2015;30:58-60. doi:10.1016/j.apnr.2015.09.004.

13. van Laer T, de Ruyter K, Visconti LM, Wetzels M. The extended transportation-imagery model: a meta-analysis of the antecedents and consequences of consumers' narrative transportation. *J Consum Res.* 2014;40:797-817.

14. Zebregs S, van den Putte B, Neijens P, de Graaf A. The differential impact of statistical and narrative evidence on beliefs, attitude, and intention: a meta-analysis. *Health Commun.* 2015;30:282-289.

15. Houston TK, Allison JJ, Sussman M, et al. Culturally appropriate storytelling to improve blood pressure: a randomized trial. *Ann Intern Med.* 2011;154:77-84.

16. Murphy ST, Frank LB, Chatterjee JS, et al. Comparing the relative efficacy of narrative vs nonnarrative health messages in reducing health disparities using a randomized trial [published online ahead of print April 23, 2015]. *Am J Public Health.* doi:10.2105/AJPH.2014.302332.

17. Jenkins H. *Convergence Culture: Where Old & New Media Collide.* New York, NY: New York University Press; 2006.

18. Wang H, Singhal A. *East Los High:* transmedia edutainment to promote the sexual and reproductive health of young Latina/o Americans. *Am J Public Health.* June 2016;106(6):1002-1010.

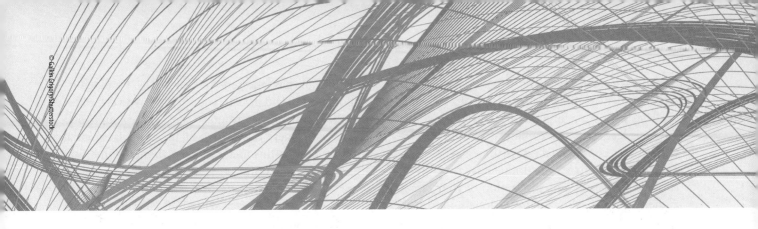

CHAPTER 7

Planning Health Communication Interventions

Sarah Bauerle Bass and Claudia Parvanta

LEARNING OBJECTIVES

By the end of this chapter, the reader will be able to:

- Weigh the pros and cons of forming partnerships to plan interventions.
- Describe components in a health communication plan.
- Use the PRECEDE-PROCEED model to research audience behavior.
- Identify useful sources of primary and secondary research.
- Describe the scope of formative research.
- Describe key qualitative and quantitative methods used in formative research.
- Prepare a creative brief to inform message and media development.
- Prepare a strategy to guide communication channel selection.

▶ Introduction: Form, Storm, Norm, or Inform?

Now that you know how to develop messages and what media you can use to deliver them, the next piece of the health communication puzzle is to develop the programs in which those messages will be delivered. No matter the mix of communication channels, the key to effective interventions is the involvement of the target community. If you let them know that you are listening to them and understand what they need, they will be more receptive to your messages. We will discuss how to involve stakeholders, how to plan a health communication intervention, and how to pretest it with formative research methods to ensure that it meets the needs of your audience.

The Role of Stakeholders

As the name implies, **stakeholders** have something "at stake" (their lives, health, reputation, funding, etc.) that depends on the success of a project. (You may imagine campers holding tent stakes in place or contributors to a political campaign.) Stakeholders in a health communication intervention might include, among others:

- **Primary audience**: The target audience for behavioral change; the people you are hoping to influence with your intervention.

- **Secondary audience**: The gatekeepers to your target audience—they control access to communicating with your target audience (e.g., parents, religious leaders, block captains, community service groups, commercial establishments).
- **Tertiary audience**: The influencers who have earned the respect and admiration of your target audience (e.g., healthcare professionals, local personalities such as local news anchors, respected politicians, other opinion leaders, national figures such as health authorities or celebrities), if they have a reason to be concerned.

Although these people are all important to the intervention development process, it is also important to think about them as actual "players" in your intervention. This means that they not only passively provide input on the intervention but also are actively involved in its development and implementation. This can be difficult to achieve, but program planning using this model is inherently more sustainable.[1] Stakeholder-led interventions tend to work best when the group has been functioning for some time in various partnership roles, so that much of the initial "forming, storming, and norming" has taken place and the group can "perform" at its peak. **FIGURE 7-1** shows the well-known team development model first proposed by Tuckman in 1965.

How do you get from having the idea that you want to do a health communication project to forming a team, or coalition, to put it in place? You should strive to find partners who share your vision, have experience in the community or with an approach, and possess skills that complement your own. If you or your organization has assessed your strengths, weaknesses, opportunities, and threats, you should have a clear idea of your comparative advantage (i.e., where your group shines) and where you need to fill in gaps. It is essential to be honest in this analysis, even though some find this assessment painful.

Having defined your own strengths and weaknesses, you would be well served in selecting partners who have knowledge, skills, resources, or connections to a target audience that you lack. You can choose partners who are in the same field as you or your organization, but also look outside your domain to others that serve the same constituencies, including the private sector, as potential partners. In addition, keeping opportunities and threats in mind, if you are aware of an organization planning something that pertains to your issue, begin by offering to help them with their project first. To paraphrase Ralph Waldo Emerson, the best way to have friends (in health communication) is to be one.

BOX 7-1 lists the numerous benefits as well as some barriers to consider before involving others in your project.

Why Do This Now?

There are good reasons to gather your stakeholders together *before* conducting your initial planning:

- Your partners may have already collected some of this information and would be willing to share it for a common cause.
- They may be able to facilitate recruiting participants for focus groups and other formative research tasks.

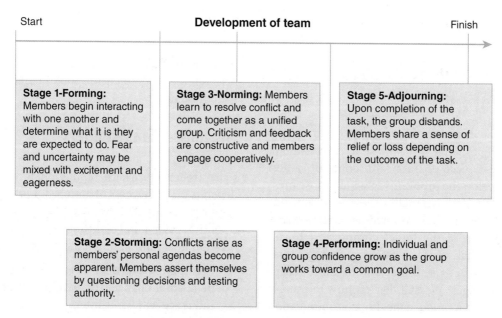

FIGURE 7-1 Stages of team or group development: the Tuckman model.

Data from Tuckman BW. Developmental sequence in small groups. *Psychological Bulletin*. 1965;63(6):384-399; Tuckman BW, Jensen MA. Stages in small group development revisited. *Group and Organisation Studies*. 1977;2:419-427.

BOX 7-1 The Pros and Cons of Health Communication Partnerships

There are several possible benefits to working with partners on health communication programs. Coalitions with multiple partners can be helpful in one or more of the following ways:

- Coalitions bring diverse representation, not just racial/ethnic diversity, but political, professional (e.g., providers, patients), and skill diversity.
- Diverse organizations that partner to achieve a common goal often go beyond their organizations' individual contributions.
- Help sustain programs by expanding public support.
- Provide organizations and individuals the opportunity to have a voice in community and statewide issues and participate in the strategic planning.
- Lead policy change efforts and campaigns when other partners may be limited. Coalitions also can enlist political and constituent support.
- Help change community values through systems change by eliminating influences and heightening pro-health influences.
- Establish greater credibility because they represent several organizations and individuals focused on community betterment.
- Amplify state resources by involving broad community representation, mobilizing members' talents, and engaging the community to develop public support. Through collaboration, resources can also be conserved by minimizing duplication of efforts and services.

Consider the following potential problems when deciding if a partnership model is the best way to accomplish your goal. For a successful coalition, partners need to:

- Identify stakeholders.
- Define the community capacity for a coalition and identify potential barriers.
- Recruit members – include substantive representation from all identified stakeholders; community representation is KEY.
- Formalize rules, roles, procedures, and responsibility (e.g., bylaws, standard operating procedures, goals and objectives, memoranda of understanding).
- Set priorities based on results of needs assessment and funding.
- Select appropriate strategies to achieve coalition goals.
- Raise community awareness of coalition and problem.

To maintain:

- Coalitions must provide benefits (e.g., solidarity, appreciation, evidence of impact) that exceed costs (e.g., time, frustration) to sustain membership and momentum.
- Assign tasks based on skills and available resources.
- Define action steps that are broad enough to address funders' goals and the goals of the coalition.

You also will need to handle the difficulties that occur when groups work together. Some of these obstacles can be:

- Competition for resources.
- Lack of leadership and a clear sense of direction.
- Domination by one organization or individual.
- Inadequate participation by important groups.
- Unrealistic expectations about partners' roles, responsibilities, or required time commitments.
- Disagreements among partners regarding values, vision, goals, or actions.
- Inability or unwillingness to negotiate or compromise on important issues.

Modified from Centers for Disease Control and Prevention. Coalitions - State and Community Interventions: User Guide. CDC website. https://ftp.cdc.gov/pub/fda/fda/user_guide.pdf. Published 2007.

- They may be able to share some of the costs, particularly through in-kind donations of time, effort, or meeting space.
- If everyone shares in the formative research, they are more invested in the results and seeing them translated into an effective program.

The primary reason to *not* engage stakeholders early in planning is if you believe the target audience or communication goals are likely to change based on data that you do not yet have. In that case, it makes more sense to gather the data first and then move on to partner identification.

The rest of this chapter is written from the perspective that you have obtained partners (or decided to go without) and that you are ready to move forward with planning a health communication intervention.

▶ The Planning Cycle

The health communication phases of planning, implementation, and evaluation are often depicted as a wheel to emphasize the cyclical nature of data collection and program improvement. The National Cancer Institute[2] uses the model shown in FIGURE 7-2 as a bird's-eye view of all the phases and steps in mounting a communication intervention.

FIGURE 7-3 breaks these large phases down into smaller steps, stemming from a core of dedicated tasks. These steps can be considered in five groups:

■ Steps 1 to 3 form your **macro plan**, which includes analysis of the problem, the ecological setting, the core intervention strategy, and the affected populations.

• This stage of planning normally occurs after data demonstrate the presence of a problem affecting specific groups of people. If there is evidence that a specific intervention has worked to reduce this problem elsewhere,

feasibility testing might be conducted to adapt the intervention to the new population. The less we know about the problem, potential solution, or intended audience, the more formative research must be done before taking the next planning steps.

■ Steps 4 to 6 form the **strategic health communication plan**, which focuses on specific change objectives, audiences, messages, and media.

• Concepts, messages, materials, and media strategies are tested at this stage of planning. This "pretesting" is sometimes referred to as formative research, and at times it is considered "process" research. It should precede finalization of the implementation plan that comes next.

■ Steps 7 and 8 go into the **implementation (or tactical) plan**, which says what will be done, when, where, how, with what money, and who is responsible for every piece.

• Process research is often conducted shortly after the launch of a program to make sure

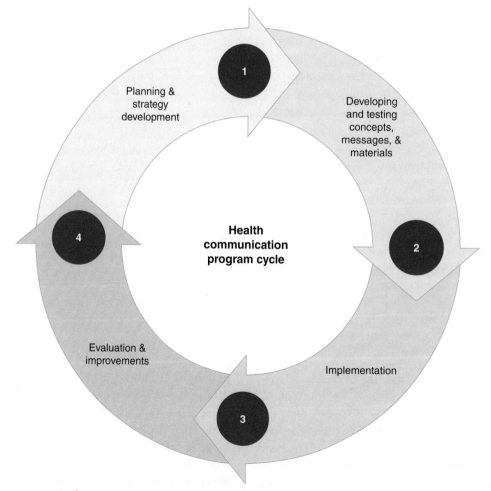

FIGURE 7-2 National Cancer Institute health communication planning cycle.

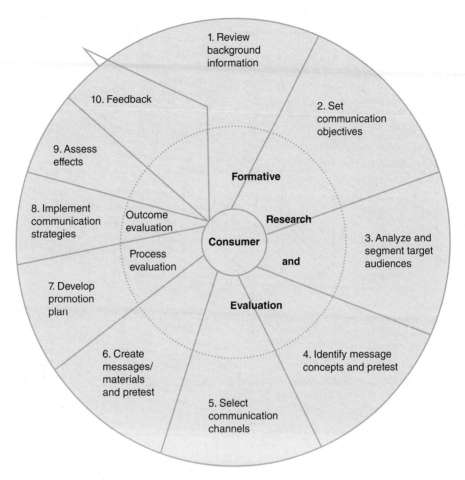

FIGURE 7-3 Health communication planning steps.

Reproduced from Roper WL. Health communication takes on new dimensions at CDC. *Public Health Rep*. 1993;108(2):179-183. Association of Schools of Public Health, SAGE Publications Inc. Journals, Superintendent of Documents, US Government Printing Office.

all operations are running smoothly and that messages are getting out and being interpreted as planned. Corrections can be made if this assessment is done early enough.

■ Step 9 makes use of an **evaluation plan**, which says what aspects of the intervention will be monitored or evaluated to determine the intervention's worth to key stakeholders. Most programs want to achieve *measurable* objectives, so baseline data often need to be collected before a program is launched. Evaluation planning must begin in the first days of program development.

■ In Step 10 you might want to form **continuation (or expansion) plans** to ensure a broader reach, diffuse expenses, and provide continuity of leadership and ownership. You might make plans for dissemination and publication, or you might look for ways to terminate your activities.

The basic steps in this sequence hold true whether you are planning a small-scale communication program, such as a campus or hospital-wide flu awareness program, or a national initiative, such as the Centers for Disease Control and Prevention's (CDC's) TIPS anti-smoking campaign.

▶ Planning Models

Many organizations involved in developing community-based programs, including health communication programs, make use of the **PRECEDE-PROCEED model** developed by Green and Kreuter.[3,4] The model works backward from a desired state of health and asks what environment, genetics, behavior, individual motivation, or administrative policy is necessary to create the healthy state. It assesses the multiple factors that shape health status and allows the planner to focus on those factors that are best targeted for intervention. **FIGURE 7-4** illustrates the model.

As the name implies, PRECEDE-PROCEED lays out an assessment phase and an implementation phase. In the assessment phase, the model asks the planner to conduct a *social* assessment, such as understanding a group's quality of life by assessing not only objective data, but also subjective data collected by working with the community to identify problems and priorities. Next is the *epidemiologic* assessment, where the planner must understand the extent of the health issue in the group, and then assess the genetics, behaviors, and possible environmental causes of the health issue.

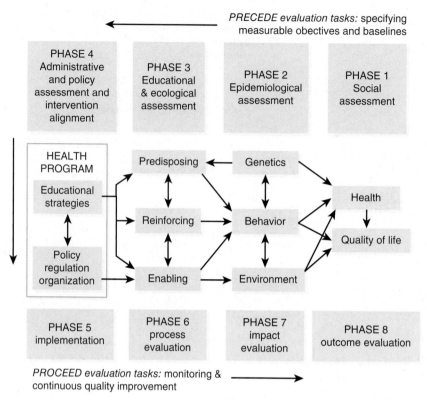

FIGURE 7-4 PRECEDE-PROCEED model.

Once the background assessment is complete, the planner can think about the predisposing, reinforcing, and enabling factors associated with the health issue. This is called the *educational and ecological* assessment. Predisposing factors are those that exist within the individuals, such as their knowledge, attitudes, beliefs, and life experiences, that might influence behavior. Reinforcing factors are those that are outside of the individual, usually in a peer group or interpersonal sphere, that may provide rewards or punishments for a behavior. This often takes the form of peer pressure or influences, social support (or lack thereof), and the vicarious reinforcement someone may receive to continue a behavior. Finally, enabling factors are those that may allow the behavior to occur at a community or societal level; often these can be societal beliefs or norms, or environmental or public policy.

The last step of PRECEDE aligns the results from the educational assessment with what might be required on a policy or programmatic level to move into implementation. **BOX 7-2** provides an example of how this could work.

PRECEDE-PROCEED is thus a general planning model that can be very helpful in developing communication interventions. What it doesn't do, however, is help you decide what exactly those messages are and whether they will actually work in your community. For that, you need to conduct formative research.

▶ Formative Research

Formative research refers to the information-gathering activities you conduct prior to developing a health communication strategy. The **BEHAVE framework**[5] provides four simple questions to be answered:

- Who are you trying to reach?
- What do you want them to do?
- What factors influence their behavior?
- Which actions will most effectively address these factors?

BEHAVE (which is not an acronym) presents these questions in the form of a statement:

> To persuade a specific target audience to perform a specific behavior, we will focus on an important benefit (something the target audience values). Our approach will address specific issues (e.g., self-efficacy, lowered barriers, enhanced health literacy) and use specific means of reaching the audience (media channels or other contact opportunities).

If you cannot answer these questions, then you must do formative research. You may be able to lay the groundwork with published literature and/or data from reliable sources, such as government agencies. More likely, you will need to conduct your own

BOX 7-2 Example of an Educational Assessment Using PRECEDE

After doing a social and epidemiologic assessment of a township in your state, you've identified that a greater number of teens start smoking before the age of 18 compared to the national or state average. You know this is important because an epidemiologic assessment shows that negative health outcomes due to smoking are higher in this area (e.g., lung cancer rates, chronic obstructive pulmonary disease), and you know that the earlier a person starts smoking, the more likely they are to continue to smoke, which leads to these negative outcomes. You also know from your social assessment that gatekeepers in the community have identified teen smoking as a significant health issue and that an intervention to address teen smoking should be implemented in the community. Based on this health issue, you work on why this is occurring by doing an educational and ecological assessment. Based on your research with teens in the township, these are the factors you've found to influence the behavior:

- *Predisposing:* (1) Teens in the township don't believe they are addicted to nicotine and believe they can stop smoking any time; (2) they don't believe that they will have negative health effects because all the ads they see about smoking and why you should stop are of "old" people; and (3) they are afraid that if they don't smoke they won't be considered "cool."
- *Reinforcing:* (1) The majority of teens in the township smoke, and peer pressure to smoke is high; (2) teens fear they will be socially ostracized if they don't smoke; and (3) many of the teens have siblings and parents who smoke, making it difficult to not be like the rest of the family.
- *Enabling:* (1) It's easy to buy cigarettes at local convenience stores, where the teens are not frequently asked for identification; (2) cigarettes are relatively cheap and easily accessible; and (3) the local high school allows students to smoke in a designated space.

Based on this assessment, you know that your communication intervention should address these factors. For example, you could have a social media campaign that addresses some of the personal beliefs of the teens, as well as the concept that "everybody does it." Perhaps you also could have health education activities at the school with key, respected students to change the beliefs about smoking and its "rewards," and train them as peer educators to do communication activities in the school. And perhaps you could have a poster campaign aimed at local convenience stores that reminds them of penalties for selling tobacco to underage students and for parents to raise awareness about the issue. Though changes to policy are not really in the purview of most health communication interventions, you could develop materials aimed at the school district leadership, do community forums discussing how to address convenience stores' lax ID checks, or have ads in the local paper addressing these findings.

qualitative or quantitative research with the target audience to get the information needed to create a communication strategy. Representatives of the target audience must guide concepts, messages, and materials as well as choice of media channels to give your intervention the best chance of success. Formative research is done to *develop* an intervention. Often it includes three different activities:

1. Using quantitative and qualitative methods to develop intervention/message concepts, devise an audience segmentation strategy, and research appropriate communication channels.
2. Testing your concepts/messages with your audience(s).
3. Pretesting your initial materials with your intended users. In the case of mHealth or other types of interactive media, user testing may also be conducted to assess whether the mechanics of the tool are easy to use and accessible to your audience.

The main point in formative research is that your audience is integrally involved in the development process. When proactively involved, you ensure that you are creating health communication that is acceptable to your audience and addresses their risk perception, barriers, and other factors that may impede them from healthy behavior.

Quantitative and Qualitative Methods

To address the first step—developing the messages and understanding who is your audience—you can collect both **primary data** and **secondary data**. Primary data are data you collect yourself, through methods such as surveys, interviews, focus groups, or observation. Secondary data are data you get from existing sources, such as the local health department, the CDC, the National Center for Health Statistics, or a local hospital. This data collection can use both qualitative and quantitative methods. For example, if you want to know how many children are obese, you will need *quantitative* epidemiologic data (secondary data); if you want to know the eating behaviors of children in the intended audience, you might conduct a *qualitative* observation (primary data).

When collecting quantitative secondary data, look for publicly available sources that have data on health behaviors, attitudes, and beliefs. These include the following:

- *Behavioral Risk Factor Surveillance System (BRFSS) and Youth Risk Behavior Surveillance System (YRBSS):* Managed by the CDC, these two large-scale surveillance systems use different methodologies to gather data on behaviors related to disease control and prevention. The BRFSS is a phone-based survey used since 1984. It completes more than 400,000 adult interviews annually, making it the largest continuously conducted health survey system in the world. The YRBSS surveys 9th- to 12th-grade students in public and private schools in the United States. Students fill in machine-readable answer sheets while in class. The YRBSS sampling frame is complex. Although neither of these surveys focuses primarily on health communication, each contains numerous items relevant to messaging and media options. See http://www.cdc.gov/brfss/ for the BRFSS and http://www.cdc.gov/healthyyouth/data/yrbs/index.htm for the YRBSS.

- *Health Information National Trends Survey (HINTS):* In 2015–2016, HINTS completed its fifth cycle of data collection and public release. Although focused primarily on attitudes and behaviors across the cancer continuum, HINTS asks numerous questions of a broad nature, such as health information seeking, the impact of media on decision making, patient–provider communication, and more. These data are available to researchers to analyze changes in how adults use different communication channels to access and use health information for themselves and their loved ones; obtain information about how cancer risks are perceived; and create more effective health communication strategies across different populations. HINTS is managed by the National Cancer Institute; go to http://hints.cancer.gov for more information about HINTS.

Basic quantitative data collection can also be done to understand the unique needs of your target audience. Surveys are the most common type of quantitative primary data that are collected. They can be done in-person, through the mail, or electronically by email or as a URL link. Although it is easy to use online survey sites such as SurveyMonkey to develop, disseminate, and analyze surveys, it is harder to ask the right questions, get the right people to respond, and obtain enough data to support a decision. Although 89% of Americans are now using the internet, as the Pew Research Center says, "...89% is not 100%, and surveys that include only those who use the internet (and are willing to take surveys online) run the risk of producing biased results."[6] Online surveys are also self-administered, in contrast to respondents replying to a live interviewer. This poses a few challenges, particularly for those who may have lower literacy levels, limited English proficiency, or visual impairments. However, self-administered surveys also have a lower chance of creating "social desirability bias," in which respondents feel the need to present themselves, their neighborhoods, or their peers in a positive light to a live interviewer, which may be an issue if you are asking questions in-person.

Another interesting application of the standard survey is a commercial marketing technique called perceptual mapping. This technique relies on survey data in which participants respond to questions using a Likert-type scale. In the perceptual mapping example in **BOX 7-3**, a 0- to 10-point scale is used for respondents to associate one item with another. Box 7-3 provides an example of using the technique in health communication at the Temple University Risk Communication Lab, which the lead author directs. Based on multidimensional scaling, these methods yield a graphic, three-dimensional, multicolored display of how respondents perceive the relationships among a set of elements.[7] This allows the researchers to study how framing effects, perceptions of risks/benefits, attitudes toward risk, or other factors contribute to cognitive and affective dimensions of decision making. The resulting maps reflect how the decision elements are conceptualized relative to each other and relative to "Self," a group average. These maps can then be used to develop very targeted message strategies through a technique called vector message modeling.

You may also use qualitative methods to understand how best to select audience segments and communication channels. For example, focus groups with children or interviews with key informants (such as parents) from your target audience—primary data—can help you decide if different messages and different channels are needed for different groups. Here is a list of some of the most common qualitative methods used in formative research:

- *In-depth interviews:* In-depth interviews are sometimes used to discuss highly personal topics, usually at a stage of research where the program does not yet feel sufficiently informed to use a group format. The in-depth interview requires the interviewer to create a comfortable, nonjudgmental relationship with the person being interviewed. The researcher may use a topic guide or work

BOX 7-3 Perceptual Mapping Example

Perceptual mapping techniques have a solid history as mathematical modeling tools.[a] In some disciplines (e.g., geography), the term *cognitive mapping* is used to describe the maps of geographic areas that people carry in their heads.[b,c] *Perceptual mapping* is the term used in psychology, marketing, sociology, and political science when using multidimensional scaling to model fundamental social–psychological processes. The more user-friendly versions of software for these mapping techniques have evolved since the 1970s and have been used in a variety of commercial and educational contexts,[d,e] but have not been used extensively in health and risk communication except by researchers at the Risk Communication Laboratory.[f-h] Our approach is based on the perceptual mapping methods and influence strategies initially set forth by Joseph Woelfel and Edward L. Fink[i] in the combined theory and methodology they term *Galileo*. Our computer software program converts the scaled judgments into distances and assembles the map elements into a structural whole. Input associations among the risks/benefits are derived from the interitem correlations of all elements, where the absolute values of the correlations are converted to a 0 to 10 scale base.

The software then performs a metric multidimensional scaling analysis and produces graphic arrays of the distances among the elements. The graphic plots can be displayed in two or three dimensions for visual interpretation (see **FIGURE 7-5**). The percentage of variance accounted for by each model is provided as an index of the explanatory power of the map. The resulting maps thus display the risk/benefit elements relative to each other and to "Self." Essentially, the maps provide a snapshot of the respondents' conceptualization of the situation and reveal the relative importance of different decision elements. For example, Figure 7-5 depicts how hepatitis C–positive methadone patients perceive treatment initiation.

Once perceptual maps are developed, vector analytic procedures are applied to determine a message strategy. To optimally position the target concept in the perceptual space, target vectors (dotted lines in Figure 7-5) are used to start the mathematical vector resolution process. By specifying the target vector and the number of concepts to be used in the final message, the software creates all possible vector resolutions, using the specified number of concepts, and then rank orders the solutions for best fit to the target vector. The vectors identify optimum message associations for moving respondents (the aggregated "Self") within the model. These message strategies involve the dynamics of "pulling" concepts closer together by emphasizing their association or "pushing" concepts farther apart by emphasizing their differences. The final form of the message (content, wording, imagery, and format) is then constructed to include and illustrate the concepts identified as optimal for addressing the respondent's concerns, knowledge, and perceptions of the risks/benefits. For example, in Figure 7-5 the vectors indicate that to get this group to "move" in the space toward initiating treatment, a message strategy would have to focus on the fact that hepatitis C virus (HCV) can be cured easily and quickly and that it would make someone feel "in charge" of their health. (For further details about our use of the perceptual mapping approach, see https://sites.temple.edu/turiskcommlab/.)

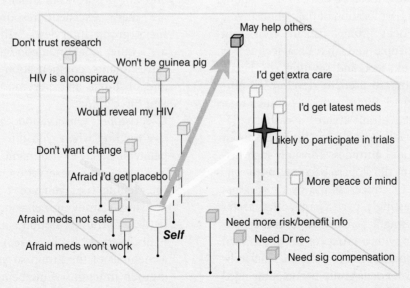

FIGURE 7-5 Perceptual map with vectors: HCV-positive methadone patients' perceptions of treatment initiation.

(continues)

We have adapted these methods to a variety of public health behaviors and decision making, with work focusing on a wide range of issues: colonoscopy decision making in low-literacy African American patients,[g,h,j] intended actions during a "dirty bomb" explosion in low-literacy urban residents,[k,l] smallpox vaccination decisions in healthcare workers,[f] perceptions of avian flu,[m] attitudes of healthcare providers who treat people with HIV,[n] and decisions related to participating in clinical trials among HIV-positive minority patients.[o] This research has shown that perceptual mapping and vector modeling methods can be used to assess group perceptions; develop tailored messages and interventions; achieve changes in understanding, attitudes, and behaviors; and evaluate outcomes in a variety of public health situations.

[a] Borg I, Groenen P. *Modern Multidimensional Scaling: Theory and Applications*. New York, NY: Springer-Verlag; 1997.

[b] Herschfeld N, Gelman S. *Mapping the Mind: Domain Specificity in Cognition and Culture*. Cambridge, England: Cambridge University Press; 1994.

[c] Kitchin R, Freundschuh S, eds. *Cognitive Mapping: Past, Present, Future*. New York, NY: Routledge; 2000.

[d] Barnett G, Boster F. *Progress in Communication Sciences: Attitude Change and Persuasion*. Norwood, NJ: Ablex; 1997.

[e] Leventhal H, Halm E, Horowitz C, Leventhal EA, Ozakinci G. Living with chronic illness: a contextualized self-regulation approach. In: Sutton S, Baum A, Johnson M, eds. *SAGE Handbook of Health Psychology*. London, England: Sage; 2004:197-240.

[f] Bass SB, Gordon TF, Ruzek SB, Hausman AJ. Mapping perceptions related to acceptance of smallpox vaccination by hospital emergency room personnel. *Biosecurity Bioterrorism: Biodefense Strat Pract Sci*. 2008;6:179-190.

[g] Bass SB, Gordon TF, Ruzek SB, et al. Developing a computer touch-screen interactive colorectal screening decision aid for a low-literacy African American population: lessons learned. *Health Promot Pract*. 2012;14(4):589-598.

[h] Ruggieri D, Bass SB, Rovito MJ, et al. Perceived colonoscopy barriers and facilitators among urban African American patients and their medical residents. *J Health Commun*. 2013. doi:10.1080/10810730.2012.727961.

[i] Woelfel J, Fink EL. *The Measurement of Communication Processes: Galileo Theory and Method*. New York, NY: Academic Press; 1980.

[j] Gordon TF, Bass SB, Ruzek SB, et al. Developing a typology of African Americans with limited literacy based on prevention practice orientation: implications for colorectal cancer screening strategies [published online ahead of print]. *J Health Commun*. 2014. doi:10.1080/10810730.2013.872725.

[k] Bass S, Mora G, Ruggieri D, et al., eds. *Understanding of and Willingness to Comply with Recommendations in the Event of a 'Dirty Bomb': Demographic Differences in Low-Literacy Urban Residents*. Washington, DC: American Public Health Association; November 2011.

[l] Bass SB, Greener JR, Ruggieri D, et al. Attitudes and perceptions of urban African Americans of a "dirty bomb" radiological terror event: results of a qualitative study and implications for effective risk communication. *Disaster Med Public Health Prep*. 2015;9(1):9-18.

[m] Bass SB, Ruzek SB, Ward S, et al. Predictors of quarantine compliance during a hypothetical avian influenza pandemic: results from a statewide survey. *Disaster Med Public Health Preparedness*. 2010;4:1-10.

[n] Matosky M, Terrell C, Gordon TF, Bass SB, Ruzek SB. Using perceptual mapping to develop HIV medical case management. Paper presented at: Annual Meeting of the American Public Health Association, San Diego, CA; 2008.

[o] Bass SB, Wolak C, Greener J, et al. Using perceptual mapping to understand gender differences in perceived barriers and benefits of clinical research participation in minority HIV+ patients. *AIDS Care*. 2015;28(4):528-536.

from very open-ended questions. An individual, in-depth interview is also easier to arrange than a focus group, because it can be done in the respondent's home, office, or location of their choosing.

- *Focus groups:* Focus groups usually consist of about 8 to 10 people and give us a feeling for what people think, feel, and say they do. Focus group discussions are used to develop hypotheses, explore broad topics, and generate ideas. A well-moderated group creates a casual environment that enables people to talk freely about feelings, beliefs, and attitudes. Through such discussions, program developers become more sensitive to the values, concerns, and needs of target audiences. Interestingly, participants often prefer discussing what might be considered embarrassing health topics with a group of people known to share their condition than alone with an individual investigator. Focus group participants need to be recruited and screened carefully, however, so that participants are representative of the target audience. For example, if you are interested in what young, white women think about a family

planning product, they need to be in your focus group, not their mothers, not their boyfriends, and not people from other ethnic groups. There are many excellent resources on conducting focus group interviews.[8] The key requirements are a quiet location, a good audio recorder, some refreshments, compensation for the participants, and, of course, an expert moderator with an excellent topic guide.

- *Observation:* Observation is a type of formative method where you directly observe ongoing behavior or an environment. Mostly this is done as "naturalistic" observation, meaning you are not intervening (i.e., you are a nonparticipant) and are simply studying behaviors that are occurring naturally. Another option is to become a "participant observer." In this case, you insert yourself as a member of the group so you can observe how a group functions while being part of it. Sending trained observers into homes and communities to watch what goes on, usually over several hours for several days in a row, helps identify behavior patterns, alternative products, or obstacles to adopting new behaviors. Observation can be very useful in understanding not only behavior, but also the context in which it occurs. For example, if you want to understand why kids choose certain foods in a school lunchroom, an observation can tell you not only which foods are chosen, but also how accessible those foods are. Accessibility may be a limiting factor in choice; observation can help you assess the effect of an environmental influence on behavior.

- *Intercept interviews:* In this technique, you go to the location where the intended audience would encounter information about a behavior or acquire a product and then invite them to participate in an interview. Shopping malls are used extensively in the United States for this kind of formative research, but so are health clinics, supermarkets, and parks. The high traffic volume of the intercept area allows you to contact large numbers of respondents in a short time. In an intercept interview you approach the individual, ask a few screening questions to determine whether they match the characteristics of the target audience, and then ask your real questions. Although the advantage of this technique is the possibility of volume, many people do not want to be bothered. You must also almost always offer incentives, such as gift cards or cash rewards, to entice people to participate.

- *PhotoVoice:* PhotoVoice is a widely used participatory method.[9] In this approach, communities are given the tools to document their own lives, problems, and possible solutions through photography. It has been used to put forward unheard voices for advocacy purposes. However, it is also a legitimate way of gathering how an affected group of people view their own situation, and it can be the precursor for a very compelling intervention to enable them to change their circumstances for the better. **APPENDIX 7A** presents a PhotoVoice project and how it was used with kids to develop plans to address unhealthy eating in Philadelphia.

One interesting adaption of qualitative methods is the use of online panels to provide information. Specific websites or online communities can be used to identify specific participants in a virtual location. These *market research online communities (MROCs)* can be used to listen to specific audience segments and explore topics in-depth, as one would with a live focus group. Advantages of MROCs include convenience for the participants, engagement with participants over an extended period of time, and greater anonymity for participants (when only audio or text responses are used). **BOX 7-4** provides a perspective on using MROCs for formative research.

Qualitative data provide the backstory for the quantitative data and may point to the need for more quantitative studies. For example, by asking many individuals or small groups of children why they hate exercising, you might learn that they feel ashamed of their bodies and are made fun of in school. They would exercise more if they could do it with other children who share their body shape, in a socially and environmentally safe environment. Do obese children feel this way? That would require another quantitative survey, and you might learn that a sufficient number feel that way, perhaps 60%, to justify a communication campaign focused on creating a safe social environment in which overweight children can play.

The combination of quantitative and qualitative research methods is referred to as a **mixed-methods approach**. **APPENDIX 7B** illustrates how these methods can be utilized to develop a program aimed at addressing teen smoking.

BOX 7-4 Market Research Online Communities (MROCs)

An organization can establish an MROC as a password-protected website where a specific group of people is recruited to take part in daily, weekly, or monthly research activities around a shared topic of interest. You could easily engage different audience segments by factors such as gender, language, and health concerns through different online communities. If you already have a social media site, such as a Facebook page or Twitter following, or an online site where, for example, new mothers or persons living with a specific illness interact, you have a way of recruiting individuals into an MROC. Or, you can work with a vendor to do the recruiting, hosting, and management for you.

Like focus groups, MROCs allow hosts to have a conversation with the participants and explore topics in depth. Like consumer panels, hosts are able to go back to the same people repeatedly over a specific period of time. An MROC project can have 50 to 500 participants and be accomplished in a week, if desired. The average cost for running an online research community through a vendor for one month is approximately $5000.

▶ Ok, Now What?

Having completed your formative research, the next step of the process is to bring everything you have learned to bear on planning the actual messages, communication tools, and health communication intervention. A very helpful document at this stage is the **creative brief**, a summary of the key features of and objectives for your health communication intervention.

Preparing a Creative Brief

The term *creative brief* comes from the advertising business, where a short document is prepared that gives details of what should be considered when something is being designed or advertised. (Less often the term is generalized to mean the entire communication strategy.) It is a clear and concise way to present the overall thinking behind a communication intervention and the issues that are most important to keep in mind during design and implementation. The basic form of the creative brief used in health communication has evolved little since it was first introduced in the 1970s. Some agencies and organizations use different elements, but the following outline reflects the consensus.

The following are the elements of a creative brief:

■ *Overview of project:* This is a short summary of the overall goals of the project and its importance to the organization(s) involved.

■ *Target audience segment:* This should be a carefully defined, unique segment with specific characteristics, such as demographic description, behavioral readiness stage, literacy level, lifestyle information, and role in the overall communication strategy (primary audience, secondary audience, etc.). When multiple audience segments are targeted, a different creative brief should be developed for each.

■ *Objectives:* What specific behavior do you want the communication to produce in the target audience? This is often phrased as what you want them to think, feel, or do, and it may be referred to as a "call to action."

■ *Obstacles:* What structural barriers, beliefs, cultural practices, social pressure, or misinformation are obstacles to your audience taking this step? Is there an audience that must be approached first in order to free your intended audience to act as desired?

■ *Benefit/key promise:* What is the single most important reward (from the audience's point of view) that will result from doing the desired behavior? Is there a secondary reward? Which is more immediate, and which will take longer to achieve? From the audience perspective, "What's in it for me?"

■ *Support statements/reasons:* These statements explain why the target audience should believe the promise of the key benefit. This may be scientific data, emotional data, or data drawn from the experience of others who the target audience admires or can relate to. Support statements should also provide solutions to the obstacles raised earlier.

■ *Tone:* What feeling or personality should your message or medium have? The tone set by the communication materials will influence how the target audience feels after interacting with the communications. Examples of tones include authoritative, family-oriented, funny, loving, modern, preachy, rural, scary, sad, and so on.

■ *Distribution opportunities:* What venues, seasons, or events increase the likelihood of reaching your audience? In what other ways might this material be used? Do you need different versions to reach audiences in different settings?

■ *Creative considerations:* What else should the writers and designers keep in mind during development? What is the intended medium and channel for this product? Will a certain style of presentation resonate more with the selected target audiences: conversational, testimonial, informational, emotional, or instructional? Will the material need to be prepared in more than one language? Will well-known spokespersons be involved (e.g., political figures or entertainers)? Are there special words or phrases to use or avoid?

■ *Other elements:* Some briefs include approval routing, timelines, and just about anything else that is needed to reach management consensus before beginning creative development.

▶ From the Creative Brief to Concepts, Messages, and Materials

We use creative briefs to organize our ideas before moving to the concept, message, and materials production phases of communication planning, but then what? When working with a creative team, either in-house (e.g., your friend the artist or yourself for a "no budget" effort, or the media/marketing department of a public health agency or voluntary organization) or with a hired agency, it is essential to keep the artists "on message" and "on strategy." It is extremely easy to let a great creative idea steal the show. But, this is where the creative brief helps you to ensure quality. Working through the creative brief, you can describe the project's overall purpose and provide all the information you have available about the intended audience. Next, you will relay the objectives of this specific communication or material.

Develop the Concept

The concepts of a health communication intervention are often large, overarching ideas of what it is you are hoping to get your audience to do or know. It might be "Wash your hands after going to the bathroom" or "Don't send your children to school when they are sick." These may not be the actual words that will be used to communicate the idea to the target audience, although they might be represented on some level. Instead, the idea—together with all the other information gathered about the audience—will generate a concept. The concept will be a creative interpretation of the information about the objectives, the obstacles, the key benefits, the support statements, the tone, and the intended media channels—as well as anything else included in the creative brief.

Concepts are gestalt interpretations; they try to grab the main idea and give it a personality. (*Gestalt* is from the German, and literally means form, shape, or general idea. Gestalt psychology emphasizes the importance of overall concepts in forming a stable mental image of the world. It sometimes also means "The whole is greater [more useful, more powerful] than the sum of its parts.") From social marketing, we have learned that the core of the concept is the most compelling benefit, surrounded by supporting information. The concept must appeal to both the head and the heart, and must communicate how this idea fits into the lives of the target audience. Does it make their life easier? Is it fun? Will it seem to be a popular thing to do (to paraphrase communications guru Bill Smith)? **APPENDIX 7C** is a good example of the development of concepts and testing for the Better Bites program from the Tweens Nutrition and Fitness Coalition in Lexington, Kentucky.

But the question remains, are the concepts and messages you have created right for the audience? Only they can answer this. Audiences and gatekeepers need to be invited to **pretest** concepts before moving on to final messages and materials for final production. In addition to gatekeepers, it is often important to consider who else might be sensitive to the ideas being put forward. When we think about how many things we try to "prevent," we should be mindful of the people who already suffer from these conditions. It might be HIV. It might be a preventable birth defect or a chronic disease. Health communicators must consider how these people, or their loved ones, will feel if their condition is portrayed as something to avoid at all costs. So, pretesting with persons who represent this audience of affected individuals is also advised.

Strategies to test concepts include most of the strategies discussed previously and can be both quantitative and qualitative in nature. One interesting application of this is the use of online panels to provide input. Amazon's Mechanical Turk (http://www.mturk.com, named after an 18th-century fake chess-playing automaton with a human inside) is a good example. It is an online "workforce" made up of people from all over the world who agree to complete online tasks. You can limit the number of respondents or have specific inclusion criteria, but for most tasks you can have literally thousands of responses in a short time. Users are paid a small amount of money (e.g., 25 to 50 cents) for each task, called a human intelligence task,[10] making the use of the panel relatively inexpensive if you limit the number.

Competing concepts can be tested against each other (i.e., A vs. B) or a new concept tested against an old concept (e.g., messages from a previous intervention or campaign compared to the new ones). Respondents can easily click on the choices on the screen and then complete a fill-in question on why they chose one concept over another. This provides concrete evidence of how your concept is being perceived and explicit feedback about why people prefer one concept over another. One issue with using these types of online forums, however, is ensuring that the respondents are truly members of your target audience. Combining this type of testing with in-person qualitative intercept interviews or focus groups is a good strategy to make sure your audience is fully represented.

From Concepts to Messages and Materials

Having tested your concepts, you will now build on that foundation to create messages and communication materials—patient–provider communication guidelines, posters, pamphlets, ads, radio scripts, social media posts—that carry your ideas to the hearts and minds of your intended audience. The channels and activities that will use your material determine the format for production, not vice versa. You can create great audio for radio spots and video material for the internet, but you will never succeed in putting video on the radio. Similarly, materials designed for healthcare providers to counsel patients are likely to be too complex for consumers at pharmacy counters or in grocery stores. Just like you tested your concept, you now must also systematically pretest your messages and materials to ensure that you have translated the concept into a format that speaks to your audience. We are looking for many of the same results as we were in concept testing, but now we need to know if we were successful in using an overall concept to produce a specific, focused, effective message.

Pretesting Messages and Materials

Creative content is ideally tested in the format in which it will be used. In other words, if an individual is meant to see a commercial spot on the television, it should be tested as if it were being shown on TV. If a patient is supposed to look at an mHealth tool on a tablet or phone, they should have the experience of using the tool on that technology. Important factors to pretest are attractiveness, understandability, and believability. Do the messages and materials engage the audience? Do they feel they would act in the intended manner after getting this information? To answer these questions, several strategies can be used, including message/user testing and usability testing. All material intended for use in a health communication intervention should be tested with the intended recipients and with the gatekeepers prior to distribution. No excuses.

Message and User Testing

In **message testing**, participants often are provided a list of messages and the context of those messages. You might create a "storyboard" or "mood board" that graphically displays the messages. This may be done prior to a more finished product to get initial input on the direction of the messages. FIGURE 7-6 is an example of a storyboard that shows the flow of screens on an mHealth tool called *mychoice*, which aims to encourage African American cancer patients to consider participating in clinical trials. This was used in message testing to get input from the audience on not only content, but also the flow of the screens. After that input, the tool was created and retested so that patients could use a tablet and get a feel for the flow of the tool, as well as how the content was presented.

In other message testing, you may want to try out similar messages in different formats; for example, one message is gain framed and one is loss framed ("When you quit smoking, you take control of your health" vs. "If you keep smoking, you lose control of your health"). In this case, you can present the different versions to see how your audience responds. Another example may be to try out a tone. If you create a humorous message, does your audience actually think it's funny? You can also check for understanding and comprehension of the message, especially if it's complicated or about a health topic or behavior that may be unfamiliar to your audience. Although many people skip message testing and do it along with user testing, if you have the time and resources, message testing can be very helpful in guiding the development of the communication materials, before you have invested resources. Some of the key questions you might ask in message testing include:

- What do you think this message is about?
- Are there any words that you would change to make it easier for others to understand?
- Please explain this message in your own words.
- Are there any words that you would find objectionable? How about others in your community?

User testing has your audience examine both the messages and the material. Usually this is done with "talk alouds," in which a small group is exposed to the material or tool and each person is asked to verbalize their reactions aloud. (For an example of this, see **BOX 7-5**.) You can also collect quantitative data through self- or interviewer-administered surveys or through larger venues such as *theater testing*, where you bring in large groups of people who respond through surveys or electronic polling using their cell phones or clickers. The primary benefits of these forms of testing are that they are relatively easy and inexpensive. You can gather the information and make corrections in your materials quickly. (The primary drawback is that participants may try to please the researcher and will say they like a message or that it will stimulate them to action, when in fact they don't and it doesn't.)

BOX 7-6 features some sample questions to use when pretesting a short piece such as a television or radio spot. You'll notice that there is some redundancy in how we ask these questions. We also ask respondents to comment on how others would feel about the pieces being tested. These are deliberate attempts to get people to speak honestly. Respondents in pretests often do not want to offend the researcher and will try to say things that they believe are the "right answers," or pleasing. By asking them what others might say, there is a better chance that they might provide some negative feedback. Remember, there is no perfect draft material. If you come back with "No changes necessary," there was something wrong with your pretest.

Usability Testing

Usability testing refers to studying how people use a finished product such as a website, mobile app, electronic game, or mHealth tool, but it can also be done with pamphlets and posters. In this type of testing, you are measuring how well an intended user can learn and use the product, as well as their satisfaction with the process. This can be done in combination with more high-tech measurements like eye tracking, which is discussed later in this section, or by observing someone and asking questions and taking notes. Some usability testing can occur off-site, meaning that someone can use a website, and their clicks and keystrokes can be collected remotely. In general, usability measures the quality of a user's experience with the product. The federal

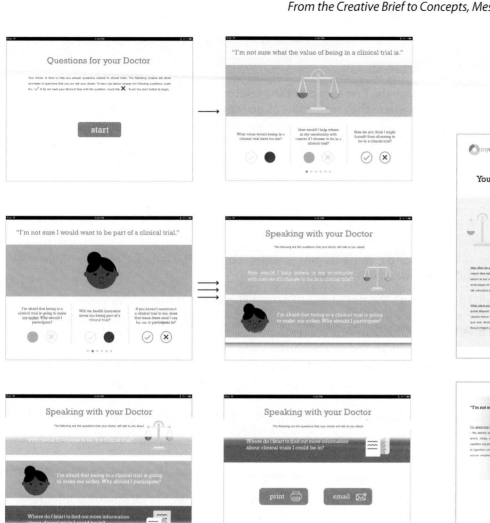
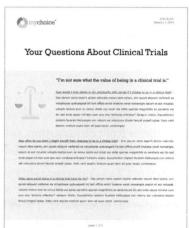
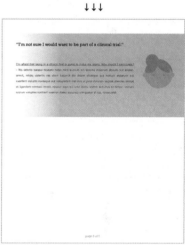
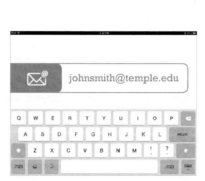

FIGURE 7-6 The mychoice storyboard.

BOX 7-5 Sample "Think Aloud" Guide for Mobile Health (mHealth) Education Tool on Hepatitis C Treatment

(Tester) Thank you for taking time to review a new educational tool that is being developed for methadone clients to help them learn more about hepatitis C treatment. The tool has a number of sections and I am going to ask you to review one section at a time. As you go through each section, feel free to make comments out loud and tell me honestly what you are doing and why. This is called think aloud and helps us to understand what someone might be thinking as they go through the site. It helps us learn what needs to be improved or made clearer. Don't worry about hurting our feelings if you don't like something. We want to know so we can help make it better.

(continues)

BOX 7-5 Sample Think Aloud Interview Guide: Mobile Apps   *(continued)*

Section 1: Ask participant to go through the first section of the educational prototype (Introduction and Section 1), exploring where they would like to go (about 10 minutes in total).

Staff will observe and document any areas of concern, questions asked, and other observations. Staff will then ask:

- Tell me what you think of the logo (including the colors and fist)?
- Tell me what you think the purpose of the tool is.
- Tell me what you think of the content. Is it too much? Is anything hard to understand?
- What messages do you remember most?
- Tell me what you think of the graphics (animations and pictures).
- Tell me what you think of the voiceover. Do you like the voice? Do you trust it?
- Does it make you want to learn more and continue?

Notes from observation, talk aloud, and comments (notes address navigation issues, potential offensive or confusing wording, or inability to understand content):

Section 2: Ask participant to go through the statements (Section 2), exploring where they would like to go. They can look at all the areas or just a few. It can be up to them (about 10 minutes to review and 5 minutes for questions). If they have not seen any of the videos, show them how they can see at least one of them. Keep track of which sections they go to and in what order.

Staff will observe and document any areas of concern, questions asked, and other observations. Staff will then ask:

- What did you think about this section? Did these sound like statements you have heard or you have made?
- What message do you most remember?
- What do you think of the content you saw? Did it answer questions you might have about hepatitis C treatment? Did you think it was hard or easy to understand?
- What did you think of the videos?
- What do you think of the pictures in the animations? Visuals? What do you think of the narrator's voice in the pictures?

Notes from observation, talk aloud, and comments (notes address navigation issues, potential offensive or confusing wording, or inability to understand content):

Section 3: Ask participant to go through Section 3 on how to talk to your doctor (about 5 minutes in total).

Staff will observe and document any areas of concern, questions asked, and other observations. Staff will then ask:

- What did you think about this section? Would you bring these questions to your doctor?
- Is the format easy to use?
- Do you think these questions would help you talk with your doctor?

Notes from observation, talk aloud, and comments (notes address navigation issues, potential offensive or confusing wording, or inability to understand content):

Section 4: Ask participant to go through Section 4 on "making the decision" (about 5 minutes in total).

Staff will observe and document any areas of concern, questions asked, and other observations. Staff will then ask:

- What did you think about this section? Did you understand how to move the phrases to the two sides of the scale? Were the instructions clear?
- Do you think this would be helpful in visualizing the pros and cons to making a decision about hepatitis C treatment?
- Are there other things you think should be on the list for people to choose from?

Notes from observation, talk aloud, and comments (notes address navigation issues, potential offensive or confusing wording, or inability to understand content):

Now that you have gone through the educational tool, we would like to get your overall thoughts and reactions.

Interviewer Questions – Interviewer will verbally ask the question.

1. How easy or difficult do you think the tool was to use? Were there any specific places you think were harder to navigate than others?
2. How might this tool influence someone's thinking about hepatitis C treatment?
3. What did you like about the educational tool?
4. What could be improved about the educational tool?
5. Would you recommend this to a friend or other methadone patients?

Reprinted with permission from Sarah Baurle Bass, MPH, PhD.

BOX 7-6 Questions for Pretesting Draft Content

1. *Comprehension:* Does the target audience fully understand and interpret the materials in the way you intend? Some questions that assess comprehension include:
   a. In your opinion, what is the message of this (television spot, radio spot, print piece)?
   b. Are there any words that you would change to make it easier for others to understand? Which are they?
   c. Please explain this message to your neighbor in your own words. (Have the respondents do so.)
   d. (Indicate a particular image.) Can you tell me what this is and why it might be in this picture?

2. *Attractiveness:* Taste obviously varies a great deal and is related to cultural factors as well as the changing times. While you are testing a rough cut of material, you should strive to make this as close as possible to the finished piece. If it is a radio spot, have someone with a good voice do the recording. If it is a storyboard for a video or a home video version of the script, still strive to be as professional as possible to prevent the low production value from distracting the audience. For print, you can probably produce a near-finished piece with today's simple graphics programs. Some questions that assess attractiveness include:
   a. What do you like the most about this piece?
   b. What do you dislike?
   c. How would you change this piece?
   d. What do you think others in this community would say about this piece?

3. *Acceptance:* This factor has more to do with the norms, attitudes, and beliefs of the target audience. Can they believe the information? Is it congruent with the community's norm? Does it require a major change of opinion to act on the information? Some questions that assess acceptance include:
   a. Is there anything about this piece that you find objectionable?
   b. How about others in this community? What would they say?
   c. Do you know any people like this, or have you seen a situation like this?
   d. (Indicate a particular aspect of the piece.) Is this believable to you?
   e. Can you think of anyone else, such as a religious leader or important community leader, who we should show this to before distributing it widely?

4. *Involvement:* The target audience should be able to recognize themselves in the materials. Based on the elaboration likelihood model, if the target audience is already concerned about the issue, then it might not be necessary to match up the imagery with their stylistic preferences. But, if you need to first focus their attention on the fact that this information is meant for them, then featuring spokespersons and images that the target audience would like to see is important. Some questions that assess involvement include:
   a. (If using noncelebrities) Whom does this piece represent? Are these people like you?
   b. (If using celebrities) Who is this? What do you feel about having [name] speak to you about [topic]?
   c. Do you feel that this piece is speaking to you? Why or why not?
   d. If this isn't meant for you, who do you think it is speaking to?

5. *Inducement to action:* All materials need a call for action. Because we have tried to identify a behavior, attitude, or change that we think is feasible for the target audience to embrace, now is the last chance to test whether this piece will prompt them to make it. Even if we are just trying to raise awareness of a problem, we want to prompt the audience to seek more information or tell others about what they have learned. Some questions that assess call to action include:
   a. What does this piece ask you to do?
   b. How do you feel about doing this?
   c. Would you need to do something else before you could do this?
   d. How would you explain this to a friend?
   e. How would they respond to this piece?

Modified from AED Toolbox, Question 18:19–21. http://www.globalhealthcommunication.org/tool_docs/29/a_tool_box_for_building_health _communication_capacity_-_question_18.pdf.

government has a project called usability.gov that helps people developing websites and other web-based designs to enhance the user experience. The project notes that usability testing should measure the following[11]:

■ *Ease of learning:* How fast can a user who has never seen the user interface before learn it sufficiently well to accomplish basic tasks?

■ *Efficiency of use:* Once an experienced user has learned to use the system, how fast can they accomplish tasks?

■ *Memorability:* If a user has used the system before, can they remember enough to use it effectively the next time, or must the user relearn everything?

■ *Error frequency and severity:* How often do users make errors while using the system, how serious are those error, and how do users recover from these errors?

- *Subjective satisfaction:* How much does the user like using the system?

High-Tech Pretesting

Physiological Effects Testing

There are a number of techniques that could be used to assess the actual physical response people have to health communication materials. These strategies can show whether the person is responding in the ways you would expect and use measures like skin temperature, eye pupil dilation, and brain waves.

Galvanic Skin Response. Popularized in crime shows as part of a polygraph lie detector procedure, or more recently as a biofeedback tool, the **galvanic skin response (GSR)** is a measure of the electrical current that passes along the surface of the skin. Because perspiration conducts electricity much better than dry skin, a minute increase in perspiration resulting from an emotional response can be detected as an increase in electrical conductance. GSR is painless and can be measured easily using uncomplicated devices and a computer display. In addition to its contribution to criminology, GSR has been used to gauge attention to and emotional response to media, messages, and images. Although an emotional response can be detected with GSR, remember that there is no way to know the nature of the actual underlying emotion without asking the subject.

Pupil Dilation and Eye-Tracking Technology. The eyes may not be the literal windows to our soul, but they do give away the locus and level of our interest. **Eye tracking** is a measure of where and how long we gaze at an image (moving or still) or text. We also have an innate response of the autonomic nervous system to imminent danger or arousal that causes our pupils to dilate. Together with our blink rate (which also speeds up when we are aroused or experience fear), pupil dilation can be measured by photographic or video processes. Eye movement tracking devices can be stationary, embedded in a computer screen, or miniaturized in a pair of glasses for free moving studies. Each of these methods can also record and save real-time video to a nearby laptop. **BOX 7-7** details how eye tracking was used to test a "dirty bomb" decision aid with low-literacy adults. The results of this method showed how difficult it was for those with limited literacy to track and read high-literacy materials compared to materials designed for easy reading.

The Bottom Line on Pretesting

A quote we are fond of is "fail early, fail small." Some of what you think are your best ideas do not work with the intended audience, outrage the gatekeepers, or offend current sufferers. Having data from the audience pretesting is an important strategy for overcoming gatekeeper resistance to a message or media concept. It is much better, and cheaper, to find this out with a small group of people at the concept, message, or even materials testing stage than after a multimedia campaign has been released to the public or materials have been printed in color to distribute to patients in a hospital.

Finally, remember that you may need many different formats of your materials, conveying different parts of your message matched to the audience and the channel; for example, you can use a "badge" on an internet site that links to a complete webpage and a hotline phone number on that same webpage, as well as a billboard and posters put up in a targeted neighborhood. Ideally, each intervention strategy should be tested for concept, message, and usability. One weak link may ruin an entire health communication program.

▶ Next? Choosing Settings and Channels

You might be surprised by how much ideas change when going from concepts to communication materials, but the process is critical to your planning. Once you are certain your messages and materials are the right strategies, you can get down to the business of planning which communication platforms you will use and how you will implement your program. There are many channel options. And as you've learned about focusing on the needs of your audience by using the PRECEDE-PROCEED model, being deliberate about how you target your audience—at the predisposing, reinforcing, and enabling levels—will help ensure success. Now is the hard part of thinking through the best settings and communication channels to reach your audience with your newly crafted messages.

Settings include places where an audience must go to receive your message (e.g., a healthcare facility, shopping mall, bar or restaurant in town, or special event) and places where the media reaches them closer to home, such as radio or television programs, online environments, and the like. Timing is very important. A place that seems like a good setting for your audience might be impractical if your communication is ill-timed for reception or too late to be used; for example,

BOX 7-7 Use of Eye-Tracking and Gaze Pattern Analysis to Test Health Messages in Low-Literacy Groups

The Risk Communication Laboratory at Temple University is utilizing eye-tracking technology and gaze pattern analysis to understand how individuals with low literacy access and process health messages through visual, graphic, web, or textual message elements. Eye tracking assesses an individual's attention to visual content (e.g., print, video) by systematically monitoring eye-movement patterns through the use of high-speed cameras either mounted on a flat, stable surface like a desk or worn by the participant (e.g., using cameras mounted on a pair of glasses). New portable eye-tracking systems can also track eye movement on moving messages or video, such as when using a smartphone or tablet.

Eye movements are a powerful indicator of interest and provide an index of the input of information to more complex processing and/or reasoning.[a-e] As such, eye movement measures can provide valuable information for the design and/or refinement of health communication messages, particularly when the messages involve combinations of language processing and visual processing. Because of its ability to show interest, eye tracking has been used primarily in marketing as a way to maximize product placement and message. This technology can be especially informative when working with low-literacy populations, but has not been used appreciably to date. Eye tracking can produce vivid data that show not only gaze duration (shown in **FIGURES 7-7** and **7-8** as green dots in which the size indicates the length of the gaze), but also gaze pattern (blue line). In research done at the Risk Communication Laboratory with adults with limited literacy, eye-tracking results showed clear patterns of differential text use in a randomized pilot comparing a higher literacy–level aid from the CDC (Figure 7-7), to a literacy-appropriate decision aid on "dirty bombs" (Figure 7-8).

This study, funded by the National Institute of Biomedical Imaging and Bioengineering, was conducted to understand attention to a decision aid on sheltering in place during a radiological terror event (i.e., dirty bomb). In this study, the decision aid was developed using formative evaluation (focus groups, survey)[f-h] and then tested in a between-subjects pilot randomized controlled trial with low-literacy adults.[i,j] Participants were shown either a CDC-authored frequently asked questions on dirty bombs (control condition) or a literacy-appropriate decision aid (experimental condition). Both conditions were presented on a computer screen as a series of slides. The experimental literacy-appropriate decision aid included visual cues and less information, and was written at a sixth-grade reading level. Subjects were recruited through community-based agencies (food bank, senior services, federal services, churches, community centers), and literacy screening occurred in person using the Rapid Estimate of Adult Literacy in Medicine—Short Version (REALM-R)[k] or over the phone using the Single Item Literacy Screening.[l]

Fifty participants were randomized to the control and experimental conditions. The mean REALM-R score was 2.11 out of a possible 8 (range 0 to 5), confirming the inclusion of low-literacy adults. Eye tracking was performed

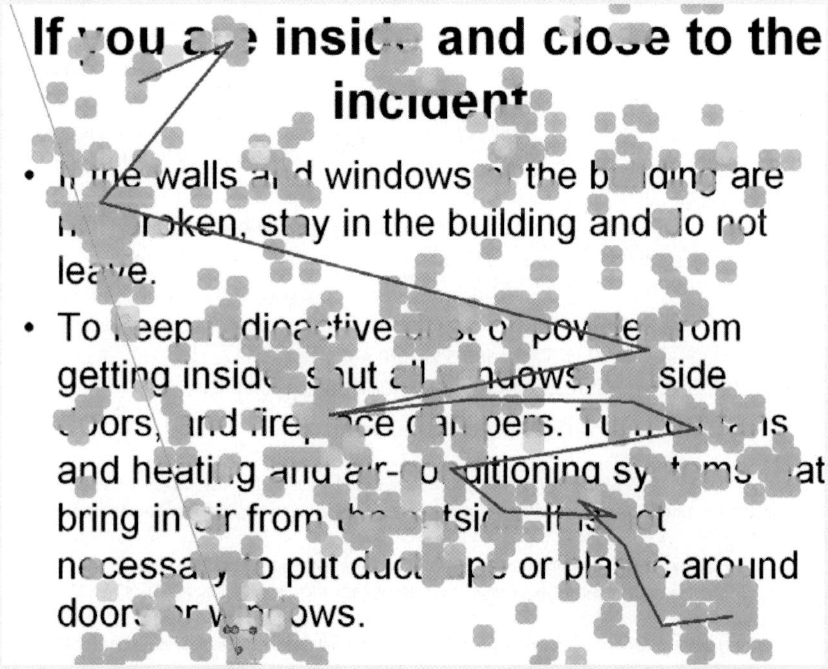

FIGURE 7-7 Eye tracking of high-literacy "dirty bomb" education in participant with limited literacy.

(continues)

BOX 7-7 Use of Eye-Tracking and Gaze Pattern Analysis to Test Health Messages in Low-Literacy Groups *(continued)*

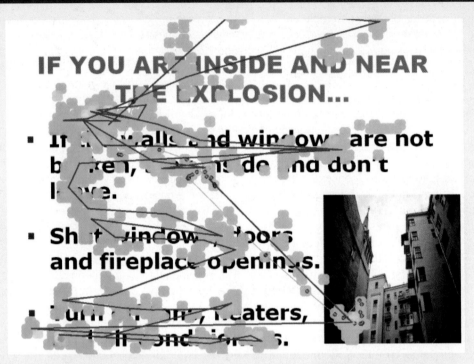

FIGURE 7-8 Eye tracking of literacy appropriate "dirty bomb" education in participant with limited literacy.

with an Applied Science Laboratory stationary eye tracker (Eye Trac 6000), and the Eyenal software program was used for analysis. In addition, a five-point subjective rating scale was developed and tested by the author to characterize gaze patterns. Interrater reliability was excellent, with coefficients for scores of participants' ability to accurately track written text of 0.90 [Pearson] and 0.99 [Spearman]. As illustrated in Figure 7-8, more accurate tracking was observed for the literacy-appropriate slide. Overall, the ability to track information was higher in the experimental condition than in the control condition for three of seven content-similar slides, with an additional two slides close to statistical significance. The difficulty of participants to attend to the relatively dense text in the control condition was reflected in significantly longer pupil fixation and gaze duration. Participants spent more time in the experimental condition looking at individual words (four of seven slides) and more time overall (all seven slides). As a consequence, participants in the experimental condition were also more likely to be "certain of what to do," had higher self-efficacy on their ability to protect themselves and their family, and were more likely to agree that they would stay home if a dirty bomb exploded. The results of this study clearly indicated that eye tracking is a viable and important method for understanding how low-literacy groups attend to health-related information and its association with comprehension.[i,j]

Eye tracking was thus found to be especially helpful in understanding how best to design materials for low-literacy groups, providing tangible evidence of how tracking of text is directly related to comprehension as well as intended or actual behavior. Eye tracking output can clearly differentiate whether an individual is reading text as expected or if they instead have to read and then reread sections because of literacy ability. If presented with material that is above literacy and/ or numeracy levels, eye tracking can be used to show areas where individuals have difficulty accessing the content, which can then be related to other outcome measures. The Risk Communication Laboratory is continuing to use these methods to test developed health communication messages to ensure that they meet the needs of individuals with all literacy abilities.

[a] Beatty J. The papillary system. In: Coles G, Donchin E, Porges S, eds. *Psychophysiology: Systems, Process, and Applications.* New York, NY: Guilford Press; 1986:43-50.

[b] Beatty J. Pupillometric signs of selective attention in man. *In: Donchin E, Galbraith G, Kietzman MD, eds. Neurophysiology and Psychology: Basic Mechanisms and Clinical Applications.* New York, NY: Academic Press; 1988:138-143.

[c] Granholm E, Asarnow RF, Sarkin AJ, Dykes KL. Pupillary responses index cognitive resource limitations. *Psychophysiology.* 1996;33(4):457-461.

[d] Bradley, MM, Miccoli, L, Escrig, MA, Lang, PJ. The pupil as a measure of emotional arousal and autonomic activation. *Psychophysiology.* 2008; 45(4):602-607. https://doi .org/10.1111/j.1469-8986.2008.00654.x.

[e] Steinhauer S. Pupillary responses, cognitive psychophysiology and psychopathology. http://www.wpic.pitt.edu/research/biometrics/Publications/PupilWeb.htm. Updated 2016. Accessed March 13, 2018.

[f] Bass S, Mora G, Ruggieri D, et al., eds. *Understanding of and Willingness to Comply with Recommendations in the Event of a 'Dirty Bomb': Demographic Differences in Low-Literacy Urban Residents.* Washington, DC: American Public Health Association; 2011.

g Bass SB, Greener JR, Ruggieri D, et al. Attitudes and perceptions of urban African Americans of a "dirty bomb" radiological terror event: results of a qualitative study and implications for effective risk communication. *Disaster Med Public Health Prep.* 2015;9(1):9-18.

h Bass SB, Gordon T, Maurer L, et al. How do low-literacy populations perceive "dirty bombs"? Implications for preparedness messages. *Health Security.* 2016;14(5):331-344.doi:10.1089/hs.2016.0037.

i Bass SB, Gordon TF, Gordon R, Parvanta C. Using eye tracking and gaze pattern analysis to test a "dirty bomb" decision aid in a pilot RCT in urban adults with limited literacy. *BMC Health Informat Decision Making.* 2016;16:67. doi:10.1186/s12911-016-0304-5. http://www.biomedcentral.com/1472-6947/16/67.

j Greener J, Bass SB, Morris JD, Gordon TF. Use of emotional response modeling to develop more effective risk communication for limited literacy adults: evaluation of a "dirty bomb" decision aid. *Int J Commun Health.* 2016;8:10-21. http://communicationandhealth.ro/upload/number8/JUDITH-GREENER.pdf.

k Bass PF, Wilson JF, Griffith CH. A shortened instrument for literacy screening. *J Gen Intern Med.* 2003;18(12):1036-1038.

l Chew LD, Griffin JM, Partin MR, et al. Validation of screening questions for limited health literacy in a large VA outpatient population. *J Gen Intern Med.* 2008;23(5):561-566.

Reprinted with permission of Sarah Bauerle Bass, MPH, PhD.

most people cannot remember phone numbers or other information given out during drive-time radio shows or on the back of buses. The credibility of the setting to the audience is also important. A middle-aged man may be wary of getting information about colon cancer in a bar from a poster, but would be receptive in a healthcare clinic in a conversation with a nurse. But bars may be an appropriate setting for other audiences and topics, such as the dissemination of sexually transmitted disease (STD) prevention information in the bathrooms of bars and restaurants to younger people (the intended audience). They may find this setting more credible than being warned about the negative effects of STDs by their parents at home.

It is easy to confuse *settings* with **channels**. Think of your home or your dorm room as a setting, but there are many media channels that can come into that setting, such as television, the internet, mobile apps or streaming services, direct mail, radio, and so on. These are all channels. But these channels can also be received in other settings, like the public library. Or other communication channels such as billboards, transit ads, posters, or even good old-fashioned health education might occur in other places, like when you are traveling, in your doctor's office, or at a community organization you belong to. How you react to the same message conveyed by the same channel might vary depending on whether you see it in the privacy of your home or in a public setting like a library. Think about which settings and which channels make the most sense. Consider this example: You have developed and pretested messages around safer sex techniques in young adults. You believe they will be effective in changing attitudes about safer sex, using a variety of different communication channels. To decide how to best reach your audience, you need to find out where these young adults congregate and how to effectively reach them. You can decide on the setting (bars, gyms, homes, healthcare clinics) and the channels (posters, social media posts, app to identify where to get condoms, peer educators, entertainment at bars) to reach the

group and then segment by demographic characteristics to further refine your strategy, which may include more specialized channels or settings. In general, you can think of communication channels in three broad categories: interpersonal, community, and media.

Interpersonal Channels and Groups

Interpersonal channels include healthcare providers, clergy, teachers, and others who will interact with the intended recipient in person. The strength of interpersonal channels is that people tend to trust the spokesperson and will possibly be ready to listen to what they say. Face-to-face channels are most effective when trying to help someone learn a skill, such as how to test their blood sugar or how to safely perform an exercise therapy; they need to trust the spokesperson before adopting a new attitude or belief. On the other hand, two-way discussion is necessary to cement a behavioral intention. Interpersonal approaches can also be used with groups, particularly if discussion among group members is part of the communication strategy. (Think about weight loss or smoking cessation support groups.) To ensure the quality of health communication using interpersonal channels, it is often necessary to develop training modules for the communicator and media supports for the audience, such as accompanying brochures or handouts. The major limitations of this channel are its reach (it reaches only small numbers of people at a time) and the resources required (it requires intense use of people and time).

Organizational or Community Channels

Compared to other group communication channels, business organizations, voluntary agencies, or religious groups have more formality and structure. They can be very effective partners for disseminating advocacy messages or health communication that is not too detailed. Bringing health communication into a trusted setting also reinforces the credibility of the message and lends a sense of community norms to the suggested behavior. Normally you would develop a whole "kit" to support working with partners such as businesses or other community groups to keep messages focused and align the timing of dissemination to coincide with mass media, if used. It might also involve the training of people in that setting who would deliver the health communication. A good example of that is training a *lay health advisor* who is a congregant of a church to counsel other congregants on a health topic, such as breast cancer screening, high blood pressure, or prenatal care.

Mass Media or Social Media

Media that reach large populations, either individually or in huge markets, have become increasingly diverse in recent years. Mass media and social media outlets are channels that are known to be effective in raising awareness and knowledge, prompting health information seeking, and changing attitudes. This can especially be true with the use of social media platforms that are mostly low in cost and potentially reach a vast number of people in a very short time.

When entertainment approaches are used, such as using drama or incorporating health messages in gaming, mobile apps, or established pop culture, health communicators are often able to achieve vicarious learning, outcome expectancy, and self-efficacy through thoughtful use of role models demonstrating good behaviors and rewards or bad behaviors and negative consequences. But remember that these channels also have their pros and cons and often require financial resources, knowledge of how to produce materials for the medium, and/or expertise in technology.

APPENDIX 7D illustrates how a social marketing approach was used to develop a program that addressed an audience's information and communication channel needs, reaching out to mothers and families eligible for the Special Supplemental Nutrition Program for Women, Infants, and Children.

▶ Final Thoughts

Planning models can substantially increase the effectiveness of your health communication program, but only if you thoughtfully and systematically go through each step. Using formative research strategies, developing messages based on a creative brief, pretesting those messages, and using a communication channel strategy are the keys to success in reaching an audience with the right messages using the most effective channels. For an in-depth look at how these methods are used, see APPENDIX 7E, which outlines the development and testing of an mHealth mobile app to address adolescent asthma.

Key Terms

BEHAVE framework	Macro plan	Secondary data
Channel	Message testing	Setting
Continuation (or expansion) plan	Mixed-methods approach	Stakeholders
Creative brief	PRECEDE-PROCEED	Strategic health
Evaluation plan	model	communication plan
Eye tracking	Pretest	Tertiary audience
Formative research	Primary audience	Usability testing
Galvanic skin response (GSR)	Primary data	User testing
Implementation (or tactical) plan	Secondary audience	

Chapter Questions

1. What is the purpose of the health communication wheel? What steps make up this process?
2. How can the PRECEDE-PROCEED model be used to better understand audience behavior?
3. What is the purpose of formative research?
4. What are primary and secondary data, and when would you use each? Give an example of each data type.
5. Briefly describe the process of transforming a creative brief into a concept.
6. Describe at least two concept/message testing techniques, and explain their purpose in pretesting.

References

1. Perrin KM. *Essentials of Public Health: Planning and Evaluation*. New York, NY: Jones & Bartlett Learning; 2015.

2. Making health communication programs work. National Cancer Institute website. https://www.cancer.gov/publications/health-communication/pink-book.pdf. Accessed March 13, 2018.

3. Green LW, Kreuter MW, Deeds SG, Partridge KB. *Health Education Planning: A Diagnostic Approach*. 1st ed. Mountain View, CA: Mayfield; 1980.

4. Green LW, Kreuter MW. *Health Program Planning: An Educational and Ecological Approach*. 4th ed. New York, NY: McGraw-Hill; 2005.

5. CORE Group. http://www.coregroup.org/index.php?option=com_content&view=article&id=52&Itemid=1. Accessed March 13, 2018.

6. Keeter S, McGeeney K, Weisel R. Coverage error in internet surveys: who web-only surveys miss and how that affects results. Pew Research Center website, http://www.pewresearch.org/files/2015/09/2015-09-22_coverage-error-in-internet-surveys.pdf. Published September 22, 2015. Accessed March 13, 2018.

7. Borg I, Groenen P. *Modern Multidimensional Scaling: Theory and Applications*. New York, NY: Springer-Verlag; 2005.

8. Krueger RA, Casey MA. *Focus Groups: A Practical Guide for Applied Research*. 5th ed. Los Angeles, CA: Sage Publishing; 2015.

9. PhotoVoice [home page]. https://photovoice.org. Accessed December 29, 2015.

10. Introduction to Amazon Mechanical Turk. Amazon Mechanical Turk website. http://docs.aws.amazon.com/AWSMechTurk/latest/AWSMechanicalTurkGettingStartedGuide/SvcIntro.html. Published August 15, 2014. Accessed September 17, 2016.

11. What & why of usability. Usability.gov website. http://www.usability.gov/basics/ucd/index.html. Accessed March 13, 2018.

Appendix 7A

Using PhotoVoice in Formative Research

Rickie Brawer, Ellen J. Plumb, Melissa Fogg, Brandon Knettel, Margaret Fulda, Abbie Santana, Melissa DiCarlo, and James Plumb

Meaningful community involvement is crucial to effective formative assessment. Engaging the community early and throughout the process creates opportunities to identify and communicate the cultural and social assets and perspectives that may promote or undermine intervention plans. Involving the community informs decisions about priorities for programs or system improvements and encourages their involvement in addressing the problems and quality of life in their community. The community may lack the knowledge and skills needed to conduct a systematic formative evaluation; however, they are often experts in understanding and using formal and informal community networks that influence problems in their community. Equitable partnerships between the academic community and community stakeholders where formative evaluation is conducted jointly can lead to more meaningful assessments and generate impactful solutions for community problems. Using a community-based participatory approach conducted by and for those most directly affected by the issue, condition, situation, or intervention being studied or evaluated can move communities toward positive social change.[1,2]

▶ Community-Based Participatory Research

Community-based participatory research (CBPR) is a partnership approach to research that emphasizes the equitable involvement of community members, organizations, and researchers in all aspects of the research process.[3,4] In other words, it is research that is conducted by and for those most directly affected by the issue, condition, situation, or intervention being evaluated. The main goal of CBPR in public health is to identify and resolve an issue of social, structural, or physical environmental inequality and improve the quality of life of a community as a whole. The effectiveness of CBPR as a research approach is based on several key assumptions, namely that people in an affected population are more willing to communicate with researchers that they know and trust, have greater insight into and information on the effects of a particular issue of concern, and have the ability to assign differential importance to data based on their personal knowledge of their community. The partnered approach of CBPR also often leads to greater acceptance of research findings by target communities.

The CBPR research approach is best used when the research issue in question relies on the experiential knowledge of the community rather than on the academic skills of a researcher, depends on support from the community members, focuses on empowerment of community member researchers, and provides a framework for long-term partnered social change. By engaging the community in all aspects of research, the CBPR approach has the potential to break down racial, ethnic, and class barriers; help people better understand the factors that influence their lives; change participant perspectives of themselves and what they can accomplish; and move communities toward positive social change.

▶ PhotoVoice as a CBPR Methodology: "A Picture Is Worth a Thousand Words"

PhotoVoice is a CBPR approach that promotes critical dialogue and knowledge about important community issues through the use of documentary photography, storytelling, and social action.[5,6] Shown to be an effective way to link needs assessment with community participation, the PhotoVoice methodology has three main goals: enabling people to record and reflect on their community's strengths and concerns, promoting critical dialogue about important issues through large- and small-group discussion of photographs, and reaching policymakers.[6] The PhotoVoice methodology provides an important opportunity to empower participants to become cultural brokers through bringing explanations, ideas, or stories of community members into the assessment process; allows for the documentation of both the needs and assets of a community; and provides tangible and immediate benefit to community members.[7]

Furthermore, the methodology enables healthcare providers and researchers to explore the experiences and perspectives of participants across an otherwise difficult-to-access sample of behavioral, cultural, and social settings.[5] The PhotoVoice method has been used to examine a range of public health concerns from chronic health problems[8] to political violence[9] and in all age groups from early adolescents to seniors.[10]

The PhotoVoice process includes partnership building and community participation, photographic training, facilitated small- and large-group discussion, and participatory analysis.[6] Consistent with CBPR, PhotoVoice recognizes that participants are best able to define and articulate their own needs and are the most capable of designing public health efforts to address those needs. The "who" of PhotoVoice projects are typically those individuals or communities that have identified an interest in improving their health. Facilitation of the projects usually includes inside and outside facilitators. Although there are some components of training for PhotoVoice projects that are dependent on the specific goals and culture of the engaged community, all trainings aim to address the key issues around ethics and photography as well as technical and mechanical camera training. Some important points of discussion that are posed during photographic training include acceptable ways to approach people to take their picture and using photographs of people without their knowledge. During facilitated small- and large-group discussions, participants discuss and contextualize selected photographs using the SHOWED approach (bolded letters in **BOX 7A-1**).

Participatory analysis of the photographs involves three phases: selection of photographs that best reflect community needs and assets, contextualizing or narrating the photographs, and codifying the photographs into emerging themes. In addition to the photographic image data, the large- and small-group discussions produce a different type of data for analysis. The

---

BOX 7A-1 SHOWED Approach

1. What do you **S**ee happening here?
2. What is really **H**appening here?
3. How does this relate to **O**ur lives?
4. **W**hy does this situation, concern, or strength exist?
5. How could this image **E**ducate the community?
6. What can we **D**o about it?

---

triangulation of these different types of data enhances research findings and helps drive action.

With its focus on empowerment and advocacy, the PhotoVoice methodology is an effective approach to use when trying to publicize a group's situation or particular issue of importance or when a group needs a powerful way to influence policymakers. As the saying goes, "a picture is worth a thousand words" in its potential impact. Additionally, PhotoVoice can be used to conduct community assessment, to perform program evaluation, and to document a way of life or situation that is threatened. Vulnerable populations who lack a voice and power in society are most likely to benefit from the PhotoVoice methodology, including homeless populations; persons who suffer with mental health issues, physical disabilities, and/or chronic disease; members of racial, ethnic, linguistic, religious, or cultural minorities; and people who are discriminated against because of class, way of life, or poverty.

The following case study describes how PhotoVoice was used to empower and address health concerns of a vulnerable community in the city of Philadelphia. It demonstrates formative research using a CBPR approach and the PhotoVoice methodology.

▶ Case Study: The Philadelphia Urban Food and Fitness Alliance: Engaging Youth in a Needs Assessment and Advocacy Program Related to Physical Activity and Healthy Eating

In 2008, the Philadelphia Urban Food and Fitness Alliance (PUFFA) was one of nine communities in the

United States to receive a 2-year planning grant from the W.K. Kellogg Foundation Food & Fitness initiative. The purpose of the funding was to support development of a comprehensive community action plan that recommended system and policy interventions to reduce the impact of childhood obesity, including diabetes and high blood pressure. These recommendations were to focus on four key priorities:

- Transforming school food systems
- Improving community food environments
- Promoting active living and routine physical activity
- Sustaining and expanding the growing national movement for healthy food and active living

The grant stipulated that planning had to be community driven, reflect community preferences, and focus on vulnerable children (defined as children who live in unsafe neighborhoods, live in unhealthy conditions, come from single-parent–headed households, are children of color, or come from segregated communities). At the end of the 2-year planning grant, grant recipients were eligible to apply for an additional 5 years of funding to implement their plan.

At the time of the grant, 65% of adults and 47% of children in Philadelphia were overweight or obese. PUFFA envisioned addressing the obesity issue by reconnecting Philadelphians to the surrounding land and to food, developing social capital within neighborhood communities, and forming lasting systems changes that supported physical activity and healthy eating habits among youth. PUFFA's mission was to "create vibrant Philadelphia communities that support access to locally grown, healthy and affordable food and safe places for physical activity and play—for everyone."[11]

To accomplish their mission, a community-led delegate assembly, spearheaded by the Health Promotion Council of Southeastern Pennsylvania, the Philadelphia Department of Public Health, White Dog Community Enterprises, and Thomas Jefferson University and Hospital, was created to drive PUFFA's comprehensive community assessment and planning phase. Action teams were formed to address specific topics related to local, healthy foods; nutrition; and physical activity and to ascertain the community's attitudes, behaviors, barriers, and preferences related to access to healthy, affordable food and safe places for physical activity for vulnerable children in Philadelphia.

Formative evaluation was integrated into all action team discussions under the guidance of PUFFA's evaluation team, led by researchers from Thomas Jefferson University and Hospital. The evaluation team, a partnership of community and academic members, developed multiple assessment strategies designed to fully engage youth in the community assessment and planning process. In partnership with the evaluation team, a community-based organization in each of four neighborhoods of interest was recruited to supervise youth during the assessment process. These neighborhoods were chosen based on disparities related to obesity, diversity of the neighborhood, and readiness to change. Youth were trained by the evaluation team to conduct a survey with adults in their neighborhood and to assess local parks and playgrounds. Youth also participated in a PhotoVoice project to document what helps and prevents them from eating healthier and being more physically active in their specific neighborhood. More than 50 youth aged 13 to 18, 150 adults, and 20 organizations participated in at least one component of the assessment process, completing 667 surveys in 21 zip codes, 26 playground assessments, 7 focus groups, and 4 PhotoVoice projects. Youth and community-based organizations involved in conducting the assessments received payment for their services.

PhotoVoice Process

Why PhotoVoice?

PhotoVoice was chosen as an essential community assessment strategy because it is a dynamic tool for conducting formative research, focuses on advocacy, and is effective in engaging youth. Using the PhotoVoice process ensured that the voice of Philadelphia youth in the target communities was heard and informed the community action plan that would be developed. It was critical to the success of PUFFA that youth perceptions and leadership were respected and integrated into the assessment and planning process. We also hoped that youth involved would become advocates for change by raising awareness about how their neighborhood environment supports or prevents healthy eating and physical activity. The details of the PhotoVoice process developed specifically for the PUFFA project were shared with Carolyn Wang, PhD for her expertise and comment.

How Did Youth Get Involved?

Youth were recruited for the PhotoVoice project from four lead community-based organizations (United Communities of Southeast Philadelphia, the 52nd Street Business Association, the East Park Revitalization Association, and Nu Sigma Youth Services) representing the West, North, South, and Bridesburg-Kensington neighborhoods of Philadelphia. Recruitment strategies varied and were headed by the lead organization in each neighborhood. In general, recruited youth were involved in activities that the lead organization or its partners sponsored during the school year or summer program. Approximately 15 youth aged 14–18 from each neighborhood agreed to participate in the PhotoVoice project.

All PhotoVoice procedures were submitted and approved by the institutional review board at Thomas Jefferson University. The parents of the youth involved were required to sign a consent form stating that they were allowing their children to take photos and participate in discussions with audio recording. In addition, youth were required to sign an assent form stating that the study was explained to them and that they had a chance to ask questions.

What Did Youth Do as Part of PhotoVoice?

Training. Youth participants took part in three to four PhotoVoice sessions that involved about 20 hours of interaction. The first session introduced youth to the concept of PhotoVoice and the techniques involved. Using photographs taken in Kenya by one of the researchers, a simulated PhotoVoice process that explored the impact of the environment and culture on access to healthy food and physical activity was presented and the SHOWED model was explained. One of the most important points made during this introduction was the rules of the picture-taking process. For safety reasons, the evaluation team and lead community-based organizations required that photography be confined to within a 10- to 13-block radius of the lead community-based organization. The designated areas were predominantly residential and included schools, businesses, playgrounds, parks, recreation centers, healthcare facilities, murals, farmers' markets, and gardening projects. In addition, the following safety precautions were implemented: (1) photo sessions were conducted in groups with an adult leader, (2) all participants were required to wear t-shirts that identified the PUFFA project, and (3) PhotoVoice trainings stressed not taking pictures of individuals' faces or of situations that might put them in danger (such as gambling in the park). To illustrate unsafe situations, youth were encouraged to take a picture of something that could represent the problem but keep them safe at the same time.

The first session also included instruction from an experienced photographer on digital camera use and how to take a good photograph. This was followed by a brainstorming session designed to introduce youth to the PhotoVoice research question: What helps or prevents you from eating healthy and being physically active in your community? Four questions were posed on flip charts around the room to engage youth in thinking about the types of pictures they might want to take to illustrate their perceptions about the question. These questions were: (1) What do you do to be physically active and eat healthy? (2) How often are you physically active? (3) Where do you go to be physically active and eat healthy? (4) What do you want to see in your community in order to be more physically active and eat healthier? This activity was followed by a practice photo session. Youth were divided into groups of two to three with at least one adult supervisor and instructed to take photos for 30 minutes, after which the groups reconvened and discussed their pictures with the larger group using the SHOWED model. At the conclusion of the session, the youth were asked to think about the types of photos and places where they would like to take pictures for the next session.

Get Out and Take Pictures, Discuss, and Choose Meaningful Photographs. The second PhotoVoice session involved a two- to three-hour photography session, after which photos were downloaded onto computers. Each group then chose 20 photos they wanted to discuss with the whole group using the SHOWED process. Individuals shared what the photo meant to them and why they took it. Discussion was then opened up to the entire group to gain other perspectives about the photographs and how they might influence policymakers and the public. During the discussion, the group facilitator kept notes on a large flip chart and used member checking in order to ensure the accuracy of the notes. Additionally, two staff members took notes, and the session was audio recorded. At the completion of the second session, students were asked to choose three to five of their pictures and write a short meaningful caption for each.

In the third PhotoVoice session, youth were encouraged to discuss the photo captions individually with the researchers and lead organization staff. Selected pictures and captions were then placed into a PowerPoint presentation and printed out to facilitate thematic analysis by the youth. Youth were asked to group the pictures into themes or similar groups and to then title each group of photos to reflect the theme. Once the themes were finalized, the discussion moved toward advocacy. The group leader addressed each theme and asked the youth what they felt should be done, what they could do, and what they would be willing to do to advocate for change or address the issues. The discussion was audio recorded and transcribed. **TABLE 7A-1** illustrates the selected themes and examples of photo captions.

TABLE 7A-1 Selected Themes and Captions	
Theme	**Caption**
Options	
Food availability (photos of empty shelves and rotten vegetables; **FIGURE 7A-1**)	"This corner store has empty shelves and spoiled vegetables. The empty shelves could be filled with healthy food. Fresh fruits and vegetables should be delivered to stores every day."
Food affordability (photos of juice, milk, and soda and the prices of each)	"If you sold sugar for $5 and apples for $.50, people would eat the apples!"
Marketing	
Promotion and placement (photos of fast food windows)	"On Snyder Plaza I feel as though the plaza has no places where there is something healthy for you to eat, the only thing you see is bars and junk food. Subway was one of the only places that you might be able to get something healthy for you, but instead of advertising healthy food in the window, they put a steak up instead, which I feel is wrong."
Aesthetics	
Trash (photos of garbage in neighborhood; **FIGURE 7A-2**)	"It takes a sign on a house for people to use their common sense. I think without the trash the neighborhood would be prettier and more kids would play outside because they wouldn't have to play in the trash."
	"No one should have to tell people where they shouldn't throw trash. They should automatically know to throw stuff in the trash can. The trash makes people not want to do physical activities because they don't want to run in litter."
Beautification (photos of murals inspire and activate people when they walk)	"Murals enhance the neighborhood, causing the people to take care of the community more often. Murals also send messages to encourage youth and adults to live life positively."
Safety	
Equipment and conditions (photos of playgrounds in disrepair)	"Playgrounds in some communities have poor quality equipment."
	"Playgrounds that are trashed, torn apart, and have drug-related problems are rarely used."

This Corner Store has empty shelves and spoiled vegetables. The empty shelves could be filled with healthy food. Fresh fruits and vegetables should be delivered to stores every day.

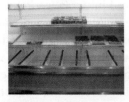
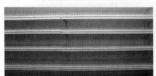
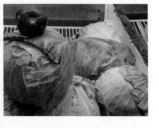

FIGURE 7A-1 PhotoVoice image of produce at corner store.

It takes a sign on a house for people to use their common sense. I think without the trash the neighborhood would be prettier and more kids would play outside because they wouldn't have to play in the trash.
Teen – age 16

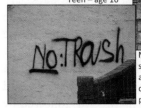

No one should have to tell people where they shouldn't throw trash. They should automatically know to throw stuff in the trash can. The trash makes people not want to do physical activities because they don't want to run in litter.
Teen – age 14

FIGURE 7A-2 PhotoVoice image of trash in neighborhood.

Sharing Findings. The final PhotoVoice session brought youth from all four participating communities together to present their PhotoVoices to each other and participating adults. The teens were then asked what similarities and differences they had noticed across the communities. The PhotoVoice team then posted premade flip charts that listed all of the suggestions the teens had put in their presentation for "What needs to be done" and "What teens can do." The list was reviewed, and youth were asked for additions to the list. Once the teens felt the list was complete, they were given dots of each of the following colors—red (1 point), yellow (2 points), and green (3 points)—and instructed to vote for "What needs to be done" and for "What teens can do." Points were summed to prioritize advocacy efforts and roles for youth in the community action plan. Priorities included the following:

- Aesthetics of the environment and food access issues have an influence on youth's ability to choose healthy behaviors. They felt that youth could help keep their community clean by picking up trash, participating in community clean-ups, and advocating for more trash cans and more frequent trash pickup.
- In addition to improving the built environment and access to healthy affordable food, youth recommended raising community awareness about healthy eating and being physically active. Youth could educate younger children about healthy eating and the importance of being physically active and promote youth activities and opportunities to advocate for community change through development of a youth council and the use of social media.
- Youth pictures and discussions highlighted the need for more equitable playgrounds and parks, improved facilities, and options for physical activities that allow children of all ages and families to be active. Community gardening projects were recommended as a great way to both engage people in physical activity and provide fresh produce. Vacant lots could be transformed into gardens, which would also beautify the community and make it feel safer.
- Youth felt that enforcing current regulations and laws such as not littering, not drinking alcohol in parks, and other illegal acts (public gambling, illegal drug use, and prostitution) would improve perceptions of community safety and encourage people in their neighborhood to be more physically active.

At the conclusion of this meeting, the teens were invited to join the PUFFA Youth Action Team and to present their findings to the full PUFFA Alliance to increase consciousness about the issues from the teens' point of view and to celebrate their achievements. Each of the partner community-based organizations was given an electronic copy of the photos, captions, and the group's slide show at completion of the project. Youth were given a framed copy of one of their photographs.

The Evaluation Team and adult leaders then reviewed notes and transcripts from each of the PhotoVoice sessions to inform thematic analysis across all PhotoVoice projects. An initial coding scheme was developed and refined based on coding conducted individually and through group coding conferences. Triangulation was used to resolve conflicts and improve validity.

Microsoft Excel was used to sort common themes and determine the frequencies of themes within groups and across sites. Cross-cutting themes included Community Safety, Community Beautification and Cleanliness, Community Mobilization and Engagement (volunteerism, building relationships, responsibility, initiative), Affordable Food and Transportation, Facility Improvement, Neighborhood Equity, Programming Enhancements, and Marketing (promotion of programs/services/resources and promotion/placement of food).

Finally, the four presentations and final recommendations from the youth were integrated into a single presentation for the larger community that used a storytelling approach and combined PhotoVoice themes and related pictures with survey data and focus group findings and quotes. Youth and adult leaders from the lead organizations enacted the scripted story while the PhotoVoice pictures were shown in the background. This was followed by a community discussion of the findings and recommendations.

From PhotoVoice to Action

As a result of the PhotoVoice projects, youth in one community identified a play structure that had a sliding board that was misaligned and a potential fall hazard. Youth, with their site leader, contacted the city recreational center responsible for that city park, and the slide, which had been this way for more than a year, was fixed within a week. This early advocacy success by the youth set the stage for reconnecting the community to the park and the city rec center and spurred the formation of a Friends of the Park group.

Thematic priorities identified during the assessment process were integrated into a 5-year action plan of system and policy changes to improve access to healthy food and safe places for physical activity in Philadelphia. Philadelphia received funding from the W.K. Kellogg Foundation to implement the plan. Key activities in the plan included:

- Increasing the number of children eating breakfast and lunch in Philadelphia schools
- Improving the nutritional quality of food served at breakfast and lunch
- Effecting change in the sedentary culture
- Increasing the number and quality of available space through active physical involvement in neighborhood revitalization efforts
- Increasing the purchasing power of families with children by maximizing enrollment and benefit levels in the Supplemental Nutrition Assistance Program and the Special Supplemental Nutrition program for Women, Infants, and Children
- Advocating for policy changes to increase acceptance of Electronic Benefit Transfer cards among vendors selling farm-fresh produce
- Supporting the expansion of a wide variety of food outlets serving affordable local produce by linking them to the Common Market and other food distribution initiatives

The funding also allowed for the development of the PUFFA Youth Action Team and the Advocacy Institute, which continues to provide advocacy training for youth in Philadelphia. PUFFA youth developed public service announcements and videos with WHYY (a local public television station) and MEE Productions to support healthier behaviors among teens. PUFFA Youth Action Team members created Students Advocating for Lifestyle Transformation (SALT), and then they and PUFFA teens were sent to advocate and speak out for more quality food in schools; access to healthier food in communities; and more safe, open spaces for play and physical activity. Social media (Facebook, Twitter, blogging) were used to encourage lifestyle changes and to promote unique activities such as PUFFA's dance mob held in Love Park. Youth also presented at local and national conferences about their efforts in Philadelphia.

At the conclusion of the PUFFA grant, SALT and PUFFA youth were encouraged to join Food Fit Philly (part of the Philadelphia Department of Health's Get Healthy Philly: Working Together for a Healthy, Active and Smoke-Free City initiative) and Get HYPE Philly!, a citywide initiative led by the Food Trust and a collective of 10 nonprofit organizations to empower Philly's young people as leaders, preparing them to live healthier lives and create healthier communities.

Overall, the project was successful in empowering students. There were a number of "lessons learned," however, in how the project was implemented, as discussed in the following.

Evaluate: Lessons Learned

- Need to be flexible in the number and timing of PhotoVoice sessions based on site needs.
- Following the completion of the first site Photo-Voice project, youth and staff felt that additional time and assistance were needed prior to initiating the photo session. Prior to implementing the project in the other communities, an interactive activity was created to encourage teens to think about what in the community they would like to photograph. This activity, conducted at the beginning of the second session, asked teens to draw a picture on newsprint that answered the question, "If teens ruled the world and could design a vacant lot, what would you put there?" In addition, instead of working with the teens individually to develop captions, the teens were split into their photo groups to develop captions and create slides for their group PowerPoint presentation. In many cases the group decided to take specific pictures; therefore, writing the caption needed to be a group effort. In addition, this allowed for more interaction and less time spent waiting for everyone to finish. Working in groups encouraged more conversation during the development of the captions as well as full group discussions following the creation of the presentations.
- Youth are effective at advocacy efforts to promote healthy lifestyle changes. Sustaining youth engagement and leadership can be problematic given competing priorities and graduation from high school. For successful engagement, consideration should be given to student schedules, interests, and time available for participation. Efforts to build leadership should be ongoing.

References

1. Kumanyika SK, Story M, Beech BM, et al. Collaborative planning for formative research and cultural appropriateness in the Girls Health Enrichment Multi-site Studies (GEMS): a retrospection. *Ethn Dis.* 2003;13:S15-S29.

2. Viswanathan M, Ammerman A, Eng E, et al. *Community-Based Participatory Research: Assessing the Evidence.* Evidence Report/Technology Assessment No. 99. AHRQ Publication No. 04-E022-1. Rockville, MD: Agency for Healthcare Research and Quality; August 2004.

3. Israel BA, Schulz AJ, Parker EA, Becker AB. Review of community-based research: assessing partnership approaches to improve public health. *Annu Rev Public Health.* 1998;19:173-202.

4. Israel BA, Schulz AJ, Parker EA, Becker AB, Allen A, Guzman JR. Critical issues in developing and following CBPR principles. In: Minkler M, Wallerstein N, eds. *Community-Based Participatory Research for Health: From Process to Outcomes.* 2nd ed. San Francisco, CA: Jossey-Bass; 2008:47-66.

5. Genuis SK, Willows N, First Nation A, Jardine C. Through the lens of our cameras: children's lived experience with food security in a Canadian indigenous community [published online ahead of print]. *Child: Care Health Dev.* 2014. doi:10.1111/cch.12182.

6. Wang C, Burris MA. PhotoVoice: concept, methodology, and use for participatory needs assessment. *Health Educ Behav.* 1997;24:369-387. doi:10.1177/109019819702400309.

7. Wang C, Burris MA. PhotoVoice: concept, methodology, and use for participatory needs assessment. *Health Educ Behav.* 1997;24:369-387. doi:10.1177/109019819702400309.

8. Oliffe JL, Bottorff JL. Further than the eye can see? Photo-elicitation and research with men. *Qualit Health Res.* 2007;17(6):850-858.

9. Lykes MB, Blanche MT, Hamber B. Narrating survival and change in Guatemala and South Africa: the politics of representation and a liberatory community psychology. *Am J Commun Psychol.* 2003;31(1-2):79-90.

10. Catalani C, Minkler M. PhotoVoice: a review of the literature in health and public health. *Health Educ Behav.* 2010;37(3):424-451.

11. Philadelphia Higher Education Network for Neighborhood Development. Philadelphia Urban Food and Fitness Alliance Open House. http://phennd.org/update/philadelphia-urban-food-and-fitness-alliance-open-house. Published June 8, 2009.

Appendix 7B

Steps in Tailoring a Text Messaging–Based Smoking Cessation Program for Young Adults: Iterative Intervention Refinement

Michele L. Ybarra

Helping young people quit smoking has both immediate and long-term impacts on smoking-associated morbidity and mortality.[1,2] Unfortunately, cigarette smoking is relatively common among 18- to 24-year-olds: 22–34% are current smokers.[3,4] Although over half would like to cut back on their smoking or quit entirely, few are successful.[5-9] This may be a result of young adult smokers underutilizing evidence-based treatments, as well as insufficient programming that is targeted toward and accessible to this group.[10-14]

Over 90% of young adults in the United States use text messaging,[15] and thus text messaging may serve as an ideal mode for delivering smoking cessation programs. Stop My Smoking USA (SMS USA) is a mobile health (mHealth) smoking cessation program that was tailored for young adult smokers in the United States. The content was originally developed as a smoking cessation program for adult smokers in Ankara, Turkey[16]; however, in order to address the unique needs of young adult smokers in the United States, the content needed to be tailored to the experiences and issues of the target population.

The SMS prototype was evaluated via user-based assessments and usability testing. Four activities were implemented: a needs assessment with young adults to gain a better understanding of their smoking behaviors and past attempts at quitting, as well as to determine the acceptability of possible program components; a content advisory team to verify acceptability, tone, and understandability of messages; and two beta tests of the intervention program to ensure the technological and programmatic logistics of the intervention. The development activities were completed in just over one year, from November 2009 to December 2010.

In order to be eligible for participation in this study, individuals had to be 18–25 years of age, smoke at least 24 cigarettes per week (at least 4 per day on at least 6 days per week), own a cell phone with texting capabilities, be enrolled or intend to enroll in an unlimited texting plan, agree to have their smoking cessation status verified by a significant other, and be able to read and write in English.

▶ Activity #1: Needs Assessment Focus Groups

In order to complete a needs assessment, two focus groups were conducted. The focus groups explored participants' reasons for smoking, triggers for smoking, and awareness and interest in smoking cessation. The acceptability of two proposed program components was also examined—*Text Crave*, which provides immediate text responses to help deal with cravings in the moment, and *Text Buddy*, in which two smokers going through the quit process are paired to provide support for one another.[17]

The focus groups were conducted online by Cruz Research, a survey research firm experienced in conducting online focus groups. A script of questions was used as a guide for the moderator's questions and included some of the following:

- What would you say are key reasons why you smoke?
- Describe when it's most difficult for you *not* to smoke.

- If you tried to quit smoking, would you use a quitting aid like the nicotine patch?
- What would keep you in a 6-month-long smoking cessation program?

Participants were divided into focus groups according to their school status, based on the belief that young adults in and out of a university setting may have different smoking patterns and quitting experiences. Nineteen individuals participated in the in-school focus group and 16 in the nonschool focus group. In each group, participants visited an online bulletin board two to three times per day for 3 days and responded to the moderator's questions and the comments posted from other participants. Transcripts of the focus group discussions were coded using a priori and emergent codes using ATLAS.ti.

Overall responses suggested that participants were highly addicted to nicotine. Many participants were unaware of or had mixed opinions about the use of pharmacotherapy, and expressed concerns about the cost and understanding of the cessation options. Participants were interested in quitting smoking because of immediate and long-term health consequences, social negatives, smell, and cost. Although participants were seriously considering quitting smoking within the next month, they generally lacked a clear plan of how they would quit; many seemed to want their willpower to get them through the quitting process. Participants' responses showed a strong social component to their smoking; thus, they associated smoking with many of their day-to-day activities. Smoking cues included alcohol, stress, driving, ending a meal, needing to focus, being bored, and as a way to take a break. Participants had favorable perceptions of both the Text Crave and Text Buddy program components.

After the needs assessment phase was completed, the information derived was integrated back into the program. Messages regarding concerns and triggers for young adults were added into the program's content. For instance, "Quitting nicotine with nicotine seems strange, but it really does work to help you learn to break the habit of smoking without the initial withdrawal." Messages were also developed that focused on common triggers for young adults in order to prepare them for those situations. For example, because going to bars was a common trigger, "When you go out with your friends to the bar, watch the nonsmokers. What do they do? What will you do as a nonsmoker? Have a plan and you'll be successful." Based on the literature, it also was important to help young adults develop a plan to quit; this provided structure rather than just a process that one hoped to "get through."

Activity #2: Content Advisory Team

Acceptability of specific program messages was confirmed by the content advisory team. They also tested the recruitment plan for the proposed randomized controlled trial.

Twenty young adults were recruited online primarily through Facebook and Craigslist. Each participant received 20% of the proposed text messages spanning the entire program and were given one week to provide feedback on the content. Participants provided qualitative reactions to the messages by answering such questions as: Do the messages energize you/turn you off? Is the message clear? What thoughts would go through your mind if a friend intercepted and read one of the messages on your cell phone? Participants were also asked to engage in a 2-day online bulletin board discussion with other members of the content advisory team to discuss their thoughts and reactions to the messages. This activity provided an opportunity for the group to come together on the salience and tone of the messages.

Although only 50% of participants provided content feedback, feedback was provided by at least one participant for each of the proposed text messages. Overall, participants preferred positive, encouraging messages rather than those that were negative or shocking, and did not like those that seemed condescending or lecturing. There was also a preference for messages that did not specifically use the word *smoking* or refer to their previous smoking behavior because they felt both might serve as a trigger. Additionally, they did not like messages that discussed the physical withdrawal of quitting or the use of the word *medication* when discussing pharmacotherapies.

After the intervention text messages were reviewed and themes of perceptions discerned, the text messages were revised. The researchers took care to balance the preferences of the content advisory team with the need to ensure that the content was evidence-based. For instance, text messages that asked people to think about their previous quit attempts were reframed. Rather than saying, "Think back to your past attempts to quit," the message was changed into a more general statement: "Some people may feel like a failure from unsuccessful quit attempts. Most smokers try to quit 6–7 times before they quit for good." Content that could be perceived as negative was made more positive. Also, lecturing messages (e.g., "Don't think you can have just one cigarette. Stay smoke-free. For now, stay clear of situations where you are most likely to want a cigarette.") were reframed to be more supportive (e.g., "Continue to stay clear of situations where you are most likely to want a cigarette. You've put a lot of effort into preparing for and actually quitting. Look how long you've been smoke-free.")

▶ Activity #3: Beta Test 1: Confirming Initial Technological Feasibility

Next it was necessary to confirm that the intervention would be technologically feasible to implement. Beta Test 1 was used to confirm functionality of the program's components, including the randomization process, the Text Buddy and Text Crave components, and the recruitment protocol.

Twelve participants recruited online (75% from Craigslist) were randomized to either the intervention group or the attention-matched control group that received messages about improving fitness and sleep patterns. Participants received the first week of their respective study arm's prequit messages. Each participant was paired with a Text Buddy with whom they were to send two text messages per day. They were also told to use the Text Crave feature at least once during the 1-week field period. Individual interviews were conducted to discuss any challenges and identify areas for program improvements.

The text messaging software functioned properly, as did the randomization program. Participants received their arm's text messages, received on-demand Text Crave messages, and communicated with their Text Buddy without incident. However, some smaller cell phone providers were incompatible with the program software. Participants found the Text Buddy component to be helpful and liked receiving the on-demand Text Crave messages. Participants preferred Text Crave messages that were behavioral-focused (e.g., "Distract yourself: Text someone a text with exactly 140 characters.") rather than cognitive-focused (e.g., "Focus on not allowing yourself a single puff. This is the fastest way through the cravings.") They also preferred Text Crave messages that were unrelated to smoking because they felt they were less

likely to reinforce the desire to smoke. Prequit messages that encouraged the maintenance of a smoking diary were perceived as "too time consuming" or something that others, but not themselves, would find helpful.

As a result of Beta Test 1, additional behavioral messages were added to the pool of Text Crave messages. A new eligibility requirement was also included to ensure that participants' cell phone providers were compatible with the intervention program's software. Any references to a smoking "diary" were changed to refer to a "log." Using an online recruitment strategy was deemed optimal.

▶ Activity #4: Beta Test 2: Confirming Technological Feasibility of the Full Program

Beta Test 2 was unanticipated, but necessary to assess any technological challenges occurring later in the 6-week program. In contrast with the 1-week Beta Test 1, participants received all 6 weeks of the intervention text messages. Research suggests that quit attempters are most likely to relapse within the first 7 days of quitting,[18] so intervention participants were contacted via text messaging at 2 days after quit day and 7 days after quit day to assess whether they were smoking. Based on their responses, they were pathed to different content (e.g., to relapse messages in order to help them recommit to quitting if they indicated they were still smoking). Consequently, a key purpose of Beta Test 2 was to verify proper pathing of intervention participants.

Twenty-eight participants were recruited online, primarily through Craigslist, and randomly assigned to either SMS USA or the control arm. Intervention participants were paired with a Text Buddy and given access to Text Crave. Follow-up data were collected at 4 weeks by text messaging, at 12 weeks by phone and online, and at 1 year by text messaging. Follow-up response rates were high: 71% completed the 4-week text messaging–based follow-up survey, 64% completed the 12-week online survey, and 68% completed the 1-year text messaging–based survey.

The registration and baseline survey, which were conducted over the phone, took 45–60 minutes to complete, which participants felt was too time-consuming. The timing was therefore an impediment to enrollment. Most candidates preferred being contacted by text message rather than by phone or email. Significant technological issues, including cell phone access (e.g., participants had unlimited text messaging, but had a smaller cell phone provider that was not compatible with the program) and programming issues (e.g., participants in the intervention group were not pathed correctly at 2 days and 7 days postquit) were also encountered. Problems occurred in the sections of the program that had not been tested in Beta Test 1.

As a result of Beta Test 2, the enrollment process was adjusted so that the registration portion was conducted over the phone, but the participants were then emailed a link to complete the baseline survey online. The significant technological problems were thoroughly addressed and tested before the pilot randomized controlled trial was launched. Indeed, once technology issues were attended to, a final internal team tested the intervention program from quit date through the final pathing stage (i.e., 7 days after quit day) to ensure all problems were resolved.

▶ Lessons Learned

Refinement of SMS USA to ensure its saliency for young adults in the United States was iterative and provided important experiences about testing a new intervention. Five steps to refining an mHealth program were identified:

1. Conduct needs assessment focus groups with your target audience to better understand their decision making around the risk behavior and trying to affect behavior change, and to confirm acceptability of program components.

2. Integrate findings from the focus groups into the draft of the program content.

3. Test the acceptability of drafted content, ideally with a two-stage focus group that allows for direct feedback on each specific text message, as well as global feedback on the content as a whole.

4. Integrate findings into the final content pool.

5. Confirm the technological feasibility of the entire intervention before fielding the planned trial.

Specific examples of how to integrate user feedback into the content of an intervention demonstrate how participatory research designs are important for ensuring that the content is salient to the target population and will be used by them, in addition to remaining adherent to behavior change theory. Iterative intervention refinement work is time consuming and costly; however, it increases the likelihood that the final product will be useful and acceptable to the target audience.

Acknowledgments

With acknowledgment to Tonya L. Prescott and Jodi Summers Holtrop, who contributed to the original study and publication from which this case study was created.

References

1. Centers for Disease Control and Prevention. Quitting smoking among adults—United States, 2001–2010. *MMWR*. 2011;60:1513-1519.

2. U.S. Department of Health and Human Services. *Preventing Tobacco Use Among Youth and Young Adults: A Report of the Surgeon General, 2012*. Atlanta, GA: Author; 2012. https://www.surgeongeneral.gov/library/reports/preventing-youth-tobacco-use/index.html. Accessed March 13, 2018.

3. Centers for Disease Control and Prevention. Vital signs: current cigarette smoking among adults aged 18 years—United States, 2009. *MMWR*. 2010;59:1135-1140.

4. Substance Abuse and Mental Health Services Administration. *Results from the 2010 National Survey on Drug Use and Health: Summary of National Findings*. NSDUH Series H-41 ed., Vol. 2012. Rockville, MD: Author; 2011. http://www.samhsa.gov/data/NSDUH/2k10NSDUH/2k10Results.htm. Accessed March 13, 2018.

5. Lamkin L, Davis B, Kamen A. Rationale for tobacco cessation interventions in youth. *Prev Med*. 1998;27(5 Pt. 3):A3-A8. doi:10.1006=pmed.1998.0386.

6. Reeder AL, Williams S, McGee R, Poulton R. Nicotine dependence and attempts to quit or cut down among young adult smokers. *N Z Med J*. 2001;114:403-406.

7. Stone SL, Kristeller JL. Attitudes of adolescents toward smoking cessation. *Am J Prev Med*. 1992;8:221-225.

8. Centers for Disease Control and Prevention. Smoking cessation during the previous year among adults—United States, 1990 and 1991. *MMWR*. 1993;42:504-507.

9. Centers for Disease Control and Prevention. Cigarette smoking among adults—United States, 2000. *MMWR*. 2002;51:642-645.

10. Curry S, Sporer AK, Pugach O, Campbell RT, Emery S. Use of tobacco cessation treatments among adult smokers: 2005 National Health Interview Survey. *Am J Public Health*. 2007;97:1464-1469. doi:10.2105=AJPH.2006.103788.

11. Solberg LI, Asche SE, Boyle R, McCarty MC, Thoele MJ. Smoking and cessation behaviors among young adults of various educational backgrounds. *Am J Public Health*. 2007;97:1421-1426. doi:10.2105=AJPH.2006.098491.

12. Bader P, Travis HE, Skinner HA. Knowledge synthesis of smoking cessation among employed and unemployed young adults. *Am J Public Health*. 2007;97:1434-1443. doi:10.2105=AJPH.2006.100909.

13. Lantz PM. Smoking on the rise among young adults: implications for research and policy. *Tobacco Control*. 2003;12(suppl 1):i60-i70. doi:10.1136=tc.12.suppl_1.i60.

14. Murphy-Hoefer R, Griffith R, Pederson LL, Crossett L, Iyer SR, Hiller MD. A review of interventions to reduce tobacco

use in colleges and universities. *Am J Prev Med.* 2005;28:188-200. doi:10.1016=j.amepre.2004.10.015.

15. Smith A. Americans and text messaging. Pew Internet & American Life Project website. http://pewinternet.org/Reports/2011/Cell-Phone-Texting-2011/Main-Report/How-Americans-Use-Text-Messaging.aspx. Published September 19, 2011. Accessed March 20, 2018.

16. Ybarra ML, Holtrop JS, Bagci Bosi T, Emri S. Design considerations in developing a text messaging program aimed at smoking cessation. *J Med Internet Res.* 2012;14(4):e103. doi:10.2196=jmir.2061.

17. Rodgers A, Corbett T, Bramley D, et al. Do u smoke after txt? Results of a randomised trial of smoking cessation using mobile phone text messaging. *Tobacco Control.* 2005;14:255-261. doi:10.1136=tc.2005.011577.

18. Zhu SH, Strecher VJ, Balabanis M., Rosbrook B, Sadler G, Pierce JP. Telephone counseling for smoking cessation: effects of single-session and multiple-session interventions. *J Consult Clin Psychol.* 1996;64:202-211. doi:10.1037=0022-006X.64.1.202.

Appendix 7C

Better Bites

Brian J. Biroscak, Ashton Potter Wright, Anita Courtney, and Carol A. Bryant

Social marketing as a discipline seeks to develop and integrate commercial marketing concepts with other approaches to influence behaviors that benefit individuals and communities for the greater social good.[1] As demonstrated by its frequent usage throughout this text, social marketing can add value to many aspects of public health communication. For example, one benchmark criterion of successful social marketing interventions is the use of all elements of the marketing mix (product, price, place, and promotion) to bring about behavior change.[2] The Community Preventive Services Task Force, based on strong evidence of effectiveness for producing intended behavior changes, recommends health communication campaigns that use multiple channels (one of which must be mass media), combined with the distribution of free or reduced-price health-related *products*.[3] Furthermore, recent systematic reviews have demonstrated the effectiveness of social marketing for influencing a wide range of behaviors.[4-6] Here we illustrate the use of formative techniques for strategy development within a social marketing context.

The term *formative* has been defined as: "Serving to form something, especially having a profound and lasting influence on . . . development."[7] Although formative research and formative evaluation are often used interchangeably, they are not one and the same. From a social marketing perspective, *formative research* is at the core of the approach and has been defined broadly to include any primary research that is carried out before a social marketing initiative is undertaken[8] (e.g., to identify potential solutions, to determine priority audiences, and to help create, communicate, and deliver exchange offerings that target audiences will value).[9] In contrast, *formative evaluation* is the use of evaluation strategies and techniques (e.g., reflective practice sessions) to improve and enhance initiatives already underway.[10] Next, we provide an example of formative research for social marketing strategy development, followed by an illustration of formative evaluation.

Formative research is another benchmark of successful social marketing because it identifies *actionable insights* such as motivational drivers and barriers that inform strategy development.[2] We used formative research to develop a social marketing strategy for an initiative designed to surround children with healthy foods in their homes, schools, and communities. Specifically, recreational venues (e.g., parks, pools, etc.) represent a promising setting for making healthy eating the default among younger patrons, but cities have been slow to make changes in parks and recreation vending and concessions.[11-13] The Tweens Nutrition and Fitness Coalition (TN&FC) in Lexington, Kentucky, partnered with the Department of Parks and Recreation to pilot the addition of healthier menu items to the parks' traditional, unhealthy fare at aquatic facility concession stands. The new options, branded as *Better Bites*, offer alternatives to calorie-dense, nutrient-poor items that dominated concessions offerings (see FIGURE 7C-1).

Due to its affiliation with the CDC-funded Florida Prevention Research Center at the University of South Florida—a national leader in social marketing research, education, and practice—the TN&FC engages in extensive formative research before it designs a program, policy, or other intervention. Following the completion of a successful program initiative (VERB Summer Scorecard[14]), the TN&FC decided to undertake policy development. The goal it determined would give it the best return on investment was to increase the amount of healthy foods available at venues sponsored by the local government in Lexington, which eventually became the

Typical Menu	
• Drinks 1.25 (Pepsi, Diet pepsi, Mt. Dew, 7-up, Dr. Pepper) • Water 1.50 • Gatorade 2.00 • Pizza 2.00 • Candy 1.00 • Chips .50 • Popcorn 1.50 • Slushies 1.25	• Nachos 2.00 • Fries 2.00 • Hot dog 1.50 • Hamburger 2.50 • Grilled cheese 1.50 • Nuggets 3.00 • Basket 4.00 • Freeze pop .50 • Ring pops .75

Snack Strong: Healthy, Fun Choices	

**SANDWICHES
AND SUCH**
• **Grilled chicken sandwich** 3.50
• **Chicken salad sandwich** 2.50
• **Grilled chicken wrap** 3.00
• **Cheese quesadilla** 2.25
• **Cheese quesadilla with salsa** 3.00
• **Grilled cheese** 2.00
• **Veggie burger** 2.50
   Hamburger 2.50
   Hot dog 1.50
   Pizza 2.50
   Chicken nuggets 3.50
   Chicken nugget basket 4.50
   Nachos with cheese or salsa 2.50
 	
DRINKS
• **Bottled water** 1.00
   Gatorade 2.00
   Pepsi products 1.25
	SWEET STUFF
	• **Grapes** .75
	• **Apple** .75
	• **Banana** .75
	• **Frozen yogurt** 2.00
	• **Popsicle** .75
	• **Chocolate banana
	   dipper** 1.50
	   Candy 1.25
	
	**SNACKS
	ON THE SIDE**
	• **Veggie dippers** 1.50
	• **Popcorn** 1.50
	• **String cheese** .75
	• **Salsa** .75
	   Baked chips .75
	   Pretzel 2.00
	   French fries 2.50

FIGURE 7C-1 Unhealthy vs. healthy menus.

Better Bites initiative. Prior to launch, however, the TN&FC used a variety of formative research techniques, including observational research, intercept interviews, and surveys, to develop an effective social marketing strategy. Today, Better Bites menu items have grown from representing 9% of concessions sales to 37%. Better Bites has spread to Kentucky state parks, after-school shops, restaurants, youth groups, and other recreational facilities. During the summer of 2014, fruit outsold chicken nuggets by a ratio of 3:1 at the pool concession stands. This community-based social marketing initiative demonstrates that healthier options can be effectively incorporated into concessions and serves as a model for practitioners looking to improve the food environment at recreational facilities.

The TN&FC uses the Florida Prevention Research Center's community-based prevention marketing (CBPM) planning framework, which combines the local wisdom, connections, and influence of a community coalition with sophisticated social marketing tools.[15] Since 2009, the CBPM framework has been adapted and expanded with the intention of enhancing community coalitions' capacity to select, tailor, promote, monitor, and evaluate evidence-based public health policies. This revised framework, CBPM for policy development (**FIGURE 7C-2**), provides coalitions and their research partners with a marketing-driven, systematic planning framework and toolkit to select and promote evidence-based policy changes at the organizational, local, or state level. CBPM for policy development is composed of the following eight steps: (1) build a strong foundation for success; (2) review evidence-based policy options; (3) select a policy to promote; (4) identify priority audiences among beneficiaries, stakeholders, and policymakers; (5) conduct formative research with priority audiences; (6) develop a marketing plan for promoting the policy; (7) develop a plan for monitoring implementation and evaluating impact; and (8) advocate for policy change.

As noted previously, formative research and evaluation are not the same thing; we are using the latter to improve the design of the CBPM for policy development framework via computer simulation. This represents formative evaluation because, with some additional improvements and testing, we are planning to market the CBPM for policy development framework for use by community coalitions, social marketers, and other potential customers. Whereas formative techniques within social marketing traditionally have been classified into two broad categories, quantitative and qualitative,[16] simulation has been described as "a third way of doing science."[17] One approach for gaining a better understanding of the determinants of public health problems prior to intervening is to apply an ecological perspective. There now seems to be sufficient recognition, however, that public health interventions are attempted within complex systems. Thus, another strategy for helping to manage "wicked problems" through an improved understanding of their dynamics is offered by the systems perspective—in particular, *system dynamics modeling*.

System dynamics can be characterized as the use of "systems thinking, management insights, and computer simulation to hypothesize, test, and refine endogenous explanations of systems change, and use those explanations to guide policy and decision making."[18(p241)] The Florida Prevention Research Center initiated a demonstration project to test the CBPM for policy development framework with the

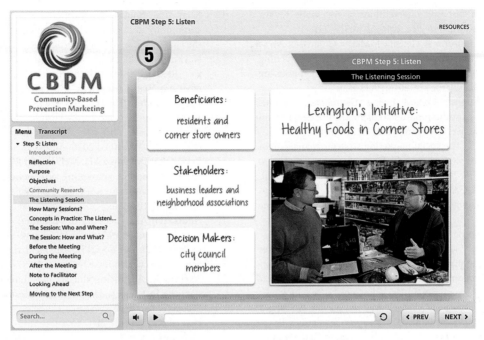

FIGURE 7C-2 Community-based prevention marketing for policy development.
Florida Prevention Research Center.

TN&FC, which generated various types of evaluation data over a period of almost 4 years. Our goal was to use those data to explicate the framework's theory of change so that its design can be improved before taking the framework to market. Results from computer model simulations show how gains in performance depend on a community coalition's initial culture and initial efficiency, and that only the most efficient coalitions may see benefits in coalition performance from implementing CBPM for policy development.

In summary, social marketing strategy development, enhanced by formative research, can add value to public health initiatives—even when used for policy and advocacy. For example, Better Bites, a policy-based initiative developed through a community coalition's use of the CBPM planning framework, continues to show evidence of success. Regarding formative evaluation, system dynamics modeling is a valuable tool in

the evaluation toolbox—as demonstrated by our application of it to decipher CBPM's theory of change—and can help the reader go beyond a traditional ecological perspective. We close with several opportunities for the reader to learn more and gain experience with the techniques described:

- Connect with other social marketers by joining the Social Marketing Association of North America (http://smana.org).
- Explore possibilities for applying formative research to policy and advocacy through learning modules available on the CBPM framework website (http://health.usf.edu/publichealth/cfh/prc/cbpm).
- Learn more about system dynamics modeling by visiting the website of the System Dynamics Society (http://www.systemdynamics.org).

References

1. The iSMA, ESMA and AASM consensus definition of social marketing. International Social Marketing Association website. http://www.i-socialmarketing.org/assets/social_marketing_definition.pdf. Published 2013. Accessed March 13, 2018.
2. Social marketing benchmark criteria. National Social Marketing Centre website. http://thensmc.com/sites/default/files/benchmark-criteria-090910.pdf. Published 2010. Accessed March 13, 2018.
3. Health communication and social marketing: health communication campaigns that include mass media and health-related product distribution. Community Preventive Services Task Force website. http://www.thecommunityguide.org/healthcommunication/campaigns.html. Published 2010. Accessed March 13, 2018.
4. Firestone R, Rowe CJ, Modi SN, Sievers D. The effectiveness of social marketing in global health: a systematic review. *Health Policy Plann.* 2017;32(4):110-124.
5. Aceves-Martins M, Llaurado E, Tarro L, et al. Effectiveness of social marketing strategies to reduce youth obesity in

European school-based interventions: a systematic review and meta-analysis. *Nutr Rev.* 2016;74(5):337-351.

6. Phillipson L, Gordon R, Telenta J, Magee C, Janssen M. A review of current practices to increase chlamydia screening in the community—a consumer-centred social marketing perspective. *Health Expect.* 2016;19(1):5-25.

7. Formative. English Oxford Living Dictionaries website. http://www.oxforddictionaries.com/us/definition/american_english/formative. Accessed March 13, 2018.

8. Andreasen AR. The social marketing strategic management process. In: *Marketing Social Change—Changing Behavior to Promote Health, Social Development, and the Environment.* San Francisco, CA: Jossey-Bass; 1995:68-96.

9. Siegel M, Lotenberg LD. Formative research. In: *Marketing Public Health—Strategies to Promote Social Change.* Sudbury, MA: Jones and Bartlett; 2007:301-354.

10. Patton MQ. Step 5. Identify and prioritize primary intended uses by determining priority purposes. In: *Essentials of Utilization-Focused Evaluation.* Thousand Oaks, CA: Sage; 2012:113-139.

11. Glickman D, Parker L, Sim LJ, Del Valle Cook H, Miller EA, eds. *Accelerating Progress in Obesity Prevention: Solving the Weight of the Nation.* Washington, DC: National Academies Press; 2012. http://www.nationalacademies.org/hmd/Reports/2012/Accelerating-Progress-in-Obesity-Prevention.aspx.

12. Khan LK, Sobush K, Keener D, et al. Recommended community strategies and measurements to prevent obesity in the United States. *MMWR Recomm Rep.* 2009;58(RR-7):1-26.

13. Naylor PJ, Bridgewater L, Purcell M, Ostry A, Wekken SV. Publically funded recreation facilities: obesogenic environments for children and families? *Int J Environ Res Public Health.* 2010;7(5):2208-2221.

14. VERB summer scorecard. Florida Prevention Research Center website. http://health.usf.edu/publichealth/cfh/prc/cbpm/verb. Published 2015. Accessed August 31, 2016.

15. Bryant CA, Courtney AH, McDermott RJ, et al. Community-based prevention marketing for policy development: a new planning framework for coalitions. *Social Market Q.* 2014;20(4):219-246.

16. Andreasen AR. Listening to customers: research for social marketing. In: *Marketing Social Change—Changing Behavior to Promote Health, Social Development, and the Environment.* San Francisco, CA: Jossey-Bass; 1995:97-140.

17. Axelrod R. Advancing the art of simulation in the social sciences. In: Conte R, Hegselmann R, Terna P, eds. *Simulating Social Phenomena.* Berlin, Heidelberg: Springer Berlin Heidelberg; 1997:21-40.

18. Richardson GP. Reflections on the foundations of system dynamics. *Syst Dynam Rev.* 2011;27(3):219-243.

Appendix 7D

Social Marketing to Increase Participation in WIC

Tiffany Neal and Virginia Department of Health

Many low-income families have limited access to healthy foods and are therefore at risk for poor health. For women, infants, and children, a federal program helps to decrease this risk. The Special Supplemental Nutrition Program for Women, Infants, and Children (WIC) provides a variety of benefits including:

- Healthy foods at no cost (milk, eggs, cheese, cereal, fruits, veggies, baby formula, and more)
- Nutrition counseling and education
- Breastfeeding support
- Referrals to other programs, such as Medicaid and the Supplemental Nutrition Assistance Program (SNAP)

Eligible participants include infants, children under 5 years of age, and women who are pregnant, are nursing, or just had a baby. In addition, their family income must fall below 185% of the federal poverty level.

By providing nutrition assistance during the critical periods of pregnancy and early childhood, WIC makes a big difference in long-term health outcomes. WIC enhances pregnancy outcomes, improves the nutritional status of women and children, and improves kids' academic skills.[1-3]

However, WIC participation has decreased nationally over recent years. One reason may be declining birth rates. Another may be the generally improving economy, in which eligible families decide that they can afford to buy all their own groceries, rather than participating in WIC to receive supplemental food. Also, many families don't realize that they qualify, especially those whose income is too high for Medicaid or SNAP but who can still use WIC. The WIC program in Virginia's Thomas Jefferson Health District received a U.S. Department of Agriculture grant to expand participation through outreach, by increasing new enrollments and decreasing attrition.

▸ Social Marketing Planning Framework

We selected a social marketing planning framework for the outreach project. This provided a strong consumer orientation and the ability to address our target audience's needs, wants, and barriers. It also allowed us to leverage limited financial resources for maximum effectiveness. The grant funded a part-time health educator, a part-time graphic designer, and production of all outreach materials (including print materials, a TV commercial, and other mass media). We planned for sustainability from the start, knowing that outreach would remain important after the funding ended. The grant allowed us to implement an initial broad campaign, as well as build a strong foundation for continued promotion activities.

As with any public health program, our first step was to conduct a needs assessment. We used the social marketing constructs of consumer analysis, market analysis, and channel analysis in the assessment.[4]

Consumer Analysis

Our target audience included current and potential WIC participants in the district, to address both retention and recruitment. Analysis of local data showed that 92% of eligible infants were enrolled in WIC, but only 55% of eligible children aged 1–4 were enrolled.[5] Therefore, we chose to focus our outreach on these older children. We conducted formative research with the target audience using surveys and semistructured interviews to explore the "four Ps" of social marketing: product, price, place/partners, and promotion.

Market Analysis

The market analysis revealed key themes of product, price, place, and partners relevant to our target audience.

- *Product:* This represents the benefits of WIC, as perceived by participants. The top product was the food benefit (worth $43 to $182 each month, depending on status). Participants also valued the recently introduced eWIC "debit" card, which makes it easy and convenient to use WIC at the grocery store.
- *Price:* Although all WIC services are free, barriers included the time and hassle spent at WIC appointments, the perceived stigma of using WIC at the grocery store, and dissatisfaction with the limited food choices.
- *Place and partners:* These potential venues for outreach included Head Start preschool programs, low-income housing complexes, community nonprofits, government assistance offices, and grocery stores.

Channel Analysis

Promotion is the final "P" of social marketing, and is the most well-known. The channel analysis was used to assess and select multilevel strategies to promote WIC to our target audience. We aimed to improve audience perception of our product while decreasing perception of the price. We reviewed the literature on WIC outreach strategies implemented in other states, and incorporated feedback from local participants and staff members. Outreach materials were designed with content at a fourth-grade reading level. They were pretested with the target audience and adapted based on consumer feedback. The project was implemented over several months in collaboration with many community partners, including the following:

- *Intrapersonal (1-on-1):* We distributed "tell-a-friend" referral cards to participants when they came in for appointments. We sent out birthday cards to current and former participants, for the children's first, second, third, and fourth birthdays to promote the benefits of continuing to participate in WIC. We canvassed low-income housing complexes with door hangers. We also mailed letters to all obstetric and pediatric clinics in our district asking providers to discuss WIC with their patients.
- *Interpersonal (small groups):* We piggybacked onto existing programs to reach small groups of mothers; for example, we attended weekly playgroups hosted by a local child development nonprofit.

- *Organizations/community:* We developed and strengthened relationships with many community partners identified in the market analysis. We asked these partners to help us distribute brochures, bookmarks, and posters. We also attended health fairs and community events, and held neighborhood "lemonade stands" with free WIC juice and promotional materials.
- *Mass media:* We produced a TV ad that was aired on local channels, as well as several radio public service announcements. We sent a mass mail postcard to targeted neighborhoods using the USPS Every Door Direct Mail service. We also put interior ads in local buses.

▸ Evaluation

Evaluation measures included reach of promotion activities, documentation of WIC referral sources, and enrollment data.

- *Reach:* We reached 257 individuals at outreach events, distributed over 6000 brochures, mailed over 10,000 postcards, and had over 300,000 impressions of the mass media ads (TV, radio, and bus).
- *WIC referral sources:* We asked new enrollees, "How did you hear about WIC?" The only referral source that showed a change over the grant period was our partner Head Start program, which doubled its referrals.
- *Enrollment data:* We analyzed enrollment data for children aged 1–4 years in our district. During the grant period (spring to fall 2015), we reversed the decreasing trend in enrollment. However, after the core outreach campaign ended, enrollment started to decline again. The percentage of enrolled children aged 1–4 years did increase from 55% in September 2014 to 61% in September 2015.[6]

The evaluation results led us to explore the challenges of this outreach project. One challenge was the evaluation itself. It was difficult to determine what else might be affecting our enrollment data (e.g., an improving economy leading more people to decline WIC, even if eligible). We cannot definitively claim that the increase in enrollment was due to our outreach activities without a deeper analysis of potential confounders. Also, when we asked new enrollees "How did you hear about WIC?," 30% of respondents did not answer, limiting our ability to determine which promotion strategies were most effective.

It was challenging to reach eligible participants who were not already enrolled in WIC. Most of the people we reached in low-income settings already were WIC participants. Some eligible participants at higher incomes expressed the sentiment that they didn't want to use WIC because others "needed" or "deserved" it more.

There were also several logistical challenges. The grant timeline was short, with only about 6 months after staff were hired. It took time to complete the consumer, market, and channel analyses, as well as to develop outreach materials, which left a relatively short time for the campaign itself. Also, governmental procurement policies led to delays in receiving and distributing materials. These policies also prevented us from purchasing ads on Facebook, which we had planned to use as an effective marketing tool to reach a specific targeted audience.

▶ Conclusion

Our next steps include continued distribution of the "tell-a-friend" cards and birthday cards, maintaining relationships with community partners, and expanding outreach to local food pantries and faith-based organizations. As discussed earlier, our evaluation results show that after the core outreach campaign ended, our enrollment returned to its declining trend. This demonstrates the importance of sustainability of outreach activities beyond the grant period.

The social marketing planning framework was effective in developing our WIC outreach project and helped us to target many eligible participants. The diversity of promotion strategies ensured a broad reach with a limited budget. We knew from the beginning that sustainability would be a challenge. Now that the grant has ended, we plan to incorporate outreach activities into the regular work responsibilities of WIC staff. This social marketing project created a strong foundation to continue promoting WIC into the future.

References

1. Gordon A, Nelson L. *Characteristics and Outcomes of WIC Participants and Nonparticipants: Analysis of the 1988 National Maternal and Infant Health Survey*. Alexandria, VA: U.S. Department of Agriculture; March 1995.
2. Rose D, Habicht JP, Devaney B. Household participation in the food stamp and WIC programs increases the nutrient intakes of preschool children. *J Nutr*. 1998;128: 548-555.
3. U.S. Department of Agriculture. *The National WIC Evaluation: An Evaluation of the Special Supplemental Food Program for Women, Infants, and Children*. Alexandria, VA: Author; 1987.
4. McKenzie JF, Neiger BL, Smeltzer JL. *Planning, Implementing, and Evaluating Health Promotion Programs: A Primer*. 4th ed. San Francisco, CA: Benjamin Cummings; 2004.
5. Virginia Department of Health. Annual reports: potential eligibles. WIC Data and Statistics, Division of Community Nutrition; 2014. http://www.vdh.virginia.gov/richmond-city/annual-report/. Accessed April 3, 2018.
6. Virginia Department of Health. Annual reports: Participation by clinic and category and potential eligibles. WIC Data and Statistics, Division of Community Nutrition; 2015.

Appendix 7E

Asthma Self-Management Mobile Application for Adolescents: From Concept Through Product Development to Testing

Tali Schneider and Jim Lindenburger

▶ Background

Asthma is the most prevalent pediatric chronic disease, affecting as many as 7 million children in the United States.[1] In 2015, 1 in 10 adolescents aged 12–18 years old reported they were told by their physician that they have current asthma.[2] In addition to the physiological symptoms, adolescents with asthma encounter challenges navigating their academic, social, and psychological environment that compromise their quality of life.[3] Similar to other chronic conditions, self-management skills are essential to asthma care. Specifically, asthma self-management education equips patients with the skills to control disease exacerbations and other related crises, and minimizes hospital emergency unit visits.[4,5] Age-appropriate self-management education for adolescents needs to take into account patients' developmental changes and their lifestyle.[6] In spite of the advances in medical care offered to control asthma, adherence to asthma treatment and self-management remain poor during adolescence, resulting in a high number of preventable asthma episodes.

In Florida, the Youth Risk Behavior Survey report demonstrated a gradual yet significant increase in lifetime asthma rates in the past decade (from 17.5% in 2005 to 23.2% in 2015).[7] Utilizing social marketing principles, an interdisciplinary team of researchers and healthcare providers at the University of South Florida (USF) collaborated to explore barriers to asthma control as perceived by adolescents, their caregivers, and their healthcare providers, as well as a potential mechanism to improve adolescents' asthma self-management skills. Social marketing uses a consumer-centered approach that taps into the needs, aspirations, attitudes, values, and lifestyles of priority populations to inform the design of a valuable product that influences a positive behavioral change.[8]

Focusing on adolescents aged 12–17 years, our research team explored a means that is "native" for this age group and comprises a "place/channel" where they spend most of their time. Social media and the use of smartphones, for example, are ubiquitous among young people and could comprise such means. According to Pew Internet Research, 94% of all teens go online daily, and 76% use Facebook, Instagram, Snapchat, or other social networking sites.[9] Virtually all teens use the internet to find information; 91% access the internet through a mobile device. Eighty-eight percent own a mobile phone of some sort; three-quarters own a smartphone.[9] Considering these rates in the use of the internet and mobile devices, it became apparent that these technologies have the potential to enhance asthma management for adolescents.

This project was composed of three phases (see **FIGURE 7E-1**). The goals were to learn from key stakeholders how mobile technologies could be utilized to improve patient–provider communication and enhance adolescents' ability to self-manage asthma.

▶ Phase I: Formative Research

The research was conducted at USF, College of Medicine Pediatric Pulmonology Clinic. Qualitative research was conducted with four key influencers of adolescents' asthma self-management: attending physicians, resident physicians, adolescents 13–18 years of age with asthma,

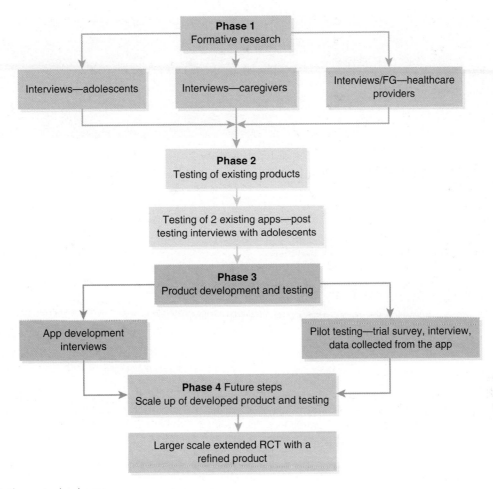

FIGURE 7E-1 Asthma study phases.

and their parents or caregivers. The research design included in-person interviews with adolescents and their caregivers and focus groups or in-person interviews with healthcare providers.

The purpose of phase I was to identify the patients', caregivers', and healthcare providers' perspectives on social media and mobile technologies, and attitudes toward the use of mobile technologies to improve asthma management among adolescents, aged 13–18 years old. Specifically, study objectives were the following:

- Explore current "standard" asthma care practices, benefits, and barriers to care.
- Explore new digital media applications to improve youth's ability to manage personal health information and communicate with healthcare providers and family members.
- Determine how to use existing social media and mobile devices to enable young people to identify peers who have asthma and participate in peer support relationships.

- Identify how pediatricians can enhance their support of asthma patients using digital media technologies and systems.

Findings

TABLE 7E-1 provides the highlights of each stakeholder group's results and a comparison of findings across the study's populations.

Adolescents with Asthma

Confirming existing literature, adolescents' use of technology (internet, mobile phones, tablets, etc.) is common. Adolescents use mobile devices primarily for entertainment and communication with members of their social networks. Mobile engagement varied; however, most adolescents used their devices to watch movies, play video games, listen to music, shoot photos, interact socially with peers through social networking sites, text, and make phone calls. Texting is

TABLE 7E-1 Phase 1: Research Design, Barriers, Benefits, and Recommended Content for the Use of New Technology in Asthma Care Across Key Stakeholders

	Healthcare Providers		Caregivers	Adolescents
	Attending	**Residents**	**Caregivers**	**Adolescents**
Methods	One focus group, one dyad, and three individual interviews	17 individual interviews	18 individual interviews	18 individual interviews
Noted benefits	■ Improve communication between asthmatic adolescents and their healthcare providers ■ Increase medication adherence ■ Develop patients' self-management skills ■ Offer a platform to deliver educational material ■ Achieve better asthma outcomes ■ Allow follow-up of asthma status between clinic visits		■ Exempt caregivers from "nagging" about medicine administration	■ One less thing to worry about ■ Early treatment of changes in asthma—prevent exacerbation ■ Connect with their healthcare provider
Noted barriers	■ Time constraints ■ Reimbursement on service ■ Protection of patient information ■ Timely response in emergency cases	■ Dependence on the system for controlling asthma ■ The complexity of operating the mobile media system ■ Sustainability of the program ■ Person assigned to manage the database system	■ Remember to perform peak flow readings and text them to the system	■ Hesitant to communicate directly with the healthcare provider
Recommended content	**Alerts** ■ Warnings about asthma condition ■ Contact the doctor ■ Verify medication use **Reminders** ■ Take controller medication ■ Purchase prescription refill ■ Clinic visits ■ Conduct peak flow readings		■ Reminders to take daily medication ■ Reminders to perform peak flow readings ■ Reminders to text values to the physician	■ Reminders to take daily medication ■ Reminders to perform peak flow readings ■ Supportive feedback ■ Weather condition and pollen count ■ Recommended treatment when asthma condition worsens

Conclusions	■ The willingness of both adolescents and healthcare providers to engage in the database system turns mobile technology that is already used broadly among teens into a viable tool in asthma care management.
	■ Potential asthma measure databases in the clinic setting seem feasible.
	■ Barriers elaborated by the physicians should be addressed.
Further exploration	■ Trial potential mobile application systems.
	■ Design a mobile application tailored to the population of interest.
	■ Conduct process and outcome evaluation.

the preferred means for connecting with others because of its immediacy and ease of use.

Adolescents reported the major barriers to asthma control are forgetting to maintain medication regimens and not carrying inhalers when away from home. They are sensitive to social stigma; they believe they are incapable of meeting their teachers', coaches', or friends' expectations, and are embarrassed by this. In spite of poor medical adherence, they acknowledge that taking medication regularly is an easy strategy to control asthma. They also noted that they were not well informed about the difference between maintenance and emergency medication, and they want more asthma education. Finally, they believe that controlled asthma would provide them peace of mind and would make them feel "normal" like their peers.

Adolescents believe an electronic asthma self-management and education tool is an optimal approach for themselves and their peers, and that the best method for delivering reminders and alerts is through text messaging via cellular phones or other portable devices such as tablets. In addition, they want the e-system to provide reminders to take their daily medication, messages on how to improve their asthma condition, reports on pollen count, notifications on weather conditions that may affect asthma status, feedback for entering their asthma peak flow values, alerts regarding changes in their asthma status (specifically changes that are very slight they may not notice themselves), and recommendations for how they can treat their asthma before the decline in asthma status becomes severe. They prefer these alerts be shared with their parents, healthcare providers, and, when appropriate, with coaches.

Healthcare Providers

Healthcare providers stress the importance of patient asthma education and asthma self-management. They note that communication with adolescent patients is not sufficient currently. Healthcare providers rarely communicate with their teen patients between clinic visits. When they do, communication occurs through patients' parents, in part because many patients are below the age of consent/authority (18 years of age). Telephone is the main communication mode, although residents believe email would provide documentation for use in patient charts. They also believe technological advances are valuable assets with which to improve asthma care, and that emerging technology can help decrease emergency department visits and school absenteeism as well as improve disease outcomes. Residents (who are typically younger in age than practicing physicians) were more inclined to use modern technologies in their daily practice. However, attending physicians and residents view the use of social media as a valuable tool to improve disease management and provide an interactive technology/channel for patient care among adolescents and their families.

Physicians also see social networking sites as an efficient way for adolescents and parents to connect with others with asthma, share their experiences, and gain support among peers. They also believe an electronic asthma self-management system where patients could input daily asthma monitoring values, generate and send daily or weekly reminders, and send alerts if patient monitoring values were out of range would be valuable. Physicians believe there is utility in an electronic system to send medication reminders, prescription refill reminders, appointment reminders, and other medical exam reminders, and to trigger avoidance messages. Such a system, however, would pose several challenges and concerns that will need to be addressed in order to make it more feasible to use. These barriers include time constraints, how reimbursement for services would occur, protection of patient health information, personalization of patient care, sustainability, and staffing. Furthermore, physicians expressed concerns over their role on-site (in the clinic) vs. their role via the electronic system, liability issues, and acceptance of/comfort with technology. Lastly, they were concerned that texting reminders and alerts in a crisis conflict with the intent to encourage adolescents to develop asthma self-management skills.

Caregivers

While being proactive in mitigating asthma episodes (e.g., eliminate exposure to secondhand smoke, maintain clean and dusted houses, and decrease exposure to allergens and other triggers), caregivers believe that the main barrier to asthma control stems from their children's poor medication adherence and failure to follow physicians' advice. They also believe social factors, such as stigma, influence their adolescents' decisions about whether to follow recommended protocols. Caregivers believe that controlling asthma has significant benefits for their adolescents and is clearly a goal for their families. They want their children to live healthy, normal, and successful lives; preventing flare-ups and attacks is key to achieving this. Their children's well-being is their top priority. This can lead to nagging their children to follow their physicians' orders, which can add stress to their relationship.

Caregivers seek asthma education mainly from their physicians, but also through nurse hotlines and internet sites (e.g., Google, WebMD, and Mayo Clinic). Caregivers believe that a mobile asthma management system with which to log asthma activity and communicate with healthcare providers would be a valuable asthma management tool for adolescents. They like features such as reminders (medications, peak flow meter readings, etc.) and alerts to adjust behaviors for certain activities or when lung capacity readings are outside the normal range. They believe this system will help adolescents to develop ownership of their condition and eliminate the need for parents to prompt their children to follow their recommended treatment regimen.

Conclusions

Physician–patient communication outside of clinic hours is limited; the time allotted for asthma education during clinic visits is restricted, which allows few opportunities for patients to learn self-management skills. Utilization of new technologies (internet, mobile devices, and web-based communication) can create learning opportunities that would improve self-management and control asthma. Physicians consider the use of such a system in clinic settings feasible and useful, with some challenges to address. The proposed system would enable physicians to track their patients' asthma status, be informed about potential asthma deterioration, and allow physicians to provide sound medical advice in a timely fashion. This system

would also provide adolescents with reminders and alerts to better treat and manage their asthma and achieve improved asthma outcomes.

This, combined with adolescents' ubiquitous use of mobile technology and their preferences for this use as a platform for health education and peer communication, offers an obvious solution; mobile phones and use of a self-management app can offer adolescents a well-suited asthma management intervention.

▶ Phase II: Testing of Existing Products

Equipped with these findings, the research team decided to explore further how a database system for asthma management would look and function. We found two mobile applications that were available on the open market and could be tested with study participants. Phase II of the study was designed for adolescents to use one of the two apps for 7–10 days and provide feedback regarding useful features, benefits and barriers to use, and ways to facilitate the use of the respective applications. Adolescents' experiences with these apps provided guidance to the research team in the design of an app that is tailored to the preferences of the priority population.

Methods

For this phase, 16 adolescents with asthma were recruited; approximately half were assigned to test one mobile app (AsthmaMD), and half were assigned to test a different one (AsthmaPulse). Each teen was given a peak flow meter and was trained to assess their lung capacity. Participants who did not have access to mobile devices were provided an iPod Touch for the trial period. Prior to the launch of the test, researchers, with participants, tested data entry and sharing capabilities of the app to ensure proper system function and to demonstrate how to perform those functions. Participants then used the asthma app independently, without instruction, as often as they wished; used the features they preferred; and shared asthma values with the pulmonologist on the research team, if they wished. After the trial, in-depth interviews were conducted with each participant using a semistructured interview guide.

Research Objectives

Interviews explored five areas relevant to adolescents' successful use of a mobile app:

■ General impressions of current asthma applications

- Barriers to using the asthma applications
- Useful features in the asthma applications
- Features that could be improved or eliminated
- Ways to facilitate/promote adolescents' use of an application

Findings

The most useful features were the peak flow readings and charts; both tested apps provided color-coded zones that represented users' asthma status, based on peak flow readings. Most participants liked the visual representation of their lung capacity over time. The ability to track changes in asthma status and view reoccurring patterns was particularly valuable. Adolescents also liked the feature that personalized asthma triggers and being able to send reports to their physician.

We discussed types of reminders for entering data, sharing information, and the preferred times for getting these reminders; similar questions were also asked about alerts. Preferred reminders are pop-up reminders, automated text messages, emails, and a notification "bubble" similar to Facebook's format, either through the application or on the mobile device. Adolescents identified in the morning before school, during the late afternoon, and early evening as their preferred times for reminders.

Adolescents' feedback was clustered around three app functions: general app usage/navigation, data entry, and sending reports. Adolescents found that one barrier to the use of the app was the need to use, or carry with them, a peak flow meter as an additional device to measure and report their lung capacity. Adolescents reported they commonly forgot to obtain and enter data; this highlighted the need to add a reminder system to prompt the users to enter data. They also had issues with successfully transmitting reports to the provider due to the lack of a "sent" notification when sharing data. Participants also had problems with wireless internet connections.

Adolescents identified many benefits in the respective asthma apps: self-awareness of daily asthma status; the ability to monitor asthma status over time; visual tracking of trends in peak flow measurements, which is helpful to link lung capacity values with the asthma triggers; and direct contact with their physicians through shared reports. This was particularly valued as a tool to keep physicians informed of their asthma patterns between appointments.

Adolescents proposed a multitude of changes and improvements for the existing apps. These included instructions for use, a symptoms feature, rearrangement of button placement for saving and entering data, colors and graphics more appropriate for their age, improvements in navigation and operation, a medication reminder, a built-in peak flow meter, a diary and notes section, and "live" recommendations from providers that would be sent to users upon entering data. Other suggestions included basic asthma facts and statistics pertinent to teenagers, informational videos on topics related to asthma in general, how to discuss asthma with others, techniques to stay calm and how to act during an asthma attack, and how to use a peak flow meter. Adolescents felt tested apps were designed for adults and were missing entertaining features (e.g., games, incentives, personal avatars, and informational video clips) that would increase the use of the app by younger users.

Conclusions

Adolescents found the tested apps useful to assist them with asthma self-management; however, it was clear they lacked elements that would inspire adolescents with asthma to regularly use them. Our next step was clear: design a consumer-tailored app that provides adolescents with their preferences for app features that would be reliable, useful, and fun to help adolescents improve asthma self-management.

▶ Phase III: App Development and Pilot Study

The objectives of phase III were the following:

- Apply the findings from phase II to the design of a new asthma app prototype for USF asthmatic teen patients and their healthcare providers.
- Pilot test the usability of the developed app with the priority population.
- Assess perceived changes in self-management skills and asthma outcome after a trial period of 3 months using the newly developed app.

Our next step was to establish an app development and product research team. An interdisciplinary team of public health, information technology, and computer design engineer professionals worked closely with the target population in three development "sprints" (app production phases). Our team followed findings from previous studies, the foundation for a consumer-driven approach. **TABLE 7E-2** presents the design elements that were incorporated

TABLE 7E-2 Adolescents' Recommended App Features (Phase II) and Implementation in Current (Phase III) and Future (Phase IV) Phases *(continued)*

Desired App Feature	Included in Prototype	Considered for Next Version
App		
Prompt to use the app (in text message format)	+	
Reminders to take medication		+
Encouraging messages	+	
Visual aids: graphs and charts	+	
Note section to add free text	+	
Gamification or avatar		+
Built-in peak flow meter		+
Asthma educational video clips/short text		+
Two-way communication with the healthcare provider		+
Interface		
Customizable font	+	
Customizable background and style	+	
Automatic progression of the data entry process	+	
Verification buttons (e.g., sent button)	+	

into the developed app in response to the adolescents' feedback. The prototype was completed (within a restricted budget) and was tested with the priority population in a 3-month trial period. Through a mixed methodology design, the study collected qualitative and quantitative data from study participants and readings from the app. Information was gathered on product usability and acceptability, as well as utilization of the specific features in the app and changes in asthma measures/outcome. We are currently completing analysis of data; however, the preliminary findings show positive results for app use and asthma self-management. With these promising results, our next step is to refine app design and functionality and conduct a randomized controlled trial to compare patient–provider communication and asthma management between app users and adolescents who receive standard/traditional treatment.

Acknowledgments

Thank you to Anthony D. Panzera, Mary Martinasek, Marisa Couluris, Laura Baum, and Amy Alman for their contributions to one or more of the phases of this project.

References

1. Akinbami LJ, Moorman JE, Bailey C, et al. Trends in asthma prevalence, health care use, and mortality in the United States, 2001–2010. *NCHS Data Brief.* 2012;94(94):1-8.

2. Reid K. Data sources and tools for action. Florida Asthma Coalition 2017 Summit; February 3, 2017; Orlando, FL.

3. Forrest J, Dudley J. Burden of asthma in Florida. Florida Health website. http://www.floridahealth.gov/diseases-and -conditions/asthma/_documents/asthma-burden2013.pdf. Published September 2013. Accessed March 14, 2018.

4. Busse WW, Boushey HA, Camargo CA, Evans D, Foggs MB, Janson SL. *Expert Panel Report 3: Guidelines for the Diagnosis and Management of Asthma.* Washington, DC: U.S. Department of Health and Human Services, National Heart Lung and Blood Institute; 2007.

5. Wagner EH. The role of patient care teams in chronic disease management. *BMJ.* 2000;320(7234):569.

6. Valerio M, Cabana MD, White DF, Heidmann DM, Brown RW, Bratton SL. Understanding of asthma management: Medicaid parents' perspectives. *Chest J.* 2006;129(3):594-601.

7. High school YRBS: Florida 2005–2015 results. Centers for Disease Control and Prevention website. https://nccd.cdc .gov/youthonline/App/Results.aspx?TT=L&OUT=0&SID =HS&QID=H87&LID=FL&YID=YY&LID2=&YID2 =&COL=S&ROW1=N&ROW2=N&HT=QQ&LCT =LL&FS=S1&FR=R1&FG=G1&FSL=S1&FRL=R1& FGL=G1&PV=&TST=&C1=&C2=&QP=G&DP =1&VA=CI&CS=Y&SYID=&EYID=&SC=DEFAULT &SO=ASC. Accessed January 15, 2017.

8. Grier S, Bryant CA. Social marketing in public health. *Annu Rev Public Health.* 2005;26:319-339.

9. Lenhart A. Teens, social media & technology overview 2015. Pew Research Center website. http://assets.pewresearch.org /wp-content/uploads/sites/14/2015/04/PI_TeensandTech _Update2015_0409151.pdf. Accessed April 13, 2018.

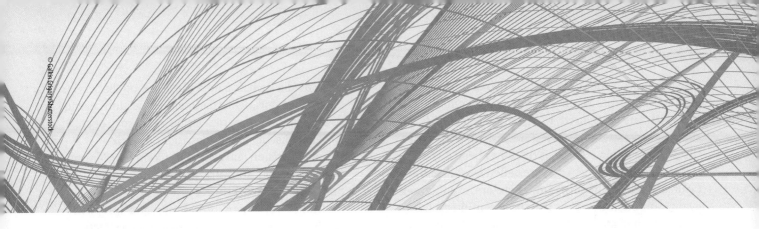

CHAPTER 8

Implementation and Evaluation

Claudia Parvanta

LEARNING OBJECTIVES

By the end of this chapter, the reader will be able to:

- Prepare a logic model for a communication intervention.
- Work with stakeholders to create a SWOTE analysis and define relevant metrics of success.
- Describe success factors for production and dissemination.
- Draft a timetable, budget, and work plan.
- Plan a program launch.
- Identify process and outcome evaluation measures and procedures.

▶ Introduction

In many health communication how-to books, when you get to the point of executing the intervention, it simply says, "Make it so," like Captain Picard from *Star Trek: The Next Generation*. The primary task at this point is to create a tactical plan that defines what will be done, when, where, how, and with what money, and who is responsible for each task or deliverable. Depending on the dissemination strategy, interventions (including media) may be released gradually using a geographic or time-based phasing. This is sometimes called a **soft launch**, in that the program planners do not call a lot of attention to initiating the intervention. With a soft launch, one or several sites may be used to test out procedures and ensure that all processes are running smoothly before expanding the program to the intended scale. Testing out the intervention in this manner is called **pilot testing**.

Regardless of the decision of whether to run a pilot test, most programs set a hard launch date (after the pilot, if one will be used) and hold a partner kickoff meeting, news event, town hall, or other activity designed to generate interest and enthusiasm in the program. Shortly after the launch, program managers will monitor all aspects of the intervention to ensure they are functioning as planned. These monitoring activities constitute **process evaluation**. In operational settings, corrections—or continuous quality improvement—can still take place. In experiments (e.g., the effectiveness trials of interventions), protocols would need to be resubmitted to institutional review boards before making major changes.

Throughout the program's implementation, program managers will want to collect and review some key metrics with stakeholders to see whether objectives are being reached. After the intervention has run for long enough to have reached a sufficiently large audience and potentially made an impact, an evaluation of outcomes can then be conducted. The evaluation design depends heavily on the logic model for the intervention, which must take opportunities and threats into consideration. Hence, two of the key tools used to build a program, the logic model and **SWOTE analysis**, are also used in its evaluation. SWOTE stands for "strengths, weaknesses, opportunities, threats, and ethics." To see if there has been a change, it is essential to collect what are called **baseline data** *before* launching the program. Therefore, even though evaluation often comes at the end of an intervention, it must be included in the design from the beginning. This chapter walks through these key tasks, preparing you to manage a basic health communication intervention. Because you will need them first, we will begin with the logic model and SWOTE analysis.

▶ Preparing a Logic Model

The W. K. Kellogg Foundation, which funds many population health activities, has produced a *Logic Model Development Guide* in which it defines a **logic model** as, "a picture of how your organization does its work—the theory and assumptions underlying the program."[1] Another extremely useful resource comes from the University of Wisconsin Extension Service.[2] As the Extension Service explains in its training,

> A logic model displays the connections between resources, activities and outcomes. As such it is the basis for developing a more detailed management plan. During the course of implementation, a logic model is used to explain, track and monitor operations, processes and functions. It serves as a management tool as well as a framework to monitor fidelity to the plan.

FIGURE 8-1 shows the bare bones of a logic model. We will add some details to those empty boxes.

Resources/Inputs

Inputs and resources range from tangible items, such as money, paid staff or volunteer hours, facilities, and equipment, to more intangible items, such as expertise, data, or the involvement of collaborators at the local, state, national, or global level. Each may play a part in contributing resources to the program.

Activities

This is a description of what the program will do. A health communication program often includes the following activities:

■ Mass media such as paid advertising, public service announcements, entertainment education events (plays, television program scripts, radio soap operas), social media, or student classroom materials

■ Patient decision aids such as computer animations, decision software, pencil and paper flipbooks, kits, or worksheets

■ Training workshops for healthcare providers, teachers, coaches, or clergy to use media effectively

■ Outreach and education activities such as health fairs, speaking engagements, trade shows, or grocery store or drugstore promotional activities

Numbers are associated with activities in terms of what is anticipated and budgeted; for example, "conduct 10 teacher training workshops" or "distribute 10,000 patient decision aids."

Outputs

Outputs describe whether the activities were delivered as planned; for example:

■ For mass media:
  · If you planned to deliver 10,000 student workbooks, how many students actually received workbooks?
  · If you bought radio and television air time, when and where did your spots air? What was the measured audience? (The television and radio stations, as well as independent media auditors, measure this.)
  · If you ran a website, how many page views, downloads, or forms were completed? How long did people interact with specific pages on the site? Can you measure the exposure?
  · If you contributed to a soap opera or primetime drama television script, when and where was it aired?
  · How many people have become your "friends" on Facebook for your program's page? How many times has your YouTube video been viewed?

■ For patients:
  · How many health facilities, practices, or individual healthcare providers have agreed to use the patient decision aids? How many patients have received them?
  · If online, how many patients have downloaded or requested the materials?

■ For intermediaries (people using the health communications materials to work with others):
  · How many workshops were implemented? How many participants completed pre- and posttests?

Inputs ▶ Activities ▶ Outputs ▶ Outcomes ▶ Impact

FIGURE 8-1 A basic logic model.

- How many materials were ordered post-training?
- How many feedback cards or website entries were posted?
- For outreach:
  - How many public appearances, speaking engagements, or health fairs were held? Where and when? Who came?
  - How many grocery stores, pharmacies, or other commercial establishments ran events with the program's materials and speakers?
  - How many trade or industry shows? Where and when? Who came and participated? Who requested more information or a follow-up?

Assessing whether your outputs were generated according to plan is an essential prelude to outcomes, as described next.

Outcomes

Outcomes are normally divided into immediate, intermediate, and long-term ranges.

Immediate outcomes for mass media might include the following:

- Next-day recall of message
- Awareness of issue
- Change in attitude or motivation to try something

These responses would be assessed through survey research. Interactive media allow recipients to respond

to website invitations, purchase, donate, or post information immediately.

Intermediate outcomes generally include changes in individual behaviors, enactment of policies, or uptake of technology or strategies by organizations. *Long-term* outcomes could include permanent changes in health behavior, statutes and laws, or environmental quality. Long-term outcomes may be identical to the impact (discussed in the next section), although the former refers more to individuals (e.g., an individual quits smoking and their life is extended) and the latter to population (e.g., the death rate from tobacco goes down).

Impact

Impact is generally measured in terms of population-level health or socioeconomic improvements. This would be reflected in reductions in age-specific mortality rates, prevalence of disease, and disease-specific mortality rates. Population measures of quality of life would improve.

Putting the Model Together

You can easily find templates to create logic models in word processing programs as well as online. FIGURE 8-2 features a logic model from the University of Wisconsin Extension Service. FIGURE 8-3 shows a worked-out example for a program to reduce alcohol consumption by minors—particularly teenagers.

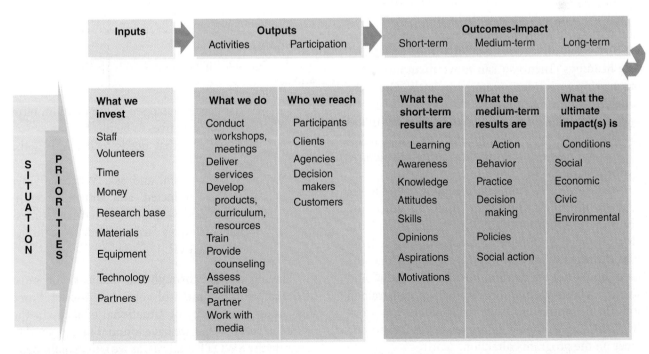

FIGURE 8-2 Logic model.

W.K. Kellogg Foundation logic model development guide. W.K. Kellogg Foundation website. http://www.wkkf.org/resource-directory/resource/2006/02/wk-kellogg-foundation-logic-model-development-guide. Published February 2, 2006. Accessed March 16, 2018.
Courtesy of W.K. Kellogg Foundation.

Input	Output *Activities*	Outcomes -- Impact		
		Short	*Medium*	*Long*
• 1.5 FTE Staff time • "Breathalyzer" Equipment • Audiovisual Equipment • Student Volunteers • Research Findings • Local business Incentives & Give-aways • SAMHSA PSAs (free)* • $10,000 grant from beverage company.	• Production and distribution of SAMHSA posters and cards to area retailers, restaurants • Farmer market tabletops • Town Hall meetings • Road Stop Alcohol Breath tests • Alcohol Free Spring Break Party • Social Media Campaign on Instagram and Twitter • Training for alcohol retailers • In-classroom activities for 6th graders • After school counselor rotations • PTA speaking engagements • Press release and staffing of warm line	↑ Awareness of < age drinking by community. ↑ Knowledge about effects of alcohol on young minds and behavior. • Commitment from parents, teachers and youth counselors to program. • Engagement through social media sites with youth. • Identification of champions for youth activities throughout school year and summer. • Five media stories published in 1 year.	↑ Compliance to alcohol laws by retailers. ↓ Arrests at road stops by police or house party raids. ↓ Parties serving alcohol to minors. ↑ Number of youth volunteering to lead school and summer activities sponsored by program. ↓ Number of youth drinking alcohol at parties or after school.	• Society not supportive of youth drinking. • Delayed average age of continued alcohol use. • Delayed average age of first alcohol use. ↓ Injuries associated with alcohol impaired behavior.

FIGURE 8-3 Logic model to reduce underage drinking.

Modified from Lisowski A. 4-H youth development educator's logic model, University of Wisconsin-Extension, 6-2009. https://fyi.uwex.edu/programdevelopment/files/2016/03/AnnieLisowskialcohol.pdf. Accessed February 15, 2017.

Note that the logic model in Figure 8-3 includes commitments of staff and volunteers; requires parents, teachers, community retailers, and counselors to participate; and includes a grant from a beverage company. The best way to create such a logic model is to invite all stakeholders potentially involved in a program to participate in its development. Your ideas can first be written on cards and stuck on the wall under basic headings. Then you can move them around as you develop your ideas more completely. Once the model is completed, it should be able to fit on one printed page. (It can be a big page.) Some say this is the only rule for logic models. Your colleagues, stakeholders, and partners will use this as the "big picture" of your program.

Because we read from left to right, we tend to see the logic model moving from inputs to outcomes. While there is no one right way to create and use a logic model, we prefer to work *backwards* from desired program impact. There is a saying that the "shoe should not tell the foot how large to grow," and therefore, planning should not initially be constrained by available resources. Your stakeholders can work toward finding all the necessary resources if everyone agrees on the program's direction.

Backwards Planning with Logic Models

Most organizations have goals, or dreams, of what they want to achieve within a specific time frame. SMART objectives (objectives that are strategic, measurable, actionable, realistic/relevant, and time-bound) represent your outcomes or even impact, depending on your time horizon.

Taking your logic model in hand, work backwards and ask:

1. What needs to happen in the medium term for these objectives to be met?
2. Before that, what needs to happen in the near term?
3. Step back again, and ask: What activities must be conducted, and with what audiences, to achieve these short-term outcomes?
4. What resources are needed to conduct these activities?

Having worked through this analysis, you must also explore the context of your logic model. Some logic models include the situational analysis in the same instrument, but we have found it more useful to separate the SWOTE analysis, as we will explain next.

SWOTE Analysis

A SWOT analysis is the standard business tool for assessment of strengths, weaknesses, opportunities, and threats. We have added an *E* to SWOT for ethical assessment, which we feel is an indispensable piece for health communication programs. Strengths and weaknesses refer to conditions that are within your control, or at least inherent to your organization's ability to implement the program. Opportunities and threats are outside of your control. You may plan for or around them, but they will happen on their own. Ethical considerations may reside inside your organization, but it is important to assess whether intentionally, or inadvertently, your program could harm someone, limit someone's rights, or promise something that cannot be delivered.

As with the logic model discussed earlier, this exercise is best conducted with those you see as partners or stakeholders in the health communication intervention. These colleagues will enable you to assess your total assets and have a 360-degree picture of opportunities and threats. Again, you can work with cards and stick them up on the wall under the big headings, moving them around as you refine your thinking. **FIGURE 8-4** shows some generic considerations for a health activity SWOTE analysis. The following is an examination of each of these areas in detail.

Strengths

There are two ways to consider strengths (and weaknesses).

- Strengths are the attributes within the organization. These include personnel capabilities, experiences, material resources, organizational commitment, time allotted, and budget.
- Strengths are the attributes of the intervention/communication campaign. These include the positioning of a product or service, its cost, its attractiveness or reputation, and so forth. If you have a great product or service to work with (e.g., a free pizza night on a college campus), that is a program strength. If you have an unpopular idea to sell (e.g., an increase in tuition), this can be a weakness.

	Positives	Negatives	Ethical
Internal • Human resources • Physical resources • Funding • Expertise • Past experiences • Reputation	**Strengths** What are your own advantages, in terms of people, physical resources, finances? What do you do well? What activities or processes have met with success?	**Weaknesses** What could be improved in your organization in terms of staffing, physical resources, funding? What activities and processes lack effectiveness or are poorly done?	What ethical issues could arise with your organization's participation in this activity? What if you do not participate?
External • Future trends - in your field or the culture • The economy • Funding sources (foundations, donors, legislatures) • Demographics • The physical environment • Legislation • Local, national, or international events	**Opportunities** What events might co-occur with your activity that could highlight or support it? What local, national, or international trends draw interest to your program? Is a social change or demographic pattern favorable to your goal? Is a new funding source available? Have changes in policies made something easier? Do changes in technology hold new promise?	**Threats** What obstacles do you face that hinder the effort - in the environment, the people you serve, or the people who conduct your work? What local, national, or international trends favor interest in other or competing programs? Is a social change or demographic pattern harmful to your goal? Is the financial situation of a funder changing? Have changes in policies made something more difficult? Is changing technology threatening your effectiveness?	Who could be harmed if you participate in this activity? Who would be harmed if you do not? What other ethical issues are pertinent in mounting this activity?

FIGURE 8-4 Generic considerations in a SWOTE analysis for a health program.

Modified from Community Health and Development. Community Tool Box: SWOT analysis: strengths, weaknesses, opportunities, and threats. http://ctb.ku.edu/en/table-of-contents/assessment/assessing-community-needs-and-resources/swot-analysis/main. Accessed February 17, 2017.

Weaknesses

As with strengths, there are two ways to consider weaknesses.

■ *Gaps within the organization:* These include a lack of knowledge, skills, experience, or material resources. Weaknesses may also be less tangible, such as a lack of leader commitment to the intervention or a nonexistent or poor reputation in the community, or within a government or other bureaucracy. Of course, insufficient funding or a rushed timeline are also program weaknesses.

■ *Weaknesses of the actual intervention:* These may include delayed or limited availability (such as seasonal flu vaccine in some years), costs to produce (if more than the market price to sell), or distribution hurdles, or it may be that the service is unattractive to consumers in some way (e.g., think about having to promote a stool blood test or colonoscopy for colon cancer screening).

Opportunities

Opportunities are positive factors related to happenings at the time and in the place you have planned for your intervention. Partners and stakeholders may provide critical insights into opportunities (as well as threats, discussed next), which you may not know exist. Examples of opportunities include:

■ *A favorable political climate:* At the state and local levels, the governor or congressional leaders can play an important role in supporting or thwarting health promotion activities within the state or congressional district.

■ *Funding:* Funding opportunities are something of a two-edged sword. Coalitions that come together solely in response to the availability of funding often have a hard time maintaining their collaboration. When academic institutions and community-based organizations try to develop initiatives on their own, they are more successful at both obtaining new funding and implementing their programs than when the partnership is formed to "get the money."

■ *Technology development and innovation:* In the health communication area, there have been enormous changes in even the past few years in terms of what is possible, as well as reductions in cost, to reach many people with more information.

■ *Seasonal and style trends:* There are always trends (e.g., in food, clothing) and seasonal reasons that may support (or again, threaten) an intervention. You would not want to sell sunscreen, and warn about skin cancer, in winter—unless you were placing your spots in permanently sunny locales, or on a travel channel and targeting vacationers to sunny climes.

■ *Big events that draw a lot of attention:* Many, many health promotion programs (as well as commercial advertisers) have tried to link their efforts to the Olympics or other major sporting events (e.g., the World Cup for global interventions; the Super Bowl or World Series for the United States). Although these events draw huge audiences, the problem is that they are focused on making the athletes and the sport the "single overriding communication objective." Whatever time event organizers do not manage to fill with showing sports is taken up by the major commercial sponsors. It is not a good idea to try to run a 15-second spot, which will cost a small fortune, in this big venue. What does work well is to try to develop a local angle, such as an athlete or Olympic competitor from the community or state. This person can become a spokesperson and do much more for the health communication program before or after the event itself.

■ *Celebrity endorsements:* There is a somewhat ghoulish reaction by those in health promotion when celebrities announce that they, or a loved one, have a health problem. If this person is well known, and can be seen as a positive role model, efforts are made to attract the celebrity as a spokesperson. Because so many celebrities seem to seek meaning beyond their media careers, there are services that help match them up with agencies or issues for which they feel an affinity. Although the celebrity has endured a personal tragedy, there is an "opportunity" to engage that person in your health issue; many celebrities find it helps them to deal with their loss in a constructive manner.

Threats

Threats are factors that could potentially delay or prevent you from achieving your program objectives; again, they are outside your immediate control. In some ways, everything listed in the previous three sections, if turned around, can be a threat; for example:

■ *Political instability:* International work is frequently threatened by clashing political parties, including uprisings, strikes, and localized conflicts. Conflict and war have to be listed as the biggest threats, not only to the work of public health practitioners, but also obviously to the entire planet.

■ *Environmental catastrophe:* Powerful weather (e.g., hurricanes, floods) that occurs seasonally or randomly, earthquakes, and agricultural conditions (such as droughts) all jeopardize international health communication efforts. Explosions in mines (or oil rigs) not only focus local or national attention for months but also require use of resources planned for public health. They are thus tragedies on several levels.

- *Activity linked to risky funding or dependent on personalities:* In the United States, organizations, academic institutions, or even small groups can all suffer externally created losses in funding or other resources. Also, the actions of one individual may threaten the reputation of an entire organization or institution. Having mentioned the opportunities posed by celebrities, too often, they are risky business. Whatever it is that keeps them in the tabloids far too often makes it difficult to rely on them for health promotion campaigns. If you are extremely careful to match your celebrity to your target audience, and they are willing to accommodate you, then their risk-taking behavior—and negative consequences—might send the right message.

Ethical Dimensions

Ethical dimensions in public health are derived from conflicts of philosophical and societal principles and values. Four stand out:

- *Utilitarianism:* Defined as the "the greatest good for the greatest number of people," **utilitarianism** is central to public health, and much of public policy, in the United States. Utilitarianism requires forecasting results and presents the possibility that the "ends justify the means." An example of a highly utilitarian public health policy is quarantine and travel restrictions for infectious outbreaks. In this case, the rights of a few are restricted to protect the health of the many.
- *Deontological principles:* Much of public health is also based on **deontological principles** (or duty-based principles). These require following rules and principles with the notion, "Stick to honorable principles, and the outcomes will take care of themselves." Many in public health believe you cannot achieve a just outcome (or end) through unjust means. A public health program that requires participants to demonstrate economic or nutritional need is an example of a deontological system because it uses rules—and not privilege (or bribery)—to distribute resources.
- *The Golden Rule:* In the Judeo-Christian tradition, this first appears in Leviticus roughly as, "Love thy neighbor as thyself"; eventually it was popularized as: "Do unto others as you would have them

do unto you." Virtually every religion and society includes the concept of putting yourself in another's place before doing something, for good or for bad. Most public health organizations, but particularly those run by charitable organizations, put caring for individuals and their rights and feelings at the top of their core values.

- *Other rights and privileges:* From the Declaration of Independence, we remember: "We hold these truths to be self-evident, that all men are created equal, that they are endowed by their Creator with certain unalienable Rights, that among these are Life, Liberty and the pursuit of Happiness." Just how far an individual's right to liberty in the pursuit of happiness may go is often described, in common speech, as far as the end of someone else's nose (or, an application of utilitarianism to life, liberty, and the pursuit of happiness).

Any student of Philosophy 101 can come up with situations where it would be impossible to apply all four of these principles simultaneously; for example, those who suggest that street drugs should be legalized might say that, "In a free country, people should be allowed to harm themselves, as long as they do not hurt anyone else in the process." This is a complicated argument that might get into comparing the damage to society from crime associated with drug dealing versus individual harm from drug ingestion. But what about the healthcare issues associated with drugs—should society bear these costs, or not? Where do harm-reduction strategies—such as a needle exchange to offset the additional risks of human immunodeficiency virus (HIV) and hepatitis infection—fall on your moral compass?

Compared with these difficult ethical dilemmas, the ones associated with health communication might seem relatively straightforward. Some fall under the audience research and pretesting category, such as, "The communications will not stigmatize any groups" (e.g., children with birth defects, or persons with HIV) or "We will refrain from using messages that present people who engage in certain behaviors in a negative way." There is no absolute way to resolve these dilemmas, because different communities and different cultures would apply their own values and principles. In the United States, different political parties are associated with allowing or disallowing government-sponsored mass media pertaining to, for example, risks of tobacco, risks associated with private ownership of firearms, and use of condoms for prevention of sexually transmitted disease and birth control. Of course, these values and associated moral codes will vary widely in international settings.

The choice of informing versus persuading may pose an ethical dilemma in some circumstances. You might think, "If I feel strongly that this harms you, or this may help you, shouldn't I use everything at my disposal to try to convince you of this?" In addition, the very acts of selecting a population as the focus (or target) of a health communication campaign and prioritizing an issue mean that some people and some issues are left out. **BOX 8-1** features a list of ethical issues identified by the Centers for Disease Control and Prevention (CDC) in *CDCynergy* as most relevant to conducting your SWOTE for a health communications program. It is based on the framework developed by Guttman and Salmon.[3]

▶ Final Strategy Analysis

Now you have a logic model and a SWOTE analysis. What do you do with them? You think about the SWOTE in terms of when and how it might affect the process described in the logical framework.

Strengths and Weaknesses

These are most likely to affect the program's inputs.

- Is the program based on the organizational strengths and those of the intervention?
  - If not, how can these strengths be featured more prominently in the intervention?
  - How can the program fix each weakness?
- Do the strengths and weaknesses of the partners balance each other out? This can be a critical question when deciding on partner arrangements.
- Is the proposed program too far away from the core business of the organization? (e.g., If the mission of the university is to educate students, may you conduct a health communication campaign in the community?)
- Do you need to rethink the program before too much is invested?

BOX 8-1 Ethical Considerations in Public Health Communication: Bioethics

Bioethics is the branch of ethics, philosophy, and social commentary that discusses the life sciences and their potential impact on our society. A set of principles or guidelines that are based on bioethics can articulate and assess ethical and moral dilemmas. These ethical guidelines may include the following:

- The obligation to avoid doing harm through the actions of trying to help
- The obligation to do good by doing one's utmost to better the health of the intended populations
- Respect for the freedom of every person and community to make their own decisions according to what they think would be best for them
- Ensuring adherence to justice, equity, and fairness in the distribution of resources, and providing for those who are particularly vulnerable or who have special needs
- Maximizing the greatest utility from the health promotion efforts, especially when resources are limited and are publicly funded, and considering the good of the public as a whole

Ethical Considerations Through the Stages of Program Design and Implementation

Each facet of the intervention needs to be examined to determine whether it meets these precepts. The questions provided in the following sections can help facilitate the application of the precepts to each stage or facet of the intervention and the identification of ethical issues.

Goal-Setting Stage

- Who decides what the goals of the intervention should be?
- Who is targeted by the intervention, and who is excluded?
  - Why was the targeted population chosen?
  - Were populations with the greatest needs targeted, or those who were more likely to adopt the recommendations?
- Are representatives of the intervention's target population involved in goal setting?
- How will consent be obtained from the intervention's targeted populations?
- Are issues that are more relevant to mainstream populations given higher priority?

Designing and Implementation

- Collaboration:
  - Could collaboration with community or other voluntary organizations, with the idea of advancing participation and empowerment, actually serve to exploit these organizations by using their limited resources?
  - Are organizations made to feel forced to participate in the intervention's activities?

- Use of persuasive strategies and message design:
  - What kinds of persuasive appeals are used, and to what extent may they be manipulative?
  - Are the messages persuasive enough?
  - Do they unduly exploit cultural themes or symbols?
- Messages on responsibility:
  - Do messages imply that if people get an adverse medical condition, it is their fault because they did not do enough to prevent it? In other words, these kinds of messages can be viewed as potentially harmful because they may literally blame people and make them feel guilty when various circumstances prevent them from adopting the recommended practices.
  - Do the messages make it appear that one person is responsible for preventing others from taking health risks (e.g., spouse, friend, employee); that is, how much is one person responsible for others?
- Messages that may stigmatize or make people overly anxious:
  - Do messages that try to get people to avoid unwanted health conditions (e.g., AIDS, stroke, smoking) portray those who have the conditions in a negative light?
  - Does the intervention raise the level of anxiety, fear, or guilt among target populations?
- Messages that may make people feel deprived:
  - Does the intervention tell people to avoid doing certain things that give them pleasure, but not provide them with affordable and rewarding alternatives?
  - Does the campaign tell people to avoid cultural practices that are of particular significance to them?
- Messages that make promises that cannot be fulfilled:
  - Does the intervention make promises for good health when it urges people to adopt particular practices, although the promises may not be fulfilled?
  - Does the intervention contribute to increased demands on the healthcare system, which may not be able to meet the demands?
- Messages that turn health into an ultimate value:
  - Do the messages stress that health is an important value that should be vigorously pursued, and does the intervention make it sound as if those who do not pursue good health are less virtuous or have vices?
  - Does the intervention contribute to making health an ideal or a super value that people need to pursue resolutely?
- Messages that may distract:
  - Does the intervention focus on specific health topics, thus possibly serving to distract people from thinking about and pursuing activities related to other important issues?
  - Does the intervention focus on individual behavior changes and, by so doing, distract people from thinking about the importance of social factors that influence health? That is, are downstream behaviors being blamed before upstream problems for population health?
- Control of people in work organizations:
  - Do interventions that take place in work organizations, although they may be efficient, present opportunities for employers to control the private lives of their employees?

Evaluation Stage

- Who decides the evaluation criteria and the success of the intervention?
- Are the targeted populations and the intervention practitioners involved in the assessment process?

Modified from CDCynergy. Centers for Disease Control and Prevention website. https://www.orau.gov/cdcynergy/web/default.htm.
Note: Go to the program launch site to access Phase 2 Step 5, on which this box is based.

Opportunities and Threats

These tend to affect achievement of outputs as planned, or outcomes.

- How can the program exploit each opportunity?
  - What must be changed to exploit an opportunity?
  - What does it maximize: achievement of outputs or outcomes?
  - Do you need to build additional alliances to take advantage of an opportunity?
- How can the program defend against each threat?
  - How realistic are the threats, and how great a risk do they pose?
  - At what point do you need to account for the threats: between inputs and outputs or between outputs and outcomes?
  - Do you need to make additional alliances to defend against these threats?

Ethics

How can the program/organization be fair and conduct the intervention in the most ethical manner possible?

- What are the bases of these decisions?
- Again, what needs to be changed, if anything, to prioritize human rights, gender equity, or other ethical issues over short-term programmatic gains?
- Do you need to add partners to accomplish these changes?

As mentioned earlier, this analysis is best done with your partners and stakeholders. Define each of the SWOTE factors and rank-order them. Normally, you need to devote most of your attention to the top five items in each of the lists. The others should not be ignored, but they will probably not need to be addressed as you plan the launch of your intervention. Comparing the strengths and opportunities for your program against the weaknesses and threats, you will make a "go/no-go" decision. Perhaps the program needs to be postponed to allow for an opportunity, to wait out a threat, or to gather a stronger alliance and attract more resources. Or, maybe you need to move the deadline up for some of the same reasons. These strategic decisions are part of your final plan.

▶ Production and Dissemination Factors

Having considered the timing and organizational strengths and weaknesses, you can now focus on the strengths and weaknesses of your intervention itself. The following is a list of criteria that apply more broadly to production and dissemination[4]:

- **Presentability**: How many people toss the black-and-white, photocopied brochure in the trash as they exit a health clinic? In terms of producing something that people will pay more attention to, and possibly keep, quality saves money. A cliché that applies is this: Anything worth doing [including mass media, entertainment education, or counseling] is worth doing well. This does not necessarily mean that it has to be expensive, but that the time invested to get it right will pay off. One way to limit costs is to focus on specific audiences over a time schedule. Strategic communication does not try to be all things to all people. The

surest route to reaching multiple audiences with higher-quality media is to work with partners and share the expenses.

- **Expandability**: Almost anything will work in a small enough community with loving care lavished on every detail. The real challenge is bringing this to a scale where there can be a genuine public health impact. In general, mass media are used to expand the scope of an intervention. Mass media are the most effective way to reach a lot of people; however, the communication is one-directional. Now, through social media, there are multiple, inexpensive ways of scaling up communications that allow for an exchange of views. Traditionally, the most costly intervention to bring to scale is trained counselors working with clients on behavior change. Ironically, this intervention looks to be the least expensive to do in a pilot. There are ways of bringing interpersonal communication to scale, again, by working with partners or widely spread networks of practitioners. But, quality control becomes more of an issue.

- **Sustainability**: How many health programs have resourced a communication campaign for 6 months, evaluated at 1 year, and been disappointed by the amount of change? As a gentle reminder, there is always advertising for Coke and Pepsi. A strategic health communication program matches partner organizations to intended audiences and spreads the costs of a campaign broadly. This enables an intervention to have a broader reach and be something that each organization can afford. It is not pointless to do something really spectacular once or on an annual basis. But, unless it is worked into a longer-term schedule of public relations, partner counseling, or other ways of carrying the message beyond this time and place, it is not strategic.

- **Cost-effectiveness**: Public health interventions tend to have very limited budgets, certainly compared to competing commercial campaigns for products such as tobacco, soft drinks, and fast foods. So little money is spent on sustaining health communication interventions that it is almost pointless to assess their cost-effectiveness. For those with adequate budgets, newer evaluation methods go beyond "costs per impression" (an older mass media term for number of times an advertisement is run on TV, radio, or print copy) to costs per person reached. If a communication strategy can be linked to health outcomes—for example, an anti-smoking campaign examined over many years against deaths due to tobacco—then costs per deaths averted can be used. Whether the metric has a short or long time scale, strategic communication uses resources creatively and to best advantage based on audience research and process evaluation.

Now you have a clear sense of what will make your health communication program more likely to succeed. It is time to create and execute the implementation plan.

▶ The Implementation Plan

The implementation plan answers the following questions[5]:

- What will be achieved?
- Who will do the work?
- What are the expected roles and responsibilities of partners and allies?
- How much will all this cost?
- What is a realistic timeline?

What Will Be Achieved?

The implementation plan defines the activities to take place according to a schedule and sequencing; for example, you might plan to have worksites, schools, or health centers run small discussion groups, distribute small materials, and use digital signage or posters *while* you use radio and television ads to promote an overall effort. The implementation plan should explicitly include the production and delivery of materials to the sites, as well as training of personnel in their use, prior to dissemination of the broadcast media.

In addition to internal factors, the implementation plan needs to account for external events such as holidays, school or university schedules, major sporting events, or political events that could compete for time, the attention of the program's target audience(s), broadcast space, or space/facilities.

In contrast to avoiding certain times of the year, it may help to link specific activities to major events. Thanksgiving is often used to promote healthy eating; skin cancer prevention and safe swimming make more sense in the summer; and parents are thinking about immunizations around back-to-school time. The U.S. Department of Health and Human Service's Healthfinder.gov site shows an annual calendar of health observances by month and day (when relevant).[6] It took decades for people to associate October with breast cancer awareness, but there are actually about 27 other health issues vying for attention in October. **BOX 8-2** provides some ideas on how to promote a national health observance, or you can link your own activity to one of these to bring added clout to your messaging.

TABLE 8-1 lists at least one observance per month, although there are many more to choose from.

Who Will Do the Work?

Staff

Health communication activities can be done by professionals or volunteers, provided they have the right mix of skills. When managing a project, do not assume anything will be done unless everyone has agreed to their responsibilities and accountability.

BOX 8-2 Planning a National Health Observance

Each national health observance (NHO) presents an opportunity to educate the public, energize co-workers and community members, and promote healthy behaviors. The NHO toolkits have the information and tools you need to get started.

- Contact the NHO sponsoring organization several months ahead of time to request up-to-date information and materials.
- Consider enlisting the help of a community partner to help you plan and promote your event.
- Meet with those who will be valuable in your event coordination. To get started, sit down with potential partners, such as local businesses, local government agencies, key leaders, organizations, and media partners who share an interest in the NHO.
- Recruit volunteers, speakers, and community liaisons.
- Develop new or adapt existing materials to distribute at the event.
- Be sure to get them printed and/or copied in advance.
- Conduct a run-through before the event.

Reproduced from Tips for promoting a national health observance. healthfinder.gov website. https://healthfinder.gov/nho/NHOtips.aspx. Accessed March 15, 2018.

TABLE 8-1 National Health Observances by Month

Month	Major Observance
January	National Birth Defects Prevention Month
February	American Heart Month
March	National Cheerleader Safety Month National Nutrition Month
April	National Autism Awareness Month National Child Abuse Prevention Month
May	National Teen Pregnancy Prevention Month Mental Health Month
June	Men's Health Month National Safety Month
July	Juvenile Arthritis Awareness Month World Hepatitis Day
August	National Breastfeeding Month National Immunization Awareness Month
September	National Childhood Obesity Awareness Month
October	National Breast Cancer Awareness Month Health Literacy Month
November	American Diabetes Month Great American Smokeout
December	World AIDS Day National Handwashing Awareness Week

BOX 8-3 provides some questions to consider when staffing a project.

In today's world, considering who has skills in social media is essential.

Roles of Partners

When planning a health communication program with a national scope, there are potentially many partners with whom to work. The trick is usually determining how to work each stakeholder's objectives into a unified plan so that the collective communication intervention supports individual programmatic needs. This level of negotiation could take many months (or even years) to accomplish. But on a national level, it can determine the success or failure of a program. The most successful programs include several key organizations that underwrite the initial stages of an intervention, while transferring responsibilities, training, and material assets down to smaller entities to continue the project on their own. This builds a level of sustainability into what otherwise might be a relatively short burst of mass media or other communications.

For example, the CDC and the March of Dimes recruited additional organizations into the National Council for Folic Acid. The CDC contributed most of the audience research, as well as the epidemiologic data tracking. The March of Dimes provided advocacy. The costs to produce the mass media spots were shared, but air time was all donated from media outlets per the rules pertaining to public service announcements. None was paid for at the time. Print materials were initially covered by the National Council for Folic Acid, and eventually

---

BOX 8-3 Questions to Guide Health Communication Staffing

- Have team roles and levels of effort been assigned appropriately, relative to the size of the project?
  - On a large project, roles should be staffed on a full-time basis.
  - On a small project, team members should be flexible, responsive, and have the right mix of skills to perform several roles.
- Does the project team include people with previous experience and training in health communication programming?
- Does the project have adequately skilled staff for the chosen strategic approach of the project? (If the focus is on community mobilization or advocacy, do team members have the right skill sets to achieve program goals?)
- Do the skill requirements for the project match the actual skill levels that staff possess in order to achieve program goals? What shortfalls exist, and what training is necessary?
  - Is the mix between experience and junior staff skills appropriate? Is there backup support for key personnel? Are people with the right skills brought in at the right time?
- Has adequate attention been given to whether the gender balance within the work team reflects the gender balance of the health communication audience or audiences?
- Have volunteers been adequately recruited, oriented, and trained?
- How can partners help support activities?

U.S. Agency for International Development. *CModules: A Learning Package for Social and Behavior Change Communication (SBCC) Communication for Change (C-Change) Project*. Version 3. Washington, DC: C-Change/FHI 360; May 2012.

became available for partner distribution for the cost of production. The CDC and the National Council for Folic Acid covered the costs of developing a partner resource guide to mount community and other small-scale interventions and, later, a media resource guide.[6] These tools, together with the website, have allowed the folic acid program to extend well beyond the resources available to the CDC alone, by empowering any organization concerned about the issue with facts as well as outstanding communication assets.

In planning your program, **TABLE 8-2** provides a model partner asset worksheet to help you think about what different partners can contribute to implementing a large- or small-scale communication intervention.

Budgeting: How Much Will It Cost?

There are popular guidebooks available today that tell you how to do health communication and social marketing "on a shoestring." But if you want a good result (and there is no reason to do a campaign that is not of good quality), you will need to trade off time for money—and you must create a budget. There is no reason that a dedicated group of students, for example, could not mount an effective health communication campaign using internet-based media and live events, with potential coverage by local broadcast and print media, for "nothing more" than the time and effort they devote to the campaign. Out-of-pocket (OOP)

TABLE 8-2 Partner Assets Worksheet

Organization: Partnering Role(s):		
Assets	**% Time or Yes**	**Task/Objective**
People		
Leadership		
Expert staff		
Administrative support		
Students/volunteers		
Expertise		
Research		
Regulatory		
Product		
Packaging		
Shipping		
Marketing		
Communication		
Marketing facilitation		
Training		
Others		

(continues)

TABLE 8-2 Partner Assets Worksheet		_(continued)_
Organization: **Partnering Role(s):**		
Assets	**% Time or Yes**	**Task/Objective**
Relationships		
Our primary target audience		
Our secondary audience		
Donors		
Policymakers		
Community leaders/groups		
Media		
Suppliers		
Others		
Resources		
Information/data (capture)		
Public health		
Environmental		
Regulatory		
Marketing		
Public opinion		
Local knowledge		
Other		
Information (Dissemination)		
Electronic listservs/blogs		
Print/online publications		
Paid advertising		
New outreach (PR)		
Word of mouth		
Viral		

Tangibles/Products		
Food/beverage		
Ingredients		
Medicines		
IT		
Equipment		
Energy		
Transportation		
Advertising time		
Advertising creative		
Other		
Accommodations		
Meeting rooms (20–49)		
Meeting rooms (> 50)		
Project office		
Individual office		
High-profile events		
Media setup		
Storage		

Based on The Partnering Toolbook. Box 2, resource map from GAIN/International Business Leaders Forum. The Partnering Initiative (TPI) website. http://thepartneringinitiative.org/publications /toolbook-series/the-partnering-toolbook/. Accessed February 17, 2017.

expenses—such as professional talent, video and sound production, printing services, and paid placement—are what drive up costs.

Another major cost in health communication is personnel salaries for anyone with expertise that you cannot acquire for free; for example, the salary of counselors or educators is what makes the interpersonal approach relatively expensive. Your budget should cover all the costs or expenses of the intervention activities. The next sections discuss categories that are normally reflected in health communication budgets.

Direct Costs

Direct costs are the part of the budget that contributes directly to a program's outputs. This line item is made up of personnel costs and OOP costs (those associated with products and services not obtained through a salaried employee).

- *Personnel costs:* These include the salaries and benefits, or portions thereof, for the people who will work on the project. Full-time employees who will work part-time on the project should be included at the appropriate percentage of time; for example, if a research assistant will spend 20 hours per week on the project for its first year, they should be budgeted for 50% of the total salary and 50% of the fringe benefits. (Fringe benefits include Social Security taxes, health insurance, dental insurance, and other benefits that your agency provides.) Most organizations have a calculated fringe benefit rate that can be used when developing a budget. It is often in the range of 25% to 30% of the salary.

■ *OOP/nonpersonnel costs:* These are expenses connected to program outputs that are provided by vendors. Such costs may include production services, travel, equipment, office supplies, postage, telephone expenses, and the like. Some donors allow you to break out facility rental, maintenance, and insurance in your nonpersonnel costs; others expect them to be covered by your overhead.

Indirect Costs

Also called "overhead," **indirect costs** are what it costs your agency to exist, but they are not tied directly to creating the program's outputs. Examples usually include office space, environmental management (heat, air conditioning, water, custodial services, etc.), and depreciation on equipment. Indirect costs are usually calculated as a percentage of direct costs. Institutions that have worked with the U.S. government, including many universities, have an approved overhead rate. You might be shocked to learn that it can run as high as 60% or more of the direct costs. Therefore, if you are developing a grant proposal budget, for example, and you know that the total amount of the award is fixed, you must be mindful of your indirect rate to know how much money you actually have to work with. Some donors will pay only a small percentage of indirect costs. Others, such as the National Institutes of Health, provide indirect costs on top of direct costs for research projects.

In-Kind Contributions

In the nonprofit world in which public health often operates, organizations frequently consider their time, space, use of equipment, and other in-house resources as **in-kind contributions** to a project budget. These will be used to produce program outputs but are not factored into the direct or indirect costs of the budget.

Total Budget

The **total budget** is the sum of direct and indirect costs, including in-kind contributions and additional donations. If the project will run for more than one year, an annual budget needs to be prepared as well as a budget for the total time period. Sometimes you will need to separate out and track funding streams in your budget; for example, if a charitable organization wants to know how you spent its contribution, you want to be able to explain this with some precision (e.g., not just, "for 30% of the project"). In addition to a spreadsheet, you often need to provide a budget narrative that describes each expenditure and its purpose.

BOX 8-4 shows a made-up budget proposal for a small-scale, youth-oriented anti-tobacco campaign to be run in one county in southern Florida.

BOX 8-4 Tobacco-Free Kids Proposed Budget Narrative

Tobacco-Free Kids (TFK) is an activity-based program to discourage young people from beginning to use tobacco products. It will consist of a combination of school and recreational facility on-site activities for youth 9–13 years of age as well as social media exposure. The project budget will cover one year of expenses. It includes chiefly staff time, supplies, graphic design for social media, and travel. The university will provide in-kind support of computers and software for mounting social media, as well as contract support for negotiating purchasing of supplies and equipment.

A. Personnel
Project Director: This position is filled by the Director of Health Promotion at a 0.25 FTE level of effort. The Director of Health Promotion position is currently filled by Gloria Rush, MS, MPH. The allocated budget for this salary expense is $18,000, based on a $72,000 annual salary.

Youth Specialist: The Youth Specialist has the responsibility of coordinating and leading the daily afterschool and monthly weekend programs. This position is currently held by Lola Catt, BA. The allocated budget for this salary expense is $6400, based on a $32,000 annual salary and a 20% level of effort.

Graduate student assistants: Two graduate students from the Public Health Program at the University of South Florida will provide approximately 10 hours a week for 14 weeks a semester, for a total of 560 hours provided to the project. Students are paid at a rate of $15.00/hour. Students are TBN (to be named). Students will primarily manage our social media campaign, posting to Twitter, Snapchat, Instagram, and Pinterest.

B. Fringe Benefits
A total amount of $7588 is budgeted to pay for fringe benefits for the two salaried positions (Project Director and Youth Specialist) for the specified employment periods. Fringe benefits include FICA, unemployment insurance, workers' compensation, and health and disability insurance. Full-time employees (must work at least 32 hours a week) receive USF's standard health, dental, life, and disability insurance benefit package. Fringe benefits for current employees on staff are calculated at 31.1% of gross salary.

C. Travel

The total budget for travel is $2400.

Local travel: Local travel expenses include the costs of using public transportation (currently $1.75 per trip) as well as private automobiles to conduct project activities. Local travel will include sending project staff out to community centers, churches, and other after-school programs within our catchment area for special events. It also supports travel to attend off-site meetings, training, and regional conference sessions. Private automobile mileage will be reimbursed at the federally approved rate of $0.45/mile, by means of a mileage log.

The local travel budget for staff is $1200 for the 12-month project period.

Out-of-state travel: A travel budget of $600 is included for air and ground travel for two project staff to attend a professional conference related to youth smoking prevention.

Per diem and lodging: The total budget for per diem and lodging is $600. This is the estimated cost for per diem and lodging for two project staff to attend a professional conference related to youth smoking prevention.

D. Out-of-Pocket

The total budget for out-of-pocket (OOP) expenses is $3600.

The largest portion of this will be spent on activity and educational supplies. This includes staff curriculum materials, participant materials, and parent materials, as well as outreach to promote the activity in the community. We anticipate using very limited services of a graphic designer to provide a coherent look to our website and media feeds. We will purchase sports equipment, games, light refreshments, and incentive items ($5.00 or less) for the after-school and weekend programs. We are able to budget low OOP because the university will purchase educational and sporting equipment through our contracted vendors.

Tobacco-Free Kids Budget Spreadsheet

Object	% TIME	Year 1
A. Personnel		
Project Director	0.25	$18,000.00
Youth Specialist	0.20	$6400.00
Graduate student assistants 2 (10 hours/week) × 28 weeks × $15/hour	100.00	$8400.00
Total Salaries		**$32,800.00**
B. Fringe Benefits		*$7588.00*
C. Travel		
Local		$1200.00
Out of state		$600.00
Per diem and lodging		$600.00
Total Travel		**$2400.00**
D. Out-of-Pocket		
Video recording software		$200.00
Video recording devices		$300.00
Sporting equipment		$500.00
Incentives and refreshments		$1000.00
Other office supplies		$400.00

(continues)

BOX 8-4 Tobacco-Free Kids Proposed Budget Narrative *(continued)*

Object	% TIME	Year 1
D. Out-of-Pocket		
Postage		$240.00
Telephone service contract (12 months × $35.00)		$420.00
Professional services: graphics		$600.00
Total OOP		**$3660.00**
E. Total Direct Costs		*$46,448.00*
F. Indirect Costs (0.25%)		*$11,612.00*
Total Budget		**$58,060.00**

USF In-kind contribution: Computer equipment, negotiated contract support (estimated at $15,000)

BOX 8-5 Sample Project Timeline

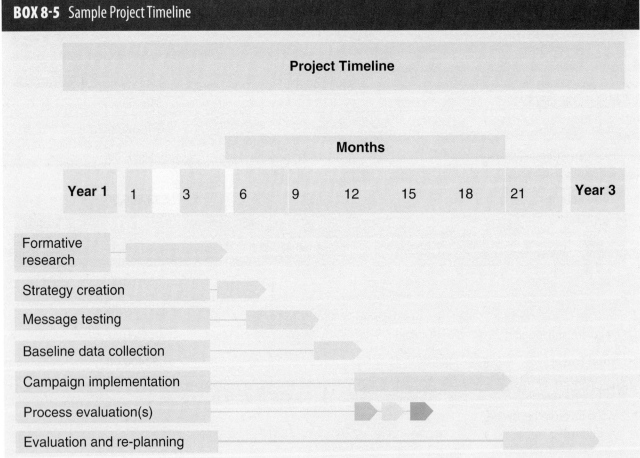

What Is a Realistic Timeline?

You will note the budget in Box 8-4 is for one year of implementation. Most larger-scale communication programs take one year to plan and produce, including conducting formative research, developing and testing materials, and readying everything for dissemination. The actual implementation depends on the strategy being used, but a campaign of less than a few months, except in an emergency situation, is not advised. It really takes time to capture the public's attention. **BOX 8-5** shows a sample timeline for a small-scale program including the formative research, production, and dissemination phases.

Advocacy

If your project is meant to garner support for a local issue, such as funding for an under-five health or education program, you might want to hold a local town hall meeting to launch your activities.

Another important element of advocacy for your program is to get the press involved and engaged. This can serve as free publicity for your program, which not only potentially raises awareness about the program in those you want to reach, but also allows you to leverage the coverage with other media involvement such as stories, interviews, and photos. Two of the most common ways to interact with members of the media are through the use of a **press advisory** (sometimes also called a media advisory) and a **press release**. **BOX 8-6** provides a quick overview of how these are written and what is included in each.

The press or media advisory is a short, one-page alert that lets media know about upcoming events. Think of it like an invitation that provides the who, what, when, where, and why of what you are doing. It will let the media know the nitty gritty of what is

happening so they can make a quick decision about whether they are interested. **BOX 8-7** shows a sample press advisory.

A press release, on the other hand, is written like an article you might find in a newspaper or news website. It has facts about the health issue and quotes from key stakeholders to stimulate pickup by news outlets to generate print and broadcast coverage. The press release creates an image and story the press can use as background when putting together a story. In smaller media markets, press releases may be published in their entirety, which ensures all the information you are trying to get out to your audience is presented. **BOX 8-8** shows a sample press release.

Managing Your Social Media

Social media and butterflies share the same life span, or so it seems. Social media blogger Nathan Ellering has studied the science of posting to social media sites. **BOX 8-9** distills his observations and 15 studies down to some guidelines. (See **FIGURES 8-5** through **8-9**.)

There are applications to manage posting to social media, which might seem to defeat the purpose of using it to interact. But, as Ellering points out, you

---

BOX 8-6 Key Elements of a Press Advisory vs. a Press Release

Key Elements of a Press or Media Advisory

- Should be brief and to the point. It is an alert to the media for upcoming events, often to provide photo opportunities.
- Should contain a headline detailing the most important information.
- Should include the five Ws (i.e., who, what, where, when, and why).
- Should include contact information for reporters to get more information.
- Format:
  - On the top, type "MEDIA ADVISORY".
  - Underneath that, put the date of the event.
  - On the right side, include your contact information.
  - At the end of the advisory, type "End ###", centered, to indicate it is over.

Key Elements of a Written Press Release

- Should be written like an actual story, in the inverted pyramid style of news writing—headline and most important information at top.
- Include quotes from key spokespeople and facts to stimulate pickup by news outlets to generate print and broadcast coverage.
- Should create an image and story that journalists can use alone or as background when writing a story.
- Format:
  - On the top, type "PRESS RELEASE".
  - Underneath that, type "FOR IMMEDIATE RELEASE".
  - On the right side, include your contact information.
  - At the end of the press release, type "End ###", centered, to indicate it is over.

BOX 8-7 Sample Press Advisory

Organization
Logo here

Media Advisory

For March 20, 2017
For Directions and information, contact:
NAME, Organization Name
222-222-2222

Local Agency Sponsors Community Event to Increase Awareness about Healthcare Access

Event to be held Monday, March 20, noon to 3 p.m.

WHAT: The ORGANIZATION NAME will sponsor a free event for community members to hear about and discuss how the repeal of the Affordable Care Act (ACA) could affect their healthcare access and what actions they can take. Speakers from local government, community members impacted by the repeal of the ACA, and local healthcare organizations will be available. Community agencies will also have booths and materials available, including food and activities.

WHEN: Monday, March 20th; noon to 3 p.m.

WHERE: Everywhere Community Center, ADDRESS

WHO: Scheduled to speak:

-Mayor XXX
-Congressman XXX
-XXX, Executive Director, ORGANIZATION
-Local citizens currently getting health care through the Affordable Care Act

PHOTO OPPORTUNITIES: After remarks, speakers will be available for photos and one-on-one interviews. Community members will be writing letters to their Congress members at the event. They will also be available to tell their stories about their experiences with the ACA.

BACKGROUND: The proposed American Health Care Act would replace the types of subsidies that people get to help them afford health insurance. This is particularly important for lower and moderate income individuals who do not have access to coverage at work and must purchase coverage directly. Currently, the ACA provides three types of financial assistance: Medicaid expansion for those with incomes below 138% of poverty; refundable premium tax credits for people with incomes 100% to 400% of poverty who purchase coverage through federal or state marketplaces; and cost-sharing subsidies for people with incomes from 100% to 250% of poverty to provide lower deductibles and copays when purchasing silver plans in a marketplace. The proposed legislation instead relies on refundable tax credits that will vary with age and will drastically reduce the number of people able to access these credits as most low income people do not have to pay income taxes and would be ineligible. The potential repeal of the Affordable Care Act could thus have devastating consequences for the 20 million people currently covered with ACA health insurance programs, including a significant number of XXX residents.

could spend all your time creating, curating, and releasing your posts; or you could use a scheduling app. If you are the one person responsible for social media, this is probably the way to go. With appropriate analytical tools (discussed next), you can respond in a timely manner.

▶ Monitoring and Evaluating Your Program

As shown in FIGURE 8-10, you collect data to guide and evaluate your program at just about every stage of planning and implementation. The information gathered through this process is necessary to make decisions about the program in process as well as what you plan to do in the future. We have previously discussed formative research and pretesting used to develop and test your messages and materials. Now you are trying to determine the following:

■ *Whether activities are functioning as planned:* This is called *process evaluation.* The term *monitoring* is sometimes used interchangeably. The key difference is that monitoring usually refers

BOX 8-8 Sample Press Release

FOR IMMEDIATE RELEASE

Date

Contact: Your name

Your phone

Your email

FAMILY FUN PLANNED AROUND CELEBRATED CHILDREN'S BOOKS!

The celebrated, inspiring, and delightful Eagle Books stories for children will come to life when <local organization/community> hosts a festival inviting families to have fun while learning how to prevent type 2 diabetes. The activities begin at <event starting time> and continue until <event ending time> on <day and date> at <location >. This Eagle Books <title of event> will include <activity>, <activity>, and <activity> with Eagle Books giveaways available to all who attend. The event is free and all ages are welcome.

<Insert a quote from planning committee representative. For example: "Type 2 diabetes is a very real and very serious disease within our community," said <name>, <title>. "The good news is that type 2 diabetes can be prevented. Our health fair includes activities that will really help families understand that they have control over everyday things that affect their health. Eagle Books show us those strengths in a fun way! We encourage the whole community to come join in the excitement."

Developed under the direction of the Native Diabetes Wellness Program, Division of Diabetes Translation, Centers for Disease Control and Prevention, in partnership with the Tribal Leaders Diabetes Committee and the Indian Health Service Division of Diabetes Treatment and Prevention, the Eagle Books are a series of four elementary-level story books in which engaging animal characters—Mr. Eagle, Miss Rabbit, and clever trickster, Coyote—connect with a young boy named Rain That Dances and his friends to explore the joys and benefits of physical activity, good eating habits, and seeking advice from their elders about living a healthy life. The story books are used in many schools, clinics, and Head Start programs and are part of the K-12 Diabetes Education in Tribal Schools: Health is Life in Balance curriculum for grades K-4.

More information is available from <local contact person> at <phone number>. Eagle Books information is available at http://www.cdc.gov/diabetes/pubs/eagle.htm.

###

Reproduced from CDC. Sample news release/press release. https://www.cdc.gov/diabetes/projects/ndwp/doc/ebsamplenewsrelease.doc.

to collection of data from the same sources over set periods of time, whereas process evaluation is often done only once or twice at the outset of a program.

- *The contribution of each activity to the overall effect:* This is based on the program's logic model and requires collecting data about the effectiveness of delivery.
- *Whether the program is effective at accomplishing its goals:* Is it reducing barriers that prevent change and increasing desired behaviors?
- *Whether unintended consequences are taking place, so that the program can be modified as needed:* For example, a health communication program aiming to increase partner testing may have the unintended consequence of increasing gender-based violence.
- Which activities should be continued and/or scaled up?

Process Evaluation

Process evaluation, or monitoring, tells you whether your project is functioning according to plan. In a logic model, this step measures your inputs and outputs. Depending on your program, you may measure dissemination, reach, training results, customer satisfaction with services or interventions, and so on.

Media Dissemination

This indicator will tell you what went "out" from your organization. You might measure:

- By media channel, number of impressions or placements of the information (occurrences in newspapers, magazines, billboards, television spots, radio announcements)
- Number of materials disseminated to intermediaries, such as teachers, community educators, clergy, and so on
- Where and when your social media posted

BOX 8-9 Best Times to Post on Social Media

- *Time zones:* Fifty percent of the U.S. population is in the Eastern Time Zone, and the Eastern and Central combined represent almost 80% of the U.S. population. For those of you who have audiences outside the United States, demographic research like this is simple enough with Google Analytics to understand where your own audience is, giving you the opportunity to target their time zones accordingly.

  There are also a few tools to help you find when your own audience is online and using the social networks you're concentrating on—which helps you understand the best times to share based on your local time zone.

- *Platform-specific guidance:* Figures 8-5 through 8-9 give some guidance on when to post to Facebook, Twitter, Pinterest, Instagram, and LinkedIn.

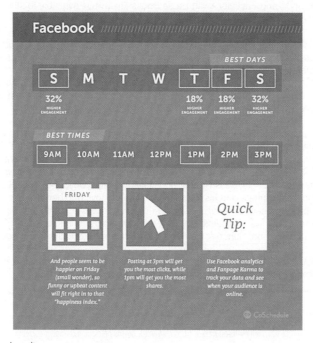

FIGURE 8-5 When to post on Facebook.

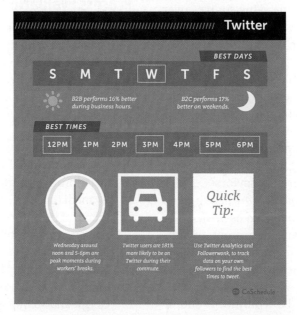

FIGURE 8-6 When to post on Twitter.

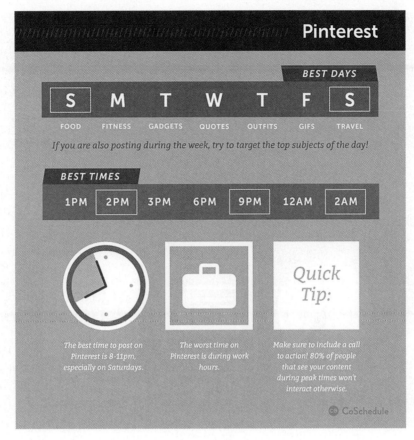

FIGURE 8-7 When to post on Pinterest.

Reproduced from Ellering N. What 20 studies say about the best times to post on social media. https://coschedule.com/blog/best-times-to-post-on-social-media/. Published October 16, 2017.

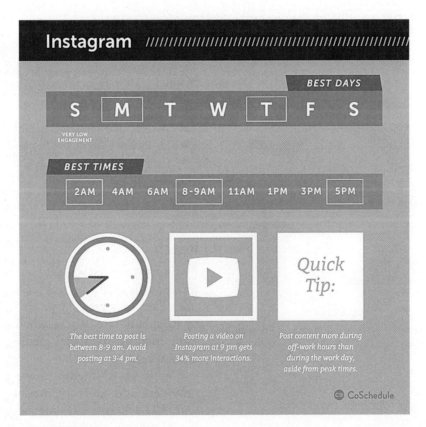

FIGURE 8-8 When to post on Instagram.

Reproduced from Ellering N. What 20 studies say about the best times to post on social media. https://coschedule.com/blog/best-times-to-post-on-social-media/. Published October 16, 2017.

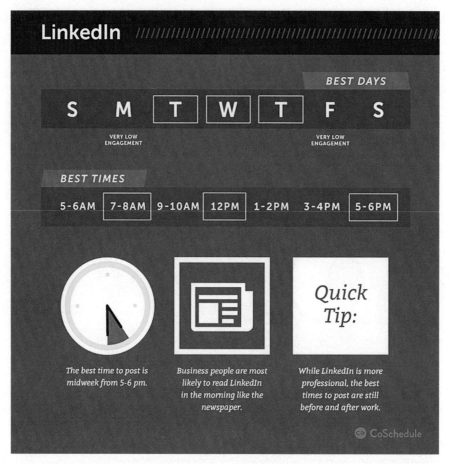

FIGURE 8-9 When to post on LinkedIn.

Reproduced from Ellering N. What 20 studies say about the best times to post on social media. https://coschedule.com/blog/best-times-to-post-on-social-media/. Published October 16, 2017.

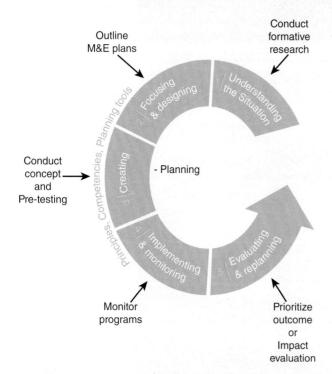

FIGURE 8-10 Monitoring or evaluation throughout the communication planning cycle.

Reproduced from U.S. Agency for International Development. *CModules: A Learning Package for Social and Behavior Change Communication (SBCC) Communication for Change (C-Change) Project.* Version 3. Washington, DC: C-Change/FHI 360; May 2012.

BOX 8-10 Key Engagement Metrics for the Most Commonly Used Social Media Platforms

- *Facebook:* Likes, shares, link clicks, and comments
- *Twitter:* Likes, retweets, and replies
- *Instagram:* Likes and comments
- *LinkedIn:* Likes, comments, and shares
- *Google+:* +1s, shares, and comments
- *Pinterest:* Likes, comments, and repins

Reach

By contrast to what was sent out, reach measures what was actually delivered or received. Many researchers use a "next day recall" type survey (usually delivered by telephone) to assess whether broadcast media were attended to. Social media provide more easily accessed data.

With social media, there are a multitude of providers and tools for measuring uptake of content. **BOX 8-10** provides metrics that are tracked by the platforms themselves or through third-party providers.

You can spend hours attempting to monitor the effectiveness of your social media across a multitude of platforms. There are many subscription-based services (many with a free entry level) that allow you to create a dashboard tracking the metrics of most use to your project. Feldman[7] recently posted a nicely structured process to use these tools in a manner consistent with process evaluation. Some of his guidelines are these:

- *Establish a baseline.* This is so obvious in every other form of evaluation that we do, but we often overlook it when using social media. Feldman notes that both Facebook and Twitter provide data that can be exported to spreadsheets, so tracking over a time period is simple.
- *Create a multichannel dashboard.* As mentioned previously, a dashboard can allow you to compare channels against each other, as well as specific content you have posted on various channels.
- *Identify the top channels with Google Analytics.* Using this free tool, you can determine which social channels drive the most traffic to a site (whether a website, Twitter feed, Pinterest site, or the like). You can also see the length of time visitors interact with content on each platform.
- *Use SMART goals for social media.* This includes measuring the number of visits, leads, and "customers" (regular users) within specific time frames.
- *Drill down on individual posts.* Consider each post as a message. You can assess immediate feedback from the audience by how they like, comment, or share it.
- *Identify your influencers.* When someone retweets or repins your stuff, thank them.
- *Use hashtags (#) to your advantage.* Some platforms (e.g., Twitter, Instagram) use them more than others. Hashtagify.me can help you identify trending hashtags to use in your posts.

Use what you learn to update your messaging strategies, personas, and overall campaign. With social media, it is always a work in progress. But unless your intervention is strictly about social media, all of this would be considered process evaluation or campaign monitoring.

Training Preparation

If you are using personnel in a project, such as health educators, patient navigators, or wellness coaches, then preparing them to deliver the intervention in a consistent manner is a necessary step. The most common way of evaluating this preparation is through a pretest of knowledge, attitudes, and confidence conducted before training, and then a similar assessment afterwards. Particularly for interpersonal communication in a healthcare setting, a supervisor or other trained specialist can use published tools for assessing the quality of interaction. The gold standard is likely the Roter Interaction Analysis System,[8] which has been used chiefly in research due to the time investment required to learn the coding system.

Other Quality Assessments

In addition to healthcare communications, you might be interested in assessing how the target audience perceives the quality of an interaction. The most common example of this is a customer satisfaction survey. As you've doubtless heard many times when calling a customer service line, "This call is being recorded for quality assurance (and training) purposes." The "quality assurance" might mean that evaluators are listening to recorded (or live) calls to make sure the interaction is going as planned.

There is also a trend to measure customer satisfaction after every encounter with a provider. This is driven by the *touch-points* process in commercial sales; that is, that any interaction with a customer contributes or detracts from a potential engagement and sale.

The largest noncommercial application of customer service research is coming from the Centers for Medicare and Medicaid Services, which has instituted the Hospital Consumer Assessment of Healthcare Providers and Systems (HCAHPS) survey.[9] Pronounced "H-CAPS," this is the first national, standardized, publicly reported survey of patients' perspectives of hospital care. Although many hospitals have collected information on patient satisfaction for their own internal use, HCAHPS is the first nationally standardized and publicly reported information about patient experience. You will note the emphasis on communication and patient understanding.

In 2016, more than 4400 general hospitals participated. (Pediatric, psychiatric, and specialty hospitals were excluded.) More than 99% of the hospitals used an approved survey vendor who contacted patients by mail (60%) or telephone (40%). **BOX 8-11** shows an abstract of the questions used in the HCAHPS in English. It is also available in Spanish, Russian, Chinese, Vietnamese, and Portuguese, as of this writing.

Outcome Evaluation

Program evaluation is a specialty field in health communication. A key reference to guide our work has long been Patton's *Essentials of Utilization-Focused*

BOX 8-11 HCAHPS Survey

HCAHPS Survey

SURVEY INSTRUCTIONS

♦ You should only fill out this survey if you were the patient during the hospital stay named in the cover letter. Do not fill out this survey if you were not the patient.

♦ Answer <u>all</u> the questions by checking the box to the left of your answer.

♦ You are sometimes told to skip over some questions in this survey. When this happens you will see an arrow with a note that tells you what question to answer next, like this:

☐   Yes
☑   No   → *If No, Go to Question 1*

> *You may notice a number on the survey. This number is used to let us know if you returned your survey so we don't have to send you reminders.*
> *Please note: Questions 1-25 in this survey are part of a national initiative to measure the quality of care in hospitals. OMB #0938-0981*

Please answer the questions in this survey about your stay at the hospital named on the cover letter. Do not include any other hospital stays in your answers.

YOUR CARE FROM NURSES

1.   **During this hospital stay, how often did nurses treat you with <u>courtesy and respect</u>?**

   ^{1}☐ Never
   ^{2}☐ Sometimes
   ^{3}☐ Usually
   ^{4}☐ Always

2.   **During this hospital stay, how often did nurses <u>listen carefully to you</u>?**

   ^{1}☐ Never
   ^{2}☐ Sometimes
   ^{3}☐ Usually
   ^{4}☐ Always

3.   **During this hospital stay, how often did nurses <u>explain things</u> in a way you could understand?**

   ^{1}☐ Never
   ^{2}☐ Sometimes
   ^{3}☐ Usually
   ^{4}☐ Always

4.   **During this hospital stay, after you pressed the call button, how often did you get help as soon as you wanted it?**

   ^{1}☐ Never
   ^{2}☐ Sometimes
   ^{3}☐ Usually
   ^{4}☐ Always
   ^{9}☐ I never pressed the call button

January 2018   1

Evaluation.[10] As the name implies, the people who need the information about a program—the intended users—have everything to do with how the evaluation will be designed and carried out. Not all programs require an extensive evaluation. The costs of collecting information from a representative sample of the population exposed to an intervention can be prohibitive. Some agencies require evaluations and build the costs into grant support mechanisms. Others are content with process indicators. The starting point for deciding to do an evaluation is the needs of the program managers and stakeholders. The evaluation demonstrates the effectiveness of the intervention. Finding this out can lead to a decision to change or stop activities, expand them, or try something new.

Outcome evaluations of health communication programs need to document impact by measuring whether program objectives have been met, barriers have been reduced, favorable attitudes and perceptions have come about in the target audience, and particular desired behaviors have increased. Different kinds of questions will produce different findings.

Description

What happened as a result of the intervention?

Is there an observable change in behavior, or a behavioral antecedent (knowledge, attitudes, social norms) from one point in time to another? You might want to use both quantitative methods (counting, measuring) and qualitative methods (interviewing participants about their experience) to answer these questions.

Causality

Can you attribute what you see as a change to the intervention? Some specific questions to ask include:

- Did the change take place *after* the health communication program began (that is, the change cannot be attributed easily to something contemporaneous, such as a change in weather for outdoor exercise or the availability of healthy foods for a nutrition education intervention)?
- Can you detect a degree of response against a "dose" of the intervention (that is, the more communication, the greater the response)?
- Can you control for confounding variables (e.g., educational level, socioeconomic status, access, etc.)?
- Was there a comparison group?
- What was the likelihood that those persons more likely to adopt the behavior were those who participated in the first place? (This is called a propensity score in statistical terms. In everyday terms, it is called preaching to the choir.)

Even when managed as a quasi-experiment, in which one group receives an intervention and another does not, it can be extremely difficult to attribute change to a communication intervention in community settings. To begin, the chance of exposure is limited, for all the reasons said previously about the oceans of competing information we encounter on a daily basis. Unless you achieved about a 50% reach, it is unlikely there was sufficient exposure for later effects such as attitude or behavior change to take place.

Second, people share information all the time, so maintaining clear boundaries on where an intervention takes place is nearly impossible. Third, other entities might be communicating about the same thing, without you being aware of it; for example, was it the local bus advertisements about colorectal cancer screening that prompted more people to call for a colonoscopy, or was it a national PSA with Ozzy Osbourne? The only real recourse is to have a tight logic model and measure along each step from inputs to outputs to outcomes.

Judgment

You have detected outcomes; for example, you increased the healthy behavior by about 15% over the baseline. (This is a pretty typical change in a one-year, education-alone program.) Are the outcomes good enough? Recalling the stages of change theoretical frameworks, it would be unreasonable to expect large changes in behavior in a population that was completely unaware of a health behavior before the campaign began. Based on diffusion theory, it would be reasonable to expect about 15% being early adopters. But, once this group adopts the behavior, with ongoing normative support, it is likely that others will follow. Can the program take credit for this level of change?

Were there unintended and negative consequences? Was a group harmed as a result of the communication program? How can that be avoided in the future?

There are a number of specific approaches and subquestions within this overall question. Most often, if a measurable outcome can be quantified, the next question will pertain to the costs of achieving it. This is called a cost-benefit analysis.

Next Steps

Should the program be continued? Expanded in geography or numbers? Tried with different groups of people? Shut down?

Depending on the nature of the evaluation question, you will select indicators as well as the tools for collecting those indicators.

BOX 8-12 Individual-Level Indicators for Measuring Outcomes in Health Communication

If Using a *Stages of Change* (Transtheoretical) Model	If Using an *Integrative* Model	If Using a *Health Belief* Model or *Parallel Process* Model
From Baseline, % Change In		
Awareness/knowledge	Beliefs	Perceived susceptibility
Contemplation	Norms	Perceived severity
Preparation	Attitudes	Perceived benefits of intervention
Trial	Self-efficacy	Reduction of barriers to performing protective steps
Maintenance	Intention to perform behavior	Awareness of cues to action
	Perceived skills and abilities	Reduced anxiety or fear
Behavior	**Behavior**	**Behavior**

Indicators for Measuring Change

Assuming a baseline survey or some other data collection has taken place (again, the time to think about evaluation is *not* at the end of the project!), the theoretical structure and logic model you have designed for the intervention will lead to selecting an indicator. **BOX 8-12** lists some indicators associated with three widely used theories of change.

When attempting to make group-level change, your indicators might examine changes in participation and engagement, social capital formation (i.e., how much individuals rely on each other and come together to solve problems), collective efficacy, resiliency, community vibrancy, and social norms.

Managing an Evaluation

Thanks to the "Better Evaluation" international collaboration, with financial support from a number of charitable organizations and agencies, there is a great

online resource that provides extensive guidance for planning and managing evaluations appropriate to health communication programs. They have broken the evaluation process into seven tasks: manage, define, frame, describe, understand causes, synthesize, report, and support use. **BOX 8-13** features the collaboration's overarching guidelines for the first task, managing an evaluation.

Getting the Word Out

When you get to the end of the evaluation, you need to write up the results and share them with stakeholders or the public. BetterEvaluation.org again has some great tips for presenting findings. These appear in **BOX 8-14**. Remember that the point of doing an evaluation is to use the results. Too many big reports sit on shelves and gather dust—if shared online, there is a better chance that someone will find them and use the results. **APPENDIX 8A** shows an example of formative, process and summative evaluation for a children's nutrition program.

BOX 8-13 Managing an Evaluation

An overview of key tasks according to Better Evaluation.org

1. Understand and engage stakeholders.

Begin by clarifying who has an interest in the evaluation in addition to the primary intended users. An analysis of the interests of different stakeholders helps in thinking about how you will keep stakeholders engaged during the evaluation.

2. Establish decision-making processes.

Specify how decisions will be made about the evaluation. Who will provide advice, who will make recommendations, and who will make the actual decisions?

3. Decide who will conduct the evaluation.

Who will actually undertake the evaluation? Will it be a group internal to the organization that is implementing a program, an external evaluator, or some combination of the two? Will the community and/or intended beneficiaries be involved in conducting the evaluation?

4. Determine and secure resources.

Identify what resources (time, money, expertise) will be needed and available for the evaluation. Consider both internal resources (e.g., staff time) and external resources (e.g., participants' time to attend meetings to provide feedback).

5. Define ethical and quality evaluation standards.

What will be considered appropriate quality and ethical standards for the evaluation and what will need to be done to ensure these standards are achieved? These decisions will be influenced by the purpose and timing of the evaluation, the level of resourcing available, and the characteristics of the intervention being evaluated.

6. Document management processes and agreements.

It is usually necessary to develop formal documents about an evaluation, including a brief, a plan, and terms of reference. Additional documents will be needed if an evaluation is externally contracted, such as an expression of interest, a request for proposal, a request for tender, and a contract.

7. Develop an evaluation plan, framework, or policy.

An evaluation plan sets out how an individual evaluation will be undertaken. An evaluation framework guides a series of evaluations.

8. Review evaluation (do meta-evaluation).

Review the evaluation process, findings, and conclusions drawn; when appropriate, it is valuable to engage stakeholders in this task.

9. Develop evaluation capacity.

How can your organization or group build on, or develop, human capital (knowledge and skills), organizational capital (technical infrastructure and processes), and social capital (supportive networks) for effectively managing, undertaking, and using evaluations?

Reproduced from BetterEvaluation.org. Manage evaluation. http://www.betterevaluation.org/plan/manage_evaluation.

▶ Conclusion

It is both challenging and fun to implement or evaluate health communication programs. An ongoing poll run by the Society for Health Communication asked the following question: Which trend do you think will most impact health communication? Here are the choices:

- Rise of social media
- Enhanced evaluation tools
- Use of mobile devices
- New communication theories
- Integration with traditional marketing

You are invited to go online and vote (http://www.societyforhealthcommunication.org), as well as see the results. (We will not give them away here.)

You will be shaping the future of health communication, inventing new ways to communicate and evaluate programs, and discovering new health-related topics about which to communicate. Go and make it so!

BOX 8-14 BetterEvaluation Report

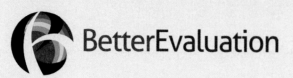

betterevaluation.org
May 2013

Report and Support use of findings

Develop and present findings in ways that are useful for the intended users of the evaluation, and support them to make use of them.

1. Identify reporting requirements
What timeframe and format is required for reporting?

Communication plan: developing a plan that outlines the strategies which will be used to communicate the results of your evaluation.

Reporting needs analysis: working with your client to determine their reporting needs.

2. Develop reporting media
What types of reporting formats will be appropriate for the intended users?

Written

Executive Summaries: including an executive summary which is a shortened version of the full report.

Final Reports: ensuring they are readable, straight to the point, and use a writing style that promotes understanding regardless who the target audience is.

Interim reports: presenting the interim, preliminary, or initial evaluation findings.

Memos and email: maintaining ongoing communication among evaluation stakeholders through brief and specific messages about a particular issue.

News media communications: sharing news relating to evaluation findings through press releases.

Newsletters, bulletins, briefs and brochures: highlighting particular findings or angles on an evaluation using shorter communications such as bulletins, briefs, newsletters, blogs and brochures.

Postcards: collecting information quickly in order to provide a short report on evaluation findings (or an update on progress).

Website communications: disseminating information such as that coming from evaluations via a range of web based tools.

> You may develop a number of reports, in different formats, for different sets of stakeholders. Work with your primary users and stakeholders to determine when and in what form they want to receive evaluation reports. Also determine who you will involve in viewing draft and interim reports.

Presentations

Conference: discussing a set topic or theme in a large group of people at a set venue.

Displays and exhibits: drawing attention to particular issues and assisting in community engagement.

Flip Charts: providing a useful way of interacting with your audience and therefore allowing you to present your own ideas and results and also to immediately record input, feedback and ideas from your audience.

Information Contacts: providing a contact person for all media and public enquiries about a project or program.

Posters: presenting your evaluation findings in the form of a poster provides a good opportunity to get your message across in a clear way while also providing opportunities for feedback.

PowerPoint: organizing and communicate information coming from evaluations in the form of a slide show which can be used at a meeting or conference.

Teleconference: facilitating discussion of evaluation findings via telephone.

Verbal briefings: providing specific information to an audience of interested participants allowing for a structured question and answer format based on that information.

Video: highly flexible and immediate medium which allows you to make an emotional meaningful connection with the audience.

Videoconference: gathering data, communicating information about an evaluation, reporting findings, receiving feedback, and planning for utilization.

Web-conference: bringing people together from around the world using the internet.

Creative

Cartoons: allowing readers to see a point differently, add humour, and break up large sections of prose.

Photographic reporting: making your report more appealing to readers and also making the key messages more memorable by including photographs.

Poetry: communicating the experience of participants can be achieved by presenting some of the findings in the form of a poem.

Reporting in pictures: presenting information in an alternative way and therefore increasing understanding of your results.

Theatre: communicating evaluation findings and engaging intended users in responding to them.

> Presenting your report in a creative manner may be the most relevant means to get your information across if the context allows for it. You may consider working with an artist or a graphic designer to produce creative displays.

Graphic design

Arrangement: Descriptive text and its related data visualization should be arranged so they appear together on a page. Narrative text should be left-justified.

Color: Blocks of background color can help group cognitively-similar items or set off reporting elements like sidebars. Text intended for narrative reading should be set in black or dark gray on a white or very light background.

Images: Written reports and presentations should always include images. Beyond just charts and graphs, photographs or drawings increase the relevancy of the material to the audience and make the report more engaging.

Type: Generally speaking, serif fonts support readability in long, narrative-style documents produced on paper. Sans serif fonts are easier to read in electronic reporting media.

Example of an infographic used as a reporting format

This graphic was developed in the 1850s by Florence Nightingale depicting causes of death in the British Army in 1854. The graph shows that by far the biggest killer was preventable disease, not battle wounds as was previously thought. This led to improved conditions in military hospitals.

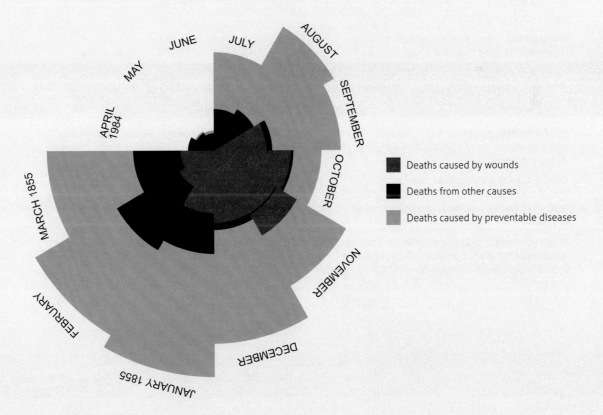

- ■ Deaths caused by wounds
- ■ Deaths from other causes
- ■ Deaths caused by preventable diseases

BetterEvaluation - Report and Support Use of findings (May 2013)
http://betterevaluation.org

(continues)

BOX 8-14 BetterEvaluation Report *(continued)*

3. Ensure accessibility
How can the report be easy to access and use for different users?

Applied graphic design principles

Simplified report layout: three different ways of simplifying the report layout are to eliminate chartjunk, emphasise headings as summary statements, and use descriptive subtitles.

One-Three-Twenty-Five (1:3:25) principle: ensuring that research findings are presented in a logical and consistent manner by allowing for a 1 page outline, a 3 page executive summary and 25 pages to present the findings and methodology.

Support users with auditory disabilities

Support users with colour blindness

Support users with visual disabilities

Use appropriate language: ensuring the language of a report is clear, concise and allows accessibility for all stakeholders.

4. Develop recommendations
Will the evaluation include recommendations? How will these be developed and by whom?

Beneficiary exchange: discussing findings between beneficiaries in order to provide feedback.

Chat rooms: setting up online spaces where findings can be discussed.

Electronic democracy: using new and emergent forms of media in order to engage community members in seeking to influence the decision making process.

External review: having external experts or anonymous reviewers provide feedback.

Group critical reflection: facilitating a group stakeholder feedback session.

Individual critical reflection: asking particular individual stakeholders for their independent feedback.

Lessons learned

Participatory recommendation screening: testing recommendations with key stakeholders.

World Cafe: hosting a group dialogue which emphasizes the power of simple conversation when considering relevant questions and themes.

5. Support use
In addition to engaging intended users in the evaluation pocess, how will you support the use of evaluation findings?

Annual reviews: reviewing major evaluation findings and conclusions based on evaluation studies completed during the preceding year.

Conference Co-presentations: evaluators and evaluation commisioners or users jointly presenting findings or discussions about processes from an evaluation.

Policy briefings: providing evaluation findings and lessons learned in an accessible manner for target audiences which can be followed up by management and staff.

Recommendations tracking: keeping a transparent record of the responses to and action from recommendations.

Social Learning: focusing on how people learn through social interactions, such as modelling, making connections, sharing experiences and resources, collaboration and self-organization.

Trade Publications: producing a non-technical version of key findigns for a publication aimed at staff who can use the findings.

Find options (methods), resources and more information on these tasks and approaches online at
http://betterevaluation.org/plan/reportandsupportuse

BetterEvaluation - Report and Support Use of findings (May 2013)
http://betterevaluation.org

Key Terms

Baseline data
Cost-effectiveness
Deontological
  principles
Direct costs
Expandability
Indirect costs

In-kind
  contributions
Logic model
Pilot testing
Presentability
Press advisory
Press release

Process evaluation
Soft launch
Sustainability
SWOTE analysis
Total budget
Utilitarianism

Chapter Questions

1. How does a logic model help in developing a communication intervention? How does the backward planning help?
2. Describe the key constituents of the logic model. Give two examples for each.
3. Justify the conditions that are within and outside your control in a SWOTE analysis.
4. Explain the ethical dimensions associated with any health communication program.
5. Describe in detail any two criteria associated with production and dissemination factors.
6. What is an implementation plan? Discuss the categories in a health implementation budget.
7. What is the importance of process evaluation in a logic model? How and when do you manage the evaluation?

References

1. W.K. Kellogg Foundation logic model development guide. W.K. Kellogg Foundation website. http://www.wkkf.org/resource-directory/resource/2006/02/wk-kellogg-foundation-logic-model-development-guide. Published February 2, 2006. Accessed March 16, 2018.
2. Taylor-Powell E, Henert E. *Developing a Logic Model: Teaching and Training Guide*. Madison, WI: University of Wisconsin Extension, Cooperative Extension, Program Development and Evaluation. https://fyi.uwex.edu/programdevelopment/files/2016/03/lmguidecomplete.pdf. Published February 2008. Accessed March 16, 2018.
3. Guttman N, Salmon CT. Guilt, fear, stigma and knowledge gaps: ethical issues in public health communication interventions. *Bioethics*. 2004;18(6):531-552.
4. O'Sullivan GA, Yonkler JA, Morgan W, Merritt AP. *A Field Guide to Designing a Health Communication Strategy*. Baltimore, MD: Johns Hopkins Bloomberg School of Public Health/Center for Communication Programs. http://www.jhuccp.org/pubs/fg/02/index.shtml. Published March 2003. Accessed February 17, 2017.
5. U.S. Agency for International Development. *CModules: A Learning Package for Social and Behavior Change Communication (SBCC) Communication for Change (C-Change) Project*. Version 3. Washington, DC: C-Change/FHI 360; May 2012.
6. Media campaign implementation kit. Centers for Disease Control and Prevention website. http://www.cdc.gov/ncbddd/folicacid/documents/MediaCampaignKit.pdf. Modified April 2002. Accessed March 16, 2018.
7. Feldman B. 12 ways to get the most out of your social analytics. Social Media Today website. http://www.socialmediatoday.com/social-business/12-ways-get-most-out-your-social-analytics. Published March 14, 2017. Accessed March 16, 2018.
8. Roter D, Larson S. The Roter Interaction Analysis System (RIAS): utility and flexibility for analysis of medical interactions. *Patient Educ Couns*. 2002;46:243-251.
9. HCAHPS: patients' perspectives of care survey. Centers for Medicare and Medicaid Services website. https://www.cms.gov/Medicare/Quality-Initiatives-Patient-Assessment-instruments/HospitalQualityInits/HospitalHCAHPS.html. Modified September 25, 2014. Accessed March 27, 2017.
10. Patton MQ. *Essentials of Utilization-Focused Evaluation*. Los Angeles, CA: Sage; 2012.

Appendix 8A

The Challenges of Evaluating a Supplemental Nutrition Education Program for Low-Income Families[*]

Kami J. Silk, Evan K. Perrault, Caroline J. Hagedorn, Samantha A. Nazione, Lindsay Neuberger, R. Paul McConaughy, and Khadidiatou Ndiaye

▶ Introduction

Effective interventions to address childhood obesity in the United States have grown as the percentage of children classified as either overweight or in danger of becoming overweight has grown substantially during the last three decades.[1,2] Many requests for action have emerged in response to the obesity epidemic,[3] resulting in numerous funded programs to communicate nutrition education information. Many initiatives aim to improve dietary practices by making behavior change the goal,[4] yet their effectiveness has not consistently undergone rigorous assessment due to the inherent challenges associated with conducting evaluations. The Grow Your Kids with Fruits and Veggies (GYK) program is one such program. It is a supplemental, pilot nutrition education program funded by the U.S. Department of Agriculture (USDA). Using a three-pronged evaluation (environmental, process, and summative evaluation procedures), we aimed to uncover whether the program was effectual, and what more could be done to increase its effectiveness in the future.

▶ The Grow Your Kids Program

The GYK program began in 2006 in two Michigan counties and has since expanded statewide. Its purpose is to educate low-income audiences about healthy food choices, specifically striving to convince mothers of the importance of increasing their children's fruit and vegetable consumption, to increase mothers' knowledge of ways to increase their families' fruit and vegetable consumption, to get children to try more fruits and vegetables, and to increase children's consumption of fruits and vegetables through educational materials. The content of GYK materials is based on USDA-tested messages for low-income mothers,[5] and materials are designed to supplement other nutrition-focused campaigns and interventions. Consequently, GYK materials are often delivered in conjunction with other government-funded programs to increase efficiency among services (e.g., in Special Supplemental Nutrition Program for Women, Infants, and Children [WIC] classrooms, at farmers' markets); for example, a mother might go to a county agency office to register for a new state program, attend a required WIC training program, and also be exposed to GYK materials, all within the same day. Evaluation of GYK materials' effectiveness has yet to be conducted, perhaps due to the challenge of assessing them as an integrated component of other nutrition programs. Due to the program's highly integrated nature, three stages of evaluation were undertaken to assess the program: environmental assessments, process evaluation, and summative evaluation.

---

[*] **Note:** This material was partially funded by the State of Michigan with federal funds from the U.S. Department of Agriculture (USDA) Supplemental Nutrition Assistance Program by way of the Michigan Nutrition Network at the Michigan Fitness Foundation. This material is based upon work supported in part by the Michigan Department of Human Services, under contract number ADMIN-10-99011. Any opinions, findings, conclusions, or recommendations expressed in this publication are those of the author(s) and do not necessarily reflect the view of the Michigan Fitness Foundation or the Michigan Department of Human Services.

▶ Evaluation Steps and Procedures

Environmental Assessment

The quality of instruction, engagement level of instructors, and other environmental factors like physical space can impact program effectiveness,[6] and low fidelity in adhering to program procedures makes it less likely participants will master program objectives. The goal of this study's environmental assessment was to uncover an understanding of how GYK materials were being used by the educators and to assess the overall interest and engagement of participants. Because materials were designed to be supplemental and flexible in their integration, these data also have the potential to reveal key strategies and barriers for program delivery.

Nine program sites were selected across seven counties in Michigan. These sites were chosen because they constituted a diverse, representative sample based on venues, geographic locations, county populations, and urban/rural settings. In the summer and fall of 2009, two researchers traveled to each site on the days the programs were delivered and independently completed evaluation worksheets. These worksheets asked the frequency, location, exposure, and activities performed during reviewers' time viewing the program. Separate worksheets were created for indoor and outdoor program sites.

Process Evaluation

Failure to detect effects is often related to deficits in program materials or delivery fidelity, which can easily be identified through evaluation with program implementers.[7] Although the environmental assessment provides some information for determining potential deficits, process evaluation of program implementers provides data to assess the utility of the program's materials and allows evaluators insight into potentially unseen barriers to program delivery.[7,8]

All 56 sites that participated in the program were contacted via email one month after the official end date of the GYK program. The email provided a link to an online survey for their most involved person to complete; 28 nutrition educators completed the survey (a 50% response rate). The survey asked questions regarding the format in which they delivered the GYK program, and about their utilization and perception of helpfulness of GYK incentives, activities, and materials.

Summative Evaluation

Commonly, summative evaluation includes only posttest data collected immediately following program exposure. More comprehensive evaluation efforts include a theoretical framework as well as repeated measures with participants. In the case of GYK, the theory of planned behavior[9] was used because the constructs of attitude, subjective norms, perceived behavioral control, and behavioral intention provided an inclusive framework to evaluate the effectiveness of GYK materials.

Generating messages that leave memorable impressions in the minds of participants can also impact future behaviors.[10] These memorable messages remain salient and are likely to be shared with other people. This message sharing can help create perceived norms and benefits (or barriers) surrounding what comprises healthy eating behaviors. In the case of GYK, health messages on incentive materials were designed based on formative research.[5] The memorability and use of these messages to encourage further communication are variables needing evaluation because the success of a program can also be determined based on whether messages were important enough to be shared with others. Communication campaigns are usually more successful when they include some type of interpersonal component.[11-13] Thus, sharing of GYK messages with others, as well as the use of GYK materials, are evidence of the program's impact beyond the intervention itself, providing a measure of effectiveness long after the program's funds have run out.

Summative data were collected via survey at two time points from program participants who attended an event or site where GYK program materials were being used and disseminated ($n = 117$ Time I [within 48 hours after attending the event], $n = 80$ Time II [two weeks after the event]). Participants (mean age = 34.47 years, range: 18–59 years) received a grocery store gift card for participating. The majority were Caucasian (96.1%), and 90% were female. More than half (56%) were married, and 94% had children ($M = 2.62$); 82% were unemployed.

Time I survey items asked participants where they received GYK materials, which GYK materials they received, what GYK activities they participated in, their evaluations of GYK program messages, and how often they used promotional items. Questions related to interpersonal communication about GYK materials were also asked (e.g., did you share any messages from the GYK materials with anyone?). Using five-point scales, measures concerning efficacy levels (five items: e.g., I feel like I can prepare healthy meals for my family), barriers (three items: e.g., I get produce, but I do not know what to do with it), attitudes (five items: e.g., It is important I provide produce for my family every day), and behavioral intentions (five items: e.g., I intend to purchase produce in the next two weeks) surrounding a healthy lifestyle were also asked.

▶ Results

Environmental Assessment

As stipulated by the program, all program sites carried through by focusing on fruit and vegetable consumption. GYK content was often presented in conjunction with Project FRESH coupon distribution, which is a program supplying coupons for produce from local farmers' markets. Common themes emerging across indoor program delivery sites were that indoor classroom events offered more time for the distribution of content as well as opportunities to field questions from participants. On the other hand, outdoor events were primarily used for taste tests and dissemination of GYK incentives and handouts.

Components Observed

Taste Testings

Taste testings were utilized at all sites. Particularly innovative examples were a comparison of fresh and dried fruits, watermelon salsa, and unconventional raw vegetables such as raw slices of sweet potatoes. The vast majority of people (over 90%) who were observed being offered a taste test accepted it.

Lecture

Every indoor classroom event included a prepared lecture, often led by multiple personnel with different areas of expertise/agency affiliations. Four of the five classroom events used a traditional, prepared lecture in a teacher–student format. The fifth lecture was less formal and was conducted based on audience interest and questions. Two of the five lectures were derived from GYK WIC educator lesson plans; both focused on "Grow Your Kids with a Rainbow of Colors" and mentioned the lesson title by name.

Physical Activity

Only two sites engaged participants in a physical activity. The low offering of physical activities may have been due to confined spaces at fairs and time constraints at classroom events.

Incentive Items and Materials

All the events observed offered incentive items. Eight of the nine sites offered reusable GYK bags filled with multiple GYK items and written materials. These bags often included more than 75% of all GYK materials available to delivery sites. Although all bags contained kitchen tools, not every event offered GYK written materials. Only about half of the events took time to highlight and explain the materials to participants. Nearly all participants observed being offered bags accepted them.

Process Evaluation

According to the responses received from program implementers, the GYK program was implemented at a wide variety of venues: 15 agencies used WIC offices, 4 were at summer camps, 3 had booths at farmers' markets, 2 were at food pantries, 2 used Department of Human Services offices, and 2 did not indicate program sites. Program implementers also stated GYK program materials were usually incorporated alongside other programs being offered at the same venue (e.g., in conjunction with Project FRESH appointments, incorporated into nutrition classes and WIC appointments). These data confirm what was observed during the environmental assessments.

Handouts

All agencies reported using GYK handouts as intended at their events. Although eight agencies indicated full satisfaction with the handouts, three recommended reducing the amount of information. Two of the agencies indicated they thought bound booklets would be effective to preserve the GYK materials.

Incentives

All agencies reported using GYK incentives in their programs. Program implementers commented the incentives attracted individuals to their displays and were catalysts for conversations. The most popular incentives were orange peelers and vegetable

TABLE 8A-1 Main Variable Frequencies at Time I and Time II ($n = 80$)

Variable	Time I Mean (SD)	Time II Mean (SD)	Paired t-test
Self-efficacy	4.10 (0.77)	3.94 (0.85)	n.s.
Attitudes	4.23 (0.70)	4.02 (0.94)	n.s.
Behavioral intentions	4.24 (0.75)	4.10 (0.96)	n.s.
Times tried new recipe	2.19 (2.13)	2.67 (5.66)	n.s.
Interpersonal communication contacts	0.39 (0.75)	0.52 (0.64)	n.s.
Number of kitchen tools owned	5.57 (3.88)	5.69 (3.99)	n.s.

Note: Self-efficacy, attitudes, and behavioral intentions were measured on five-point Likert scales where 1 indicated strong disagreement and 5 indicated strong agreement. The remaining variables were numeric open-ended questions.

scrubbers. Respondents also thought there should be more kid-friendly incentives, and there was no need to have so many items. In total, 13 types of incentive items were disseminated (e.g., reusable grocery bags, jump ropes, dry and liquid measuring cups). Respondents rated zipper pulls and mouse pads the least favorably. This is not surprising given that these items are not used to directly facilitate activities promoting the consumption of fruits and vegetables. Improving the quality of certain incentives was also mentioned; some respondents noted handouts could easily tear, grocery bags ripped, and cutting boards wore out quickly if used frequently.

Barriers to Implementation

One agency suggested that short versions of the lesson plans should be created to address time constraints associated with integrating the materials alongside other programs. Also, although all 28 agencies surveyed indicated they included a fruit and vegetable taste test as part of their program delivery, some agencies discussed difficulties obtaining food permits to allow the tastings to proceed.

Summative Evaluation

Analysis of the descriptive statistics for Time I and Time II data collections regarding self-efficacy, attitude, behavioral intentions, use of GYK recipes in the last two weeks, interpersonal interactions about GYK messages, and number and use of kitchen tools by participants are provided in **TABLE 8A-1**. Results show no significant differences *(abbreviated as n.s. in table)* between Time I and Time II using paired-samples t-tests. Therefore, the impact of the GYK program remained steady across the two-week period of time assessed. Reports also remained consistent regarding the percentage of participants who remembered a GYK-related message at Time I (33.4%) and Time II (38%). An additional 37.3% remembered more than one GYK related message at Time I, and 50% did so at Time II. Barriers, which were assessed only at Time I, were also found to be below the scale midpoint ($M = 2.31$, $SD = 0.93$), indicating few barriers were present for participants regarding their abilities to consume fruits and vegetables.

Participants indicated the GYK program materials and messages were well-liked and used regularly. They particularly liked the kitchen tools provided as incentives (see **TABLE 8A-2**). The majority of individuals reported receiving all three GYK handouts provided and participating in taste-testing activities (see **TABLE 8A-3**).

A Lack of Communication with Others

Of those individuals who could remember a GYK-related message or thought they remembered a GYK-related message (60.8%), only about 40%

TABLE 8A-2 GYK Kitchen Items Collected and Most Frequently Used at Time I and Time II ($n = 80$)

Item	Time I		Time II
	Received (%)	Most Frequently Used (%)	Most Frequently Used (%)
Measuring cups (solid)	63.3	30	30.7
Measuring cups (liquid)	51.9	10	5.3
Grocery list/pad	51.9	8.6	6.7
Measuring spoons	50.6	4.3	8
Cutting board	45.6	5.7	8
Green grocery bag	50.6	5.7	5.3
Orange peeler	48.1	1.4	1.3
Kid growth chart	48.1	0	0
Recipe book	48.1	2.9	4
Scrub brush	38	7.1	6.7
Computer mouse pad	43	1.4	2.7
Jump rope	24.1	0	0
Zipper pull	2.5	0	0

Note: The percentages for most frequently used items do not add up to 100% because 9.1% of respondents answered with more than one item, and 6.8% answered with an item not on our list during Time I.

TABLE 8A-3 Activities Participated In and Information Received When Receiving GYK Materials ($n = 117$)

Activity	Participation (%)
Taste testing of vegetables	56.5
Conversation with nutrition educator	55.1
Taste test of fruit	47.6
Classroom instruction	34
Physical activity	8.7

Information	Received (%)
GYK nutrition tip sheet	65.8
GYK fold-out brochures for parents	54.5
GYK kids' activity sheets	53.6

repeated this message to someone else, usually a friend (13.7%), child (11.8%), mother (7.8%), or spouse (5.9%). This infrequent communication with others regarding program messaging is unfortunate because developing family norms through discussion with family members about healthy eating could facilitate consumption of more fruits and vegetables. Additionally, not sharing healthy lifestyle tips with one's spouse (the person least likely to be told) could pose barriers to the implementation of healthy lifestyle practices because parenting children is often a partner activity.

Communication with others cannot even be expected to occur if people are unable to remember the messages they were taught. Although approximately one-third of participants were able to remember at least one message, the most messages a participant was able to remember at Time I or Time II was 4 out of a possible 12 program messages. Therefore, it appears it was not possible for participants to remember all of the messages the program disseminated, even if they did find these messages to be favorable. Future revisions to the GYK program should include direct efforts that encourage further communication of GYK health messages with family members, particularly spouses and partners, and reducing the number of key messages delivered to participants.

▶ Conclusion

One major challenge in evaluating the GYK program was that it was a nutrition education program intended to supplement existing programs; therefore, it was not designed to stand alone. Despite the challenges in evaluating this initiative, evaluation remains necessary because millions of taxpayer dollars are being funneled into supplemental programs like GYK with the overall goal of improving the health of families in the United States.

▶ Lessons Learned

Program observers found all participants across delivery sites accepted the incentive materials offered, thus spreading GYK messages to the participants who reported using them and remembering some messages. However, many participants were unable to discriminate between GYK messages and other competing messages that emerged as a result of other programs being delivered at the same time as GYK. Although GYK is designed as a supplemental program, it is still important for program implementers to make GYK messages as distinct from other messages as possible to ensure messages are remembered, and so outcomes can be linked back to specific program components. Although the diversity of products and messages can be considered a strength, the range of products and messages can also detract from a strong singular GYK brand concept.

GYK was also successful in introducing fruits and vegetables to children through the use of taste tests. These are an easy way to introduce new foods to families. Participants held positive attitudes toward healthier eating, felt able to feed their families healthier foods, and intended to introduce healthier foods to their families. The fact that these attitudes were maintained across time suggests the GYK program promoted and reinforced positive, stable beliefs about nutrition, and certainly did not impact them negatively. However, because of the highly embedded nature of the program with other initiatives and programs, it is difficult to precisely pinpoint which parts of the GYK program were the ones with the greatest level of utility.

Although incentives were popular among participants, nutrition educators noted that not all incentives were useful for the program's overall purpose of getting families to eat more fruits and vegetables (e.g., mouse pads for computers and zipper pulls for jackets). Novel kitchen tools seem like the most important incentive investment because they provide tangible assistance in increasing fruit and vegetable consumption; for example, nutrition educators noted some mothers reported peeling fruit as a barrier to introducing fruit into their diets—providing an orange peeler addressed that barrier. Another important insight from nutrition educators regarded the importance of providing quality kitchen tool incentives to participants, because if incentives break or wear out, program participants would not have some of the basic tools to engage in healthy lifestyle choices. It is likely that funding resources would be best spent on having a few quality incentives rather than a large range of incentives not designed for long-term use.

Recognizing GYK is not a stand-alone nutrition education program, materials need to be flexible so GYK information can be communicated effectively in any type of setting (e.g., outdoor farmers' markets, classroom settings). Different versions of lesson plans (e.g., short and long formats) might be helpful to ensure all key messages are delivered to participants regardless of time and space barriers, and to ensure consistency of the program across settings. See **TABLE 8A-4** for recommendations for future, similar programs.

TABLE 8A-4   Summary of Key Recommendations for Future Supplemental Nutrition Programs

Recommendation	Example from Evaluation
Consistent branding of messages is important.	The variety of incentives and handouts was appreciated by participants; however, only a few key messages should be used on these materials to ensure greater recall from participants. (Twelve were used in this program.)
Taste tests can be effective for introducing participants to new foods or preparations.	More than half of participants took part in food taste tests, potentially providing the self-efficacy needed to purchase and prepare healthier foods in the future.
Provide tools that people might not have (e.g., peelers).	Peeling fruits and vegetables was indicated as a barrier to participants including them in their diets. Providing tools to help individuals overcome this barrier could be helpful in increasing fruit and vegetable consumption.
Materials should be robust, of a high quality, and relevant to program goals. Resources should provide for fewer, higher-quality incentives.	This program had numerous incentives; however, many were of a lesser quality (e.g., easily torn bags, cutting boards that quickly wore out), and some were not relevant (e.g., zipper pulls).
Multiple versions of lesson plans are needed.	No two venues were the same when delivering GYK, and program lessons needed to be more flexible to ensure consistency of key messages across a variety of contexts. It could be helpful to provide both long and short programs to educators.

References

1. Ogden CL, Carroll MD, Kit BK, Flegal KM. Prevalence of obesity and trends in body mass index among US children and adolescents, 1999-2010. *JAMA.* 2012;307:483-490.

2. Wang Y, Lim H. The global childhood obesity epidemic and the association between socio-economic status and childhood obesity. *Int Rev Psychiatry.* 2012;24:176-188. doi:10.3109/09540261.2012.688195.

3. Office of the Surgeon General (US). The Surgeon General's Vision for a Healthy and Fit Nation. Rockville (MD): Office of the Surgeon General (US); 2010. https://www.ncbi.nlm.nih.gov/books/NBK44660/.

4. Contento I. Review of nutrition education research in the *Journal of Nutrition Education and Behavior,* 1998 to 2007. *J Nutr Educ Behav.* 2008;40:331-340.

5. U.S. Department of Agriculture, Food and Nutrition Service website. https://www.fns.usda.gov/tn/maximizing-message-helping-moms-and-kids-make-healthier-food-choices Accessed April 18, 2018.

6. Scheirer MA, Shediac MC, Cassidy CE. Measuring the implementation of health promotion programs: the case of the breast and cervical-cancer program in Maryland. *Health Educ Res.* 1995;10:11-25.

7. Saunders RP, Evans H, Joshi P. Developing a process evaluation plan for assessing health promotion program implementation: a how-to guide. *Health Promot Pract.* 2005;6:134-147.

8. Millstein B, Wetterhall S; CDC Evaluation Working Group. A framework featuring steps and standards for program evaluation. *Health Promot Pract.* 2000;1:221-228.

9. Ajzen I. The theory of planned behavior. *Org Behav Human Decis Processes.* 1991;50:179-211.

10. Smith SW, Nazione S, LaPlante C, et al. Topics and sources of memorable breast cancer messages and their impact on prevention and detection behaviors. *J Health Commun.* 2009;14:293-307.

11. Atkin CK. Theory and principles of media health campaigns. In: Rice R, Atkin C, eds. *Public Communication Campaigns.* Thousand Oaks, CA: Sage; 2001:49-68.

12. Grunig JE, Ipes DA. The anatomy of a campaign against drunk driving. *Public Relations Rev.* 1983;9:36-52.

13. Wallack LM. Mass media campaigns: the odds against finding behavior change. *Health Educ Q.* 1981;8:209-260.

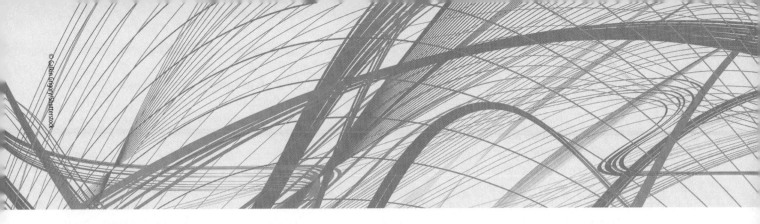

CHAPTER 9

Communication in the Healthcare Setting

Heather Gardiner

LEARNING OBJECTIVES

By the end of this chapter, the reader will be able to:

- Define effective communication.
- Describe the skills needed to communicate effectively in the healthcare context.
- Explain what is meant by *shared decision making*.
- Identify ways of developing competence in healthcare communication.

▶ Introduction

In the healthcare or clinical setting, effective communication is the cornerstone of high-quality care. Decades of research have consistently demonstrated the impact of communication on healthcare access and utilization, as well as health outcomes.[1-3] Yet suboptimal communication persists. Think about your own experiences in the healthcare setting. Can you think about a good or bad experience you have had with a doctor or other healthcare provider? All of us can tell these stories. In a recent study by Chawla and colleagues,[4] only 24% of a nationally representative sample of cancer survivors rated postdiagnosis discussions with providers as "high quality." Members of ethnic minority groups report some of the worst communication with providers.[5-7] Improving the quality of communication in healthcare settings has become a national priority, as evidenced by its inclusion as a major topic area of the Healthy People initiative. As a result, communication is now considered a core clinical skill and has become a routine component of medical training programs since the 1990s.[8,9] This chapter reviews the skills needed to engage in effective communication in healthcare settings, including some of the most challenging medical situations.

▶ Effective Interpersonal Communication

In the healthcare context, **purposeful communication** serves to exchange information and to reflect, establish, and maintain relationships between interactants in the communicative encounter.[10] Written and visual communication (e.g., patient education materials, health promotion campaigns, graphics on cigarette packages), and verbal messages (i.e., the spoken word) are the primary vehicles of information exchange. Although verbal messages can sometimes define relationships (e.g., "You're a great friend"), relational messages are largely communicated through nonverbal channels. Head nods, body orientation, gestures, tone of voice, and eye contact constitute nonverbal communication. These nonverbal messages communicate power, trust, respect, care and concern, and the full spectrum of human emotions. As such, nonverbal messages provide the context in which the verbal messages are delivered and understood. To illustrate this point, a provider's use of sarcasm during consultations can be interpreted as a lighthearted jest or as rude and mean-spirited—the interpretation is dependent on the patient–provider relationship in which the sarcastic message was delivered.

Healthcare communication is also inherently goal-driven. Patients come into the medical encounter for a reason—to obtain a diagnosis for a particular set of symptoms, to get advice about treatment options, or to obtain a prescription. Providers also have goals, including obtaining medical histories and providing recommendations and advice for improving the health and well-being of their patients. To achieve desired goals, patients and providers alike must be able to deliver verbal and nonverbal messages appropriately, with due respect for the relationship, the situation, and the setting, and in ways that ensure the messages are understood as intended.[11,12] This requires considerable skill.

Proficiency in the specific skills needed to give and gather information, and to develop and maintain relationships, is a process occurring over time. Specifically, learners are thought to traverse four stages, moving from unconscious incompetence to unconscious competence.[13] Descriptions of the four stages are provided in **BOX 9-1**.

Ideally, learners are provided with descriptions of the skills, their purpose, and examples of their appropriate use; are offered the opportunity to practice employing the skills in conversation through role-play; and receive feedback to correct errors and refine their use of the skill.[10] Alternatively, learners can engage in mindful practice.

Mindfulness is an objective, nonjudgmental approach to monitoring and correcting our own behaviors.[14] In practicing **mindful communication**, learners are fully immersed in the moment. They maintain a heightened state of awareness throughout their interactions, with the dual goals of being more conscious of their thoughts and feelings, and attending to the words used in conversation, tone of voice, gestures, facial expressions, and especially moments of silence. Employing newly learned skills in a mindful manner improves flexibility, trains learners to recognize changing situations and adapt appropriately, and helps learners identify areas for improvement and continued practice. After you review the skills outlined in the section that follows, practice using each skill mindfully in conversations. How does it feel? What is your stage of skill development? How does mindful practice differ from your approach to communication before reading this chapter?

Key Skills for Interpersonal Communication in Health Care

Two broad categories of skill are needed for healthcare providers to communicate effectively—relationship building and information exchange. These are described in the following sections, along with their associated subskills. While reading the descriptions, consider how *patients* might benefit from developing competency in each skill as well.

Relationship Building

Relationships are at the heart of all patient–provider communication. A strong, positive patient–provider

---

BOX 9-1 Four Stages of Communication Competence

1. *Unconscious incompetence:* Errors are common, but the learner is unaware of their lack of knowledge about a given skill. To advance to the next stage, the learner must identify the gap in knowledge and be motivated to fill it.
2. *Conscious incompetence:* The learner recognizes their mistakes and lack of knowledge about the skill. They also see the benefits of learning about and improving the skill.
3. *Conscious competence:* The learner has taken the steps to acquire information about and improve their execution of the skill. Engaging in the skill requires concerted effort.
4. *Unconscious competence:* The learner has practiced and now uses the skill with ease and without planning or concentration. It has become "second nature."

Data from Hargie O. Skill in theory: communication as skilled performance. In: Hargie O, ed. *Handbook of Communication Skills*. 3rd ed. New York, NY: Routledge; 2006:7-36.

relationship has been shown to improve patient satisfaction with the care received and to improve patient health outcomes.[15-18] The degree to which providers are able to establish, develop, and maintain healthy relationships with patients is largely dependent on their ability to empathize.

Empathy is understanding another person's needs, goals, desires, and emotions by perceiving the situation from their perspective.[19] Empathic providers have the emotional sensitivity to detect, understand, and accurately interpret other people's psychological and emotional states, and act appropriately and without judgment.[20] Riess and Kraft-Todd offer a useful guide for training practitioners to develop empathy (see **BOX 9-2**).[21]

In contrast, sympathy represents an attempt to vicariously experience or share in another person's condition; it is an emotional reaction in the provider and is reflected in expressions of care, concern, and pity.[19] Clinical empathy—thoughtful understanding expressed by providers as part of patient care—increases patient satisfaction, empowers patients, lowers patients' anxiety and distress, and improves patient outcomes.[22] It is also associated with increased professional growth and satisfaction, and decreased burnout and fatigue.[19] See **BOX 9-3** for more information on patient empowerment.[23]

Clinical empathy is the bedrock of relational development, pervading every step along the process. Both verbal and nonverbal skills are required to establish **rapport**, build a relationship of mutual trust and respect, and facilitate a genuine partnership.[9,11,24]

BOX 9-2 The E.M.P.A.T.H.Y. Framework

E: Eye contact
Make meaningful and culturally appropriate eye contact.

M: Muscles of facial expression
Accurately interpret facial expressions; reflect back or mirror others' facial expressions.

P: Posture
Practice open, engaging posture. Talk at eye level. This may mean sitting down and orienting the body to face and lean in toward the person you are speaking with.

A: Affect
Pay attention to emotion as expressed through verbal and nonverbal cues (affect). Use questions to confirm interpretations of other people's feelings and emotional states.

T: Tone of voice
Use tone and volume of voice to convey warmth, caring, and concern for the other person.

H: Hearing the whole person
A person's entire lived experience contextualizes the verbal and nonverbal messages sent; listen for the underlying story.

Y: Your response
Practice mindful communication—continuously reflect on the messages you send in response to the words and expressed emotions received from others to ensure your messages are appropriate and received as intended.

Modified from Riess H, Kraft-Todd G. E.M.P.A.T.H.Y.: a tool to enhance nonverbal communication between clinicians and their patients. *Acad Med.* 2014;89:1108-1112. doi:10.1097/ACM.0000000000000287.

BOX 9-3 From Paternalism to Empowerment

As keepers of medical knowledge, physicians have historically been allowed to control the communication occurring during the encounter and the resulting treatment plan. Thus, they have held the power in the clinical encounter, with patients taking a largely passive role in their own health care. This was best evidenced by physicians' decisions to filter and sometimes omit information about diagnoses and prognoses in efforts to protect patients. Over time, however, the balance of power has shifted. The paternalistic approach to care has largely been abandoned for a more collaborative approach that recognizes patients' preferences, and values and solicits patients' participation during the medical encounter. More recently, efforts have been made to further enhance patients' autonomy (patients' right to make their own medical decisions), and empower patients to take control of their health and health care.

- *Paternalism:* An approach to medical care that gives primacy to the provider. It assumes doctor knows best, allowing providers to discount and sometimes override patients' wishes in favor of their "best interest," as determined by the provider. Patients are expected to unquestioningly comply with the doctor's orders.
- *Empowerment:* The process of engaging patients in their own health care and equipping them with the information needed to make their own medical decisions and manage their health. Patients, alone, are responsible for the consequences of their decisions and behaviors.

Data from Kaba R, Sooriakumaran P. The evolution of the doctor-patient relationship. *Int J Surg.* 2007;5:57-65. https://doi.org/10.1016/j.ijsu.2006.01.005. Accessed September 20, 2016.

- *Establishing rapport:* Rapport building begins at the start of the medical encounter with greetings and introductions. As the encounter progresses, rapport-building behaviors shift to communication that supports and validates patients' thoughts, feelings, and concerns. These **confirmational messages** take the form of approvals or statements of agreement, reassurances delivered in response to expressed concerns or fears, expressions of concern for patients' well-being, and messages that legitimize patients' emotions or behaviors as being normal. Telling jokes and laughing together also help establish rapport.[25] Nonverbal behaviors are as critical to facilitating rapport as verbal messages. Making eye contact, leaning toward the patient, and demonstrating warmth through the tone and volume of voice all reinforce the verbal messages and communicate interest in and acceptance of the patient.
- *Building a relationship:* The same verbal and nonverbal messages characteristic of rapport building are essential to building a trusting, respectful relationship. Confirmational messages and nonverbal expressions of interest and concern for patients should continue to be used throughout the medical encounter as a means of developing and strengthening the relationship. Patients also want their doctors to be honest, knowledgeable, professional, and confident. Sharing thoughts and ideas by thinking aloud demonstrates knowledge and provides a rationale for behaviors that may appear unnecessary or disconnected from the rest of the encounter. Professionalism and confidence can be communicated verbally or nonverbally. Verbally, these traits are displayed through word choice and the use of clear, direct statements. A relaxed posture, smooth speech, and a confident demeanor—all elements of nonverbal communication—are critical to fostering respect and trust. In contrast, verbal messages that are unclear, confusing, or demonstrate uncertainty and nonverbal behaviors such as fidgeting, stammering (using too many "uhms" and "ahs") or mumbling, talking quickly, and using a shrill tone of voice are likely to engender distrust, dissatisfaction, and doubt in clinicians' capabilities. Additionally, providers must be attuned to patients' verbal and nonverbal messages and act appropriately. Recognizing, acknowledging, and responding to emotions in culturally appropriate ways are indicators of mindful, empathic clinical practice.

Shared Decision Making

Patient-centered care has given rise to a relatively new area for health communicators, which is the enhancement of **shared decision making (SDM)** between healthcare providers and patients. SDM is grounded in health literacy, or the patient's ease of use of information about their condition and treatment options. In addition, SDM depends on providers supporting their patient in thinking through their options and in freely expressing their preferences for treatment.

Elwyn, Frosch, Thomson, and others developed a model for SDM in clinical practice, that was later revised by Elwyn, Durand, Song, and others.[26] **FIGURE 9-1** is our interpretation of the revised model. The concept of active deliberation, in which the clinician is "expert" in the evidence and the patient is "expert" in what matters most to him- or herself, is central to SDM[27] (see Figure 9-1).

Recently, Scherer and others tested this assumption in a series of experiments. They found that although patients might feel "better" about their decisions following deliberation, the choice itself (e.g., A or B) varied little from choices made by patients giving it less thought. In fact, the authors felt that *confirmation bias* (adding arguments in favor of a preliminary decision) was the driving feature of why patients felt better about the decision.[28] Perhaps more concerning, patients might even feel better about decisions that were objectively suboptimal (i.e., would not reduce

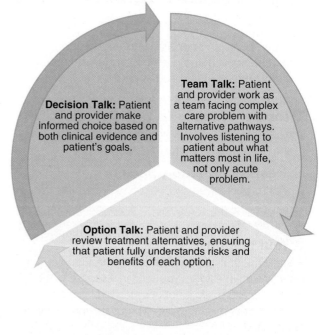

FIGURE 9-1 A three-talk model of shared decision making in health care.

Data from Elwyn G, Durand MA, Song J, et al. A three-talk model for shared decision making: multistage consultation process. *BMJ*. 2017;359:j4891

suffering or death).[9] The authors conclude that we still have a lot to learn about guiding and assisting patients in making treatment decisions.

BOX 9-4 illustrates how SDM can be integrated into a patient communication intervention to enhance decision making.[29]

Information Exchange

The information transfer, referred to as the *report* function of communication,[11] involves the solicitation and provision of information, both verbally and non-verbally. To effectively and efficiently exchange information during patient encounters, providers must employ questioning, explaining, negotiating, and listening skills.

Questioning. The skillful use of questioning is vital to opening and closing a patient encounter; soliciting information about individual and family health histories, symptom experiences, and personal explanations of illness; ensuring understanding of the information provided; and facilitating SDM. Skilled providers use **open-ended questions** and **closed-ended questions** to extract the information needed to achieve goals (e.g., give advice, diagnose illness, make treatment recommendations). Open-ended questions begin with *what*, *when*, *which*, *why*, *where*, or *how*, and prompt patients to *talk about* or *describe* their experiences. Open-ended questions allow patients to answer in any way they choose, using their own words. In contrast, closed-ended questions constrain patients' answer choices and lead to single-word answers, often yes or no. These types of questions begin with *is*, *are*,

do, *does*, *was*, or *were*. Both open- and closed-ended questions have a place during patient consultations. For instance, when assessing symptoms, a physician might start with an open-ended question like, "What kind of pain have you been experiencing? Describe it for me." After allowing the patient to talk about their pain experience, closed-ended questions might then be employed to elicit more detail: "Was it a sharp pain or a dull pain?" In addition, questioning is useful for the following:

- Confirming understanding of what the patient has said: "So, it sounds like the pain can come and go at any time, is that right?"
- Eliciting further elaboration on a response: "Would you please tell me a little more about when the pain is strongest?"
- Gauging preferences for SDM: "I'd like to come up with a plan to manage your pain together. How do you feel about that?"

It is important to avoid asking multiple questions at once, using highly technical terms or jargon that patients may not understand, or phrasing questions in ways that lead patients to a particular answer. Consider the following question: "How much of the pain medicine did you take, and how much better did it make you feel?" Questions like this, which actually ask two separate questions and elicit two distinct responses, are difficult for patients to answer. The question also assumes that the medication worked. People who prefer not to show disagreement or who want to appease others by responding "correctly" are unlikely to deviate from the response the question is leading them toward. The key is knowing what type of

---

BOX 9-4 Shared Decision Making: Decision Counseling Program© at Thomas Jefferson University

Ronald E. Myers and Anett Petrich

Important health decisions may relate to lifestyle changes, early detection tests, risk assessment, treatment, quality of life, or survivorship. Making good health decisions can be difficult for patients and providers, especially when there is a lot of information to understand and there is uncertainty about possible outcomes. Informed decision making by patients and shared decision making that involves patients and healthcare providers are recognized as hallmarks of quality medical care.

Historically, decision aids have been composed of educational handouts, booklets, or videos, all intended to deliver information to patients. Although some research suggests just providing information through decision aids can increase rates of active surveillance for localized, low risk prostate cancer, for example, a large review of the literature showed mixed results. The Decision Counseling Program developed by Dr. Ronald Myers and colleagues at Thomas Jefferson University differs from previous decision aids.

A nurse or other trained provider can use the program not only to deliver information about options, but also to identify (**FIGURE 9-2**) and weigh the effect and importance of things that matter to the patient (e.g., worry about treatment side effects, concern about developing aggressive cancer).

(continues)

BOX 9-4 Shared Decision Making: Decision Counseling Program© at Thomas Jefferson University *(continued)*

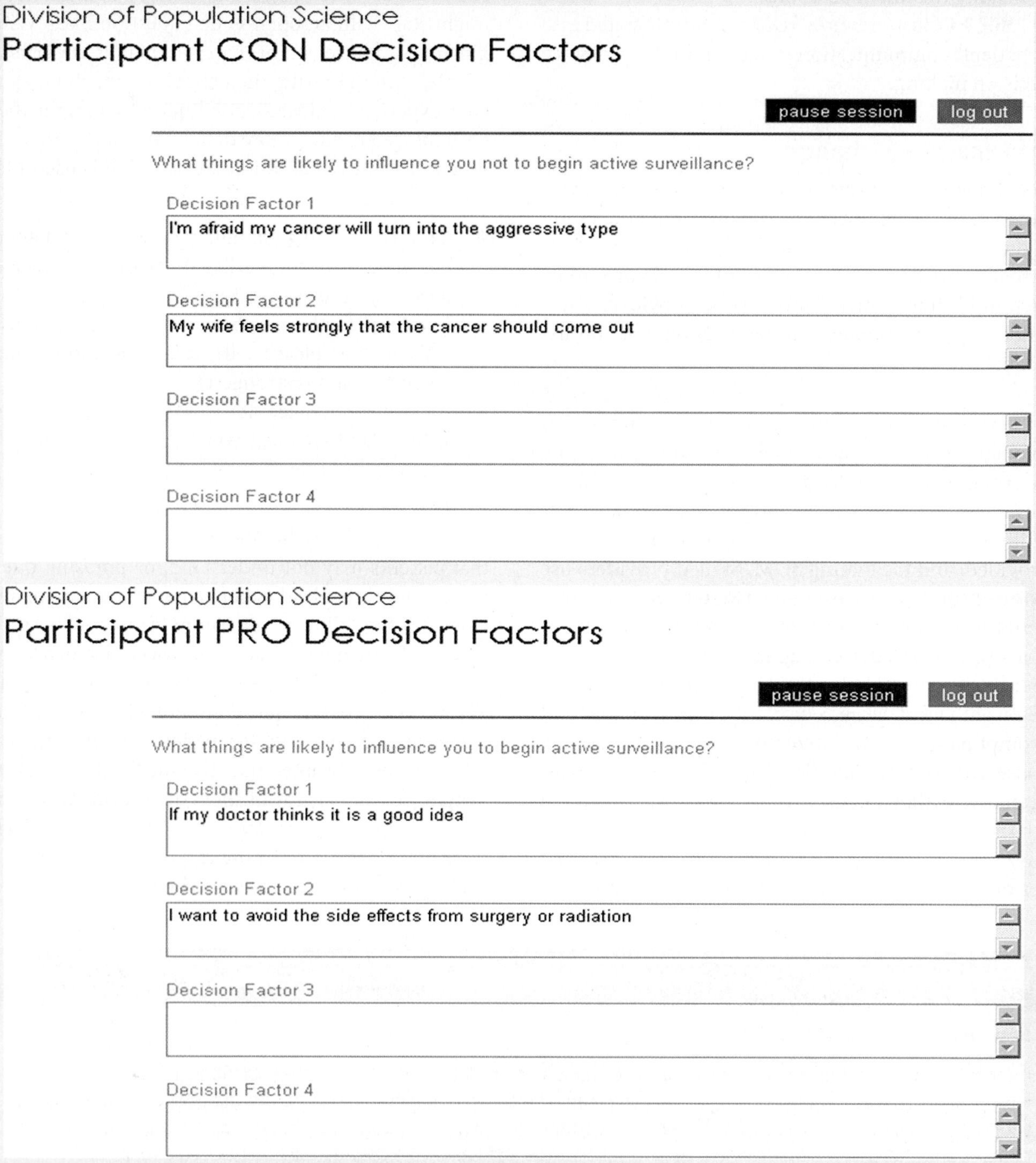

Division of Population Science
Participant CON Decision Factors

pause session | log out

What things are likely to influence you not to begin active surveillance?

Decision Factor 1
I'm afraid my cancer will turn into the aggressive type

Decision Factor 2
My wife feels strongly that the cancer should come out

Decision Factor 3

Decision Factor 4

Division of Population Science
Participant PRO Decision Factors

pause session | log out

What things are likely to influence you to begin active surveillance?

Decision Factor 1
If my doctor thinks it is a good idea

Decision Factor 2
I want to avoid the side effects from surgery or radiation

Decision Factor 3

Decision Factor 4

FIGURE 9-2 Patient-centered factors for comparing treatment options.

Reprinted by permission from Springer Nature: Springer Nature, Journal of Cancer Education, Decision Support and Shared Decision Making About Active Surveillance Versus Active Treatment Among Men Diagnosed with Low-Risk Prostate Cancer: a Pilot Study, Myers RE, Copyright 2016.

Moreover, the program clarifies the patient's preferred option and sets the stage for the patient and physician to make a well-informed choice. The Decision Counseling Program also produces a one-page summary, illustrated in **FIGURE 9-3** that the patient and their physician can use to make a shared decision that makes the most sense.

Outcomes of decision counseling may include:

- Increased patient awareness and understanding of available healthcare options
- Increased provider awareness and understanding of patient preferences
- Decreased patient worry and increased patient satisfaction with decision making
- Decreased time required by providers for patient education and support

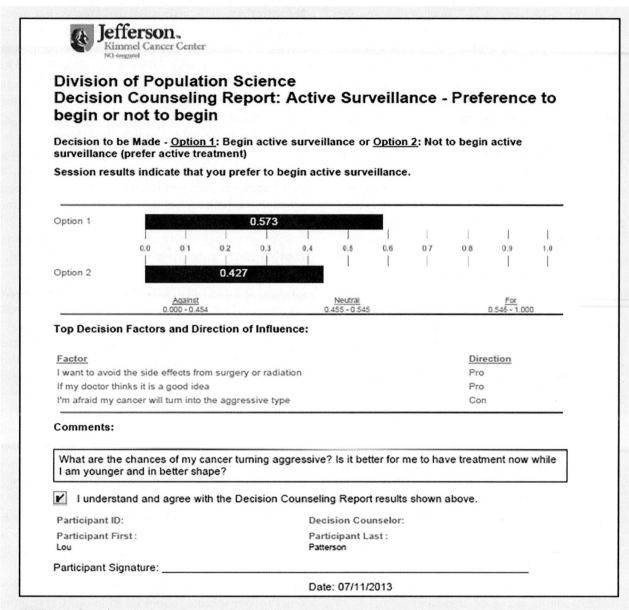

Jefferson.
Kimmel Cancer Center
NCI-designated

Division of Population Science
Decision Counseling Report: Active Surveillance - Preference to begin or not to begin

Decision to be Made - <u>Option 1</u>: Begin active surveillance or <u>Option 2</u>: Not to begin active surveillance (prefer active treatment)

Session results indicate that you prefer to begin active surveillance.

Option 1 | 0.573
Option 2 | 0.427

0.0 0.1 0.2 0.3 0.4 0.5 0.6 0.7 0.8 0.9 1.0

Against
0.000 - 0.454

Neutral
0.455 - 0.545

For
0.546 - 1.000

Top Decision Factors and Direction of Influence:

Factor	Direction
I want to avoid the side effects from surgery or radiation	Pro
If my doctor thinks it is a good idea	Pro
I'm afraid my cancer will turn into the aggressive type	Con

Comments:

What are the chances of my cancer turning aggressive? Is it better for me to have treatment now while I am younger and in better shape?

☑ I understand and agree with the Decision Counseling Report results shown above.

Participant ID: Decision Counselor:

Participant First: Participant Last:
Lou   Patterson

Participant Signature: _____

Date: 07/11/2013

FIGURE 9-3 Sample patient report.

information is needed and phrasing questions in ways that are unbiased, are easy to understand and answer, yield the necessary information, and achieve the goals of the interaction.

Explaining. Healthcare practitioners are tasked not only with explaining test results and providing diagnoses, but also with describing medical procedures, providing opinions about and recommendations for treatment, and outlining disease progression and associated prognoses. Thus, providing information is a central feature of the provider's role. Unlike the unidirectional, linear transmission of information provided through written formats, in the context of the medical encounter, explaining should be considered a transactional process whereby providers take their lead from patients, give information in a manner and at a level appropriate for the patient, assess patients' understanding of the information given, and provide additional information if needed. In addition to using plain language and other health literacy resources to improve communication with patients, providers must possess competency in the following skills:

■ *Assessing patients' prior knowledge of the subject:* Patients who already know a great deal about the topic might feel belittled if practitioners start with the most basic facts. Conversely, assuming patients have even a basic level of knowledge about a subject may lead some providers to skip the fundamentals needed to process and understand more complex or advanced information. The best approach, then, is to use questions to elicit patients' current understanding of the subject matter.

■ *Assessing patients' desire for information:* Some patients get overwhelmed and anxious when provided with detailed medical information; other patients want as much information as possible to make informed decisions about their health care. A simple open-ended question can help providers gauge patients' information preferences: "How much detail would you like about…?"

■ *Planning the presentation of the information:* A little planning ensures the information is delivered in a sequence that is logical and orderly. Preplanning also allows time to consider how best to section the information into smaller, more digestible chunks.

■ *Using visuals:* Patients differ in learning styles and abilities. Providers can accommodate for these differences by incorporating audio and visual aids, such as pictures, videos, diagrams, models, and even written information, into verbal explanations.

■ *Signaling topic changes:* Use transitional statements (e.g., "Now, I'd like to talk about…") and signposts to help patients follow along with the conversation and the information provided; for example, "There are five things you need to do to control your blood sugar. These are…"

■ *Reinforcing important information:* Use repetition and summary statements to highlight critical pieces of information, like medication schedules and treatment plans.

■ *Using the* **teach back method***:* Asking patients to repeat back what was said provides an opportunity to check their understanding, correct misunderstandings, and present the information in a different manner to help comprehension.[30]

Negotiating. It is estimated that, for various reasons, more than 40% of patients do not follow medical advice.[31,32] Nonadherence to medication schedules is also commonplace, with evidence to suggest that up to 50% of prescriptions are either not filled or not taken as directed.[33,34] Patients must not only understand the purpose of the recommendation and its expected benefit, but also be motivated to comply and believe the benefits of complying outweigh the costs. Thus, securing uptake of medical recommendations and compliance or adherence to therapeutic regimens (e.g., medication schedules) often requires the use of special communication tactics, including the use of persuasion.

A growing body of literature supports **motivational interviewing (MI)** to evoke individual behavior change and improve rates of adherence.[35,36] Born out of efforts to guide addicts through recovery, MI assumes that most people know the best course of action (i.e., to stop drinking, to quit smoking, to exercise), but experience ambivalence toward enacting behavioral changes to improve their health and well-being—they have formed arguments for and against behavior change and have become stuck in the status quo.[37] MI takes a patient-centered approach to counseling individuals toward health-promoting and disease-preventing behaviors. MI uses patients' own thoughts and feelings about the behavior in question to help patients identify personal barriers to change and strategize ways to overcome them.

As with other forms of healthcare communication, the patient–provider/counselor relationship is critical to the success of MI. In addition to exhibiting consistently high levels of respect, care, and concern for the patient, MI practitioners must develop competence in four specific communication skills: (1) asking open-ended questions, (2) providing affirmations, (3) using reflective listening, and (4) providing summary statements.[38] Descriptions of each skill along with examples of their use are provided in **BOX 9-5**.

Performed correctly, MI motivates and empowers individuals to be instruments of their own change. MI has proven effective in smoking cessation, medication adherence, adherence to self-management practices for patients with type 2 diabetes, and the management

BOX 9-5 Motivational Interviewing 101

Motivational interviewing originated in the 1980s from William R. Miller's work in substance abuse treatment. It is defined as "a collaborative, goal-oriented style of communication…designed to strengthen personal motivation for and commitment to a specific goal by eliciting and exploring the person's own reasons for change within an atmosphere of acceptance and compassion."[a(p29)]

Some of the tenets of motivational interviewing include making sure that the motivation to change comes from the patient, it is their responsibility to resolve ambivalence in their decision to act, direct persuasion is not an effective method to help a patient change, the counseling should focus on the patient's thoughts and helping them examine and understand their ambivalence, readiness to change may fluctuate over time, and the patient–provider relationship should be a partnership.[b]

MI Processes

- *Engaging:* Building and maintaining a relationship of trust, respect, and care
- *Focusing:* (Re)directing the conversation to center on change
- *Evoking:* Drawing out the patient's thoughts, feelings, and motivations for change ·
- *Planning:* Fostering a commitment to change, setting specific and achievable goals, and strategizing ways to meet the goals

MI Skills: OARS

- *Ask **o**pen-ended questions:* Phrase questions in ways that allow for further elaboration. Ask "what" or "how," and prompt for more information by asking "why." Avoid phrasing questions that can be answered with a single word or as yes/no.
- *Provide **a**ffirmations:* Affirmations validate and support patients' positive behaviors, beliefs, and accomplishments.
- *Use **r**eflective listening:* Listen actively and report back on the central message of what was said.
- *Provide **s**ummary statements:* Reiterate and highlight key points; summarize to bring closure to one topic and move on to another.

Skills in Practice

The following snippet illustrates how MI skills might be employed in practice.

MI Counselor: Hello Mr. Jones. What brings you here today? *[open-ended question]*

Mr. Jones: Well, I've been smoking cigarettes for about 15 years now and I've tried to quit, many times, but I haven't been successful.

MI Counselor: Okay. So, you're having some trouble quitting smoking. *[reflective listening]* About how many times would you say you've tried to quit?

Mr. Jones: Over the years, a lot. Maybe 10 times.

MI Counselor: And, when was the most recent attempt?

Mr. Jones: A couple of months ago.

MI Counselor: What things have you done to help you break free from smoking?

Mr. Jones: I've tried going cold turkey, the patch, the gum…what's it called…Nicorette. And, I want to quit, but I just can't seem to.

MI Counselor: First, it's really great you keep trying. A lot of people struggle to quit and those that keep persisting eventually do. *[affirmation]*

Mr. Jones: Thanks.

MI Counselor: You're welcome. So, what makes you keep trying? *[evoking]*

Mr. Jones: I know all of the things that smoking does—emphysema, COPD, the coughing, the smell. I just want to be done with it.

MI Counselor: Well, most smokers know how harmful it is, but like you find it really hard to make the changes needed to quit. So, what makes this attempt different from the others for you? *[open-ended question]*

Mr. Jones: I'm here, aren't I? And, my cousin was just diagnosed with lung cancer. She's smoked for about 30 years.

MI Counselor: You are here; that's a step in the right direction. *[affirmation]* It sounds like you've seen firsthand what the future holds, and maybe now you're even more motivated to quit. Would you say that's accurate? *[reflective listening]*

Mr. Jones: Yes.

MI Counselor: Okay. So, what do you think have been the primary reasons for not quitting in the past? *[identifying barriers]*

[a] Miller WR, Rollnick S. *Motivational Interviewing: Helping People Change.* 3rd ed. New York, NY: The Guilford Press; Copyright 2013 Guilford Press Reprinted with permission of The Guilford Press. http://lib.myilibrary.com.libproxy.temple.edu/ProductDetail.aspx?id=394471 Accessed September 20, 2016.

[b] Stewart EE, Fox CH. Encouraging patients to change unhealthy behaviors with motivational interviewing. *Fam Pract Manag.* 2011; 18(3):21-25. http://www.aafp.org/fpm/2011/0500/p21.html. Accessed March 27, 2018.

of chronic illness.[39-42] A number of studies have also explored the use of MI in primary care settings with positive effects.[43-45]

Listening. Providers cannot expect to execute the skills described with any degree of effectiveness unless they listen. Listening is more than simply hearing what another person is saying. To listen is to completely direct and focus attention on another person. Like other aspects of communication, listening is a skill that can be learned and practiced. Four discrete skills are needed to listen actively and effectively[46]:

1. *Pay attention:* First and foremost, the skillful listener stops talking and refrains from interrupting the speaker. Good listeners also demonstrate that they are paying attention by showing interest in hearing what other people have to say and allowing the speaker to set the pace of the conversation. This is primarily accomplished through nonverbal channels—smiling, head nodding, leaning toward the speaker, and maintaining eye contact signal attention and understanding. Remove distractions and focus your attention on the speaker's messages, both verbal and nonverbal, and practice mindfulness by being present in the moment.

2. *Reflect and summarize:* Another way to demonstrate attention is through reflection. Reflection consists of paraphrasing and restating the main ideas of a speaker's messages back to the speaker. Reflection statements such as, "So, what I think you're saying is…," are also a great way to confirm understanding of those messages.

3. *Clarify:* Knowing how and when to ask questions is an essential aspect of listening. Questioning not only demonstrates that listeners are actually listening, but also helps listeners gain clarity on points that were not well understood; questions also prompt speakers to continue talking.

4. *Be objective and nonjudgmental:* The listener's role is not to formulate arguments for or against the speaker or their thoughts, ideas, and feelings; rather, effective listeners demonstrate empathy, acknowledge differences, and express an intent to keep an open mind.

In addition to the relationship building, information giving, negotiation, and listening skills just outlined, providers must be attuned and responsive to patients' nonverbal communication. Engaging in mindful communication, wherein providers are continually present in the encounter and assessing their own and their patients' communicative behaviors, is an essential component of providing care. Developing **emotional intelligence**, or the ability to detect and correctly interpret nonverbal displays of emotion, and act appropriately, is necessary as well. Finally, providers must also be flexible and capable of adapting their communication as the conversation progresses. Achieving competency in the skills discussed in this section will increase the likelihood of effective patient–provider communication—that which is appropriate, reduces misunderstandings, and achieves desired goals. Honing these skills will also make communication easier, particularly in difficult or challenging situations.

▶ Communication Strategies for Difficult Conversations

Difficult or challenging conversations are commonplace in health care. In a routine medical encounter, practitioners might discuss mental illness, sexual identity and preferences, illicit drug use, marital issues, and a host of other similarly sensitive topics. Healthcare providers are also responsible for disclosing results of diagnostic procedures and tests, which all too often indicate the presence of chronic illness (e.g., type 2 diabetes mellitus, kidney disease, heart disease, HIV/AIDS) or life-threatening illness (e.g., cancer, end-stage organ failure). These discussions become even more challenging when available therapies do not work or are no longer benefiting the patient. In these instances, the conversation becomes focused on preferences for care at the end of life.

As difficult as it is to receive these messages, healthcare providers struggle with knowing how best to initiate and manage the conversations. Providers have cited feeling unprepared for the discussion, uncomfortable with the anticipated reaction from patients and their families, and unsure of the amount of detail to provide.[47] The unfortunate consequence is that providers may delay or avoid disclosing the information necessary for patients to receive the best possible care.[48] A number of tools have been developed to guide providers through the process of communicating difficult information. The **SPIKES protocol** (**BOX 9-6**) is a well-regarded framework for delivering information about diagnosis, prognosis, and treatment options.[49] Like most other protocols for the delivery of bad

BOX 9-6　The SPIKES Protocol

S: Setting

- Arrange for some privacy.
- Involve significant others.
- Sit down.
- Make a connection and establish rapport.
- Manage time constraints and interruptions.

P: Perception of Condition/Seriousness

- Determine what the patient knows about the medical condition or what they suspect.
- Listen to the patient's level of comprehension.
- Accept denial but do not confront.

I: Invitation from the Patient to Give Information

- Ask whether the patient wishes to know the details of the medical condition and/or treatment.
- Accept the patient's right not to know.
- Offer to answer questions later, if desired.

K: Knowledge: Giving Medical Facts

- Use language intelligible to the patient.
- Consider education level, sociocultural background, and current emotional state.
- Give information in small chunks.
- Check the patient's understanding of the information.
- Respond to reactions as they occur.
- Give positive aspects first.
- Give facts accurately about treatment options, prognoses, costs, and so forth.

E: Explore Emotions

- Prepare to give an empathic response.
  - Identify the emotions expressed.
  - Identify the cause/source of emotion.
  - Give the patient time to express their feelings.

S: Strategy and Summary

- Close the interview.
- Ask whether the patient wants/needs additional clarification.
- Offer an agenda for the next meeting.

Modified from Baile WF, Buckman R, Lenzi R, Glober G, Beale EA, Kudelka AP. SPIKES—a six-step protocol for delivering bad news: application to the patient with cancer. *Oncologist.* 2000;5(4):302-311. http://theoncologist.alphamedpress.org/content/5/4/302.long. Accessed March 27, 2018.

news,[50,51] SPIKES takes a patient-centered approach to information provision. Moreover, research on patient preferences for the delivery of bad news has identified four components of particular salience—the setting in which the disclosure takes place, the manner in which the information is delivered, the specific information provided and its amount, and the provision of emotional support.[52] These components align with those included in the SPIKES protocol.

As should now be evident, the communication of bad news requires the same skills and competencies as needed for providers to be effective in routine patient encounters. In both scenarios, practitioners must demonstrate empathy, build relationships, exchange information, listen actively, and negotiate courses of action. The primary difference is the degree of sensitivity with which the skills are executed. Depending on the situation, providers may need to adjust their rate of speech, volume and tone of voice, and nonverbal behaviors (gestures, eye contact) to accommodate patients' informational needs and emotional reactions when delivering bad news or discussing sensitive topics.

Clinicians should also be prepared to assess religious and spiritual preferences, particularly in end-of-life discussions. The positive impact of religion and spirituality on health outcomes has been demonstrated—religion and spirituality offer comfort and hope to many individuals at the end of life.[53] However, clinicians are often reluctant to talk about these issues.[54] The primary barriers to physicians' initiation of conversation about these topics include being afraid of offending patients, not knowing how to talk about the issues, and generally feeling uncomfortable discussing these topics.[53] Some organizations retain chaplains or other spiritual leaders to assist with conversations about religion. When faced with the task alone, healthcare providers should use confirmational messages that support and validate patients, and allow them to feel heard. Additionally, empathic communication and listening skills are needed to facilitate patient-centered care.

A number of tools are available to support providers' attempts to discuss end-of-life issues with patients, including the SAGE & THYME model, Henoch and colleagues' training in communication about existential issues, and the module of the Comskil program on death and dying.[55-57] Although these programs were developed for use with cancer patients, all patients ultimately want to feel heard and to be supported in their religious/spiritual views, even if the practitioner holds conflicting viewpoints.

▶ Competent Cross-Cultural Communication

The drastically changing profile of the U.S. populace presents unique challenges to patients and providers at all levels of the healthcare system, not the least of which are language barriers. Now, more than ever, healthcare providers must be attuned to diverse cultural belief systems, including interpretations of health and illness, and respond appropriately. Providers must strive for **cultural competence**. For instance, many Asian cultures value "saving face" or preserving dignity, honor, and respect while avoiding confrontation and the possibility of embarrassment.[58] Individuals from cultures where "face" is valued are equally motivated to protect their own face and the face of their interactional partners. This tendency to avoid "losing face" often results in answering questions in the affirmative, by saying "yes" and avoiding use of the word "no." Without an understanding of this cultural nuance, providers are likely to make the error of asking closed-ended questions that permit yes/no answers such as, "Do you understand?" or "Does that sound like a good treatment plan?" Although seemingly minor, this communicative misstep can have devastating consequences on patients' health.

Specifically, it increases the chances that patients will take the incorrect frequency or dose of a medication, fail to schedule or attend follow-up appointments, and risk further injury, illness, or even death.

This example is but one of the myriad of misunderstandings that can arise when communicating across cultures. To minimize the likelihood of similar errors, healthcare providers must work diligently to provide care in the context of patients' cultural heritage. The practice of **CulturalCare** acknowledges and respects patients' underlying beliefs about health and illness as well as the meanings patients assign to specific conditions and their preferred methods of treating disease and illness.[59] Engagement in CulturalCare represents a concerted effort to develop cultural competence or the "complex combination of knowledge, attitudes, and skills" needed to consider and appreciate patients' cultural heritage in such a way that allows them to be treated effectively and appropriately.[59]

The first step toward becoming culturally competent is to understand one's own health beliefs and accept that perceptions of health and illness vary among individuals in the same culture as well as between those from different cultures. Providers must also increase their knowledge of the belief, value, and behavior systems of different cultures. This requires both the motivation to learn about new cultures and a positive, open orientation toward cultural differences. Understanding a different culture does not need to be as formal and structured as learning a new language, though this is one way to improve cultural knowledge. Activities as simple and fun as attending cultural events, trying different foods, and socializing with individuals from diverse backgrounds can increase one's cultural sensitivity. The **Heritage Assessment Tool** (**BOX 9-7**) was developed to assist providers in understanding individual patients' background and the strength of ties to their home cultures.[59,60] (Hint: The tool can be used to assess your own cultural heritage as well.) Additionally, Purnell's handbook describing key features of over 30 different cultures and their implications on health and health care is a useful guide for the culture-conscious practitioner.[61]

To achieve cultural competence and engage in CulturalCare, practitioners must skillfully apply the knowledge about their own cultures and that of their patients to promote and improve health. Gudykunst proposes six specific skills needed to communicate competently across cultures: (1) mindfulness, (2) the ability to tolerate uncertainty or ambiguity, (3) the ability to manage anxiety, (4) empathy, (5) flexibility and the ability to adapt quickly to changing circumstances, and (6) the ability to accurately predict and interpret others' behavior.[62] Although other conceptualizations

BOX 9-7 Domains of the Heritage Assessment with Accompanying Questions

1. Childhood development occurred in country of origin or in an immigrant neighborhood of like ethnic group:
   a. Where were you born?
   b. Where were your parents, maternal and paternal grandparents born and raised?
   c. Where did you grow up?
   d. What was your neighborhood like?
2. Extended family members encouraged participation in traditional religious or cultural activities:
   a. How many siblings do you have?
   b. When you were growing up, who lived with you?
   c. Did you grow up in close contact with extended family? Do you maintain contact with extended family members? Did you and your family celebrate holidays and festivals together at home and in the community?
   d. Do you participate in church or fraternal events with family members?
3. Individual engages in frequent visits to country of origin or to "old neighborhood" in the host country:
   a. How often do you return to the country or neighborhood in which you grew up?
4. Family homes are within an "ethnic" community:
   a. What ethnic group lives in your neighborhood?
5. Individual participates in ethnic cultural events such as religious festivals or national holidays, sometimes with singing, dancing, and national costumes:
   a. Do you now participate in various ethnic or religious events, such as religious festivals, singing, dancing, costumes, and national holidays?
6. Individual was raised in an extended family setting:
   a. Who lived in your home when you were young?
   b. Did you live with grandparents, aunts, uncles, and cousins?
7. Individual maintains regular contact with the extended family:
   a. How often do you visit family members?
   b. Do you keep in close contact with those who are at a distance?
8. Individual's name has not been changed:
   a. What was your family's name when they immigrated to this country?
   b. Have they kept or changed their name? Did somebody else (immigration officials) change their name?
   c. Was the family name changed to sound more like neighbors?
9. Individual was educated in a parochial (nonpublic) school with a religious and/or ethnic philosophy similar to the family's background:
   a. Where did you go to school?
   b. What kind of a school was it?
   c. What language were you taught in?
10. Individual engages primarily in social activities with others of the same ethnic background:
    a. What is the ethnic/religious background of your spouse?
    b. Are you a member of a religious organization?
    c. Are you an active member?
    d. How often do you attend religious services?
    e. Do you practice your religion in your home?
    f. Do you prepare ethnic foods?
    g. What is the ethnic/religious background of your friends?
11. Individual has knowledge of the culture and language of origin:
    a. Have you studied the history of the people from the nation that you came from?
    b. Do you speak your native language?
    c. What language did you learn first?
12. Individual possesses personal pride about his/her heritage:
    a. How do you identify yourself?
13. Individual incorporates elements of historical beliefs and practices into his/her present philosophy:
    a. What is the history of your national group?
    b. Do you pass stories of your heritage to your children?

of intercultural communication skills exist,[63,64] providers demonstrate cultural competence when they communicate in ways that reduce misunderstandings, achieve their communicative goals, and use language (verbal and nonverbal) that is not only appropriate to the context, but also respectful of patients' cultural heritage and preferred language.

Limited English Proficiency and the CLAS Standards

As noted in Chapter 3, Title VI of the Civil Rights Act of 1964 prohibits discrimination on the basis of race, color, or nation of origin. Hospitals and other healthcare organizations receiving federal funding are thus mandated under Title VI to provide services to ensure persons with **limited English proficiency (LEP)** can meaningfully access information and receive assistance and services from federally funded programs as needed. People with LEP are individuals for whom English is not their primary language and who therefore have "limited ability to read, speak, write or understand English."[65] It is estimated that more than 300 unique languages are spoken in the United States.[66] In 2011, more than 60 million U.S. residents spoke a language other than English at home, of whom 42% reported speaking English "well," "not well," or "not at all."[67] Language barriers have been attributed to disparities in health outcomes as well as access to and utilization of healthcare services.[67-69]

Recognizing the increasing diversity of the population and a need to reduce racial/ethnic and cultural inequities in health outcomes and health care, the U.S. Department of Health and Human Services' Office of Minority Health issued the National Standards for Culturally and Linguistically Appropriate Services in Health and Health Care (**National CLAS Standards**). Upon the enactment of the CLAS Standards in 2000, healthcare organizations receiving federal funding were mandated to adopt four of the original standards pertaining to the provision of communication and language assistance services for persons with LEP.[70] The CLAS Standards were revised in 2012 to reflect progress made to improve parity in health outcomes. However, the enhanced version remains committed to ensuring that our healthcare system is responsive to the changing U.S. demography and that individuals of all backgrounds have access to and receive care that is sensitive to their cultural heritage and linguistic needs and preferences.[71] The enhanced National CLAS Standards are outlined in Chapter 3's Box 3-4. These enhanced standards offer a roadmap to help healthcare organizations in the United States plan and implement

changes to improve their ability to respond to and provide appropriate care for our country's increasingly diverse populace. Thus, the CLAS Standards represent national efforts to improve cultural competence at the organizational level and reduce disparities in health and health care.

Although none of the enhanced standards is currently mandated, federally funded healthcare organizations that fail to provide appropriate language assistance services as well as print materials in languages common to their service areas (Standards 5–8) risk censure, loss of funding, and being held in violation of Title VI of the Civil Rights Act of 1964. To help organizations meet these standards, the federal government has compiled resources on its website (http://www.lep.gov) regarding health care, immigration, voting rights, workplace safety, and other topics in numerous languages. When translating written materials (e.g., print, multimedia, signage), use of certified translation professionals is preferred. Although online translators, like Google Translate, have become widely available, the translation algorithms often fail to capture the contextual nuances of words. A human touch is needed to deconstruct the English version of a message and accurately reconstruct the message's meaning in another language.

Similarly, to meet Standard 7, only certified medical interpreters should be used when language assistance is needed. Certified interpreters have achieved a level of competence with medical terminology in their language that reduces the likelihood of translation errors and resulting medical errors. Although it may be tempting to ask bilingual individuals to serve as interpreters, there is no guarantee that these individuals will have a grasp of the language needed to accurately describe medical diagnoses and prognoses, and their recommended courses of care. Family hierarchies and cultural traditions make using minors or family members even less reliable translators. For instance, given the resistance to disclosing severe or debilitating illness, the degree to which family members of Hindu patients will provide full translations in instances where death is imminent is questionable.[61] As further illustration, asking children, particularly those of the opposite sex, to translate for adult parents will likely cause embarrassment and translational inaccuracies. Children and minors are also unlikely to be familiar enough with the medical sciences to offer accurate translations of advanced terminology. Professional medical interpreters will know how to navigate these cultural subtleties and ensure patients receive high-quality health care.[72]

Knowing when patients need language assistance services can be challenging, however. In a recent study of emergency department nurses' assessment of walk-in patients' English language proficiency, over a quarter of Spanish-speaking patients were incorrectly classified as English proficient.[73] Spanish-speaking patients in this study reported lower levels of satisfaction with the hospital's triage services than English-speaking patients did. More worrisome is the quality of care these patients likely received. There is growing evidence that **patient navigators**—people trained to help patients navigate through the healthcare system and interpret medical advice—can not only guide patients through healthcare systems, but also help reduce language barriers to LEP patients' access to necessary healthcare services.[74,75]

▶ Conclusion

This chapter has primarily focused on communication occurring in the context of the medical encounter; however, mastery of the skills outlined will prove useful in other healthcare contexts. For instance, the movement toward an integrated system of health care, which merges primary care with population health, has expanded the concept of the healthcare provider.[76,77] Today, the term applies not only to physicians, physician's assistants, nurses, and nurse practitioners, but also to individuals working in the allied health professions and public health practitioners, all of whom are responsible for communicating health information effectively. (See **BOX 9-8** for a listing.)

There is also a growing appreciation for multidisciplinary collaborations. Increasing role specialization combined with the volume of information

---

BOX 9-8 Alternative Healthcare Providers in the 21st Century

- Psychologists
- Social workers
- Genetic counselors
- Physical therapists
- Occupational therapists
- Kinesiologists
- Dieticians/nutritionists
- Diabetes educators
- Health educators
- Pharmacists
- Dentists and oral technicians
- Community outreach/field workers
- Interpreters/translators
- Family advocates
- Hospice care specialists
- Patient navigators
- Health librarians
- Chaplains

---

available has led to the development of interdisciplinary healthcare teams. Teamwork presents unique challenges, such as resolution of individual team members' conflicting needs and preferences; this necessitates application of active listening techniques, skillful information solicitation and delivery, and the development of relationships based on respect and trust. Regardless of the context, mindful, empathic communication is required to develop personal connections, minimize misunderstandings, and increase the likelihood that the dual goals of improving access and utilization of healthcare services and improving health outcomes are realized for all patients.

Key Terms

Closed-ended questions
Confirmational messages
CulturalCare
Cultural competence
Emotional intelligence
Empathy

Heritage Assessment Tool
Limited English proficiency (LEP)
Mindful communication
Motivational interviewing (MI)
National CLAS Standards
Open-ended questions

Patient navigators
Purposeful communication
Rapport
Shared decision making (SDM)
SPIKES protocol
Teach back method

Chapter Questions

1. What are the characteristics of effective communication in the healthcare setting?
2. Describe the four stages of communication competence. Explain the importance of mindfulness to communication competence.
3. What is the role of empathy in interpersonal health-related communication?
4. Define CulturalCare. What skills are needed to engage in effective cross-cultural communication?
5. What are the implications of the National CLAS Standards on health care in the United States?

References

1. Beck RS, Daughtridge R, Sloane PD. Physician-patient communication in the primary care office: a systematic review. *J Am Board Fam Pract.* 2002;15(1):25-38. http://www.jabfm.org/content/15/1/25.long. Accessed March 27, 2018.

2. Ha JF, Anat DS, Longnecker N. Doctor-patient communication: a review. *Ochsner J.* 2010;10:38-43. PMCID: PMC 3096184. Accessed September 20, 2016.

3. Henry SG, Fuhrel-Forbis A, Rogers MA, Eggly S. Association between nonverbal communication during clinical interactions and outcomes: a systematic review and meta-analysis. *Patient Educ Couns.* 2012;86(3):297-315. doi:10.1016/j.pec.2011.07.006.

4. Chawla N, Blanch-Hartigan D, Virgo KS, et al. Quality of patient-provider communication among cancer survivors: findings from a nationally representative sample [published online ahead of print]. *J Oncol Pract.* 2016. doi:10.1200/JOP.2015.006999.

5. Bao Y, Fox SA, Escarce JJ. Socioeconomic and racial/ethnic differences in the discussion of cancer screening: "between-" versus "within-" physician differences. *Health Serv Res.* 2007;42(3 Pt. 1):950-970. doi:10.1111/j.1475-6773.2006.00638.x.

6. Palmer NRA, Kent EE, Forsythe LP, et al. Racial and ethnic disparities in patient-provider communication, quality-of-care ratings, and patient activation among long-term cancer survivors. *J Clin Oncol.* 2014;32(36):4087-4094. doi:10.1200/JCO.2014.55.5060.

7. Trenchard L, McGrath-Lone L, Ward H. Ethnic variation in cancer patients' ratings of information provision, communication and overall care. *Ethn Health.* 2016;21(5):515-533. doi:10.1080/13557858.2015.1126561.

8. Kurtz S, Silverman J, Draper J. *Teaching and Learning Communication Skills in Medicine.* 2nd ed. Oxon, UK: Radcliffe; 2005.

9. Silverman J, Kurtz S, Draper J. *Skills for Communicating with Patients.* 3rd ed. Oxford, UK: Radcliffe; 2013.

10. Greene JO. Models of adult communication skill acquisition: practice and the course of performance improvement. In: Greene JO, Burleson BR, eds. *Handbook of Communication and Social Interaction Skills.* New York, NY: Routledge; 2003:51-92.

11. Watzlawick P, Beavin JH, Jackson DD. *The Pragmatics of Human Communication.* New York, NY: Norton; 1967.

12. Chou C. Building the case for communication and relationships. In: Chou C, Cooley L, eds. *Communication Rx: Transforming Healthcare Through Relationship-Centered Communication.* New York, NY: McGraw-Hill Education; 2018:3-12.

13. Hargie O. *Handbook of Communication Skills.* 3rd ed. New York, NY: Routledge; 2006.

14. Epstein RM. Mindful practice. *JAMA.* 1999;282:833-839. doi:10.1001/jama.282.9.833.

15. Peng FB, Burrows JF, Shirley ED, Rosen P. Unlocking the doors to patient satisfaction in pediatric orthopaedics [published online ahead of print]. *J Pediatr Orthop.* 2016. doi:10.1097/BPO.0000000000000837.

16. Theis RP, Stanford JC, Goodman JR, Duke LL, Shenkman EA. Defining "quality" from the patient's perspective: findings from focus groups with Medicaid beneficiaries and implications for public reporting. *Health Expect.* 2017;20(3):395-406. doi:10.1111/hex.12466.

17. Dawson-Rose C, Cuca YP, Webel AR, et al. Building trust and relationships between patients and providers: an essential complement to health literacy in HIV care. *J Assoc Nurses AIDS Care.* 2016;27(5):574-584. doi:10.1016/j.jana.2016.03.001.

18. Cobos B, Haskard-Zolnierek K, Howard K. White coat hypertension: improving the patient-health care practitioner relationship. *Psychol Res Behav Manag.* 2015;8:133-141. doi:10.2147/PRBM.S61192.

19. Hojat M. *Empathy in Health Professions, Education, and Patient Care.* Cham, Switzerland: Springer; 2016.

20. Goleman D. *Emotional Intelligence: Why It Can Matter More Than I.Q.* New York, NY: Bantam; 1995.

21. Riess H, Kraft-Todd G. E.M.P.A.T.H.Y.: a tool to enhance nonverbal communication between clinicians and their patients. *Acad Med.* 2014;89:1108-1112. doi:10.1097/ACM.0000000000000287.

22. Derksen F, Bensing J, Lagro-Janssen A. Effectiveness of empathy in general practice: a systematic review. *Br J Gen Pract.* 2013;63(606):e76-e84. doi:10.3399/bjgp13X660814.

23. Kaba R, Sooriakumaran P. The evolution of the doctor-patient relationship. *Int J Surg.* 2007;5:57-65. https://doi.org/10.1016/j.ijsu.2006.01.005. Accessed September 20, 2016.

24. Roter D. The enduring and evolving nature of the patient-physician relationship. *Patient Educ Couns.* 2000;39:5-15. https://doi.org/10.1016/S0738-3991(99)00086-5. Accessed September 20, 2016.

25. Schöpf AC, Martin GS, Keating MA. Humor as a communication strategy in provider-patient communication in a chronic care setting. *Qual Health Res.* 2017;27(3):374-390. doi:10.1177/1049732315620773.

26. Elwyn G, Durand MA, Song J, et al. A three-talk model for shared decision making: multistage consultation process. *BMJ.* 2017;359:j4891.

27. Spatz ES, Krumholz HM, Moulton BW. Prime time for shared decision making. *JAMA.* 2017;317(13):1309-1310. doi:10.1001/jama.2017.0616.

28. Scherer LD, de Vries M, Zikmund-Fisher BJ, Witteman HO, Fagerlin A. Trust in deliberation: the consequences of deliberative decision strategies for medical decisions. *Health Psychol.* 2015;34(11):1090-1099. doi:10.1037/hea0000203.

29. Myers RE, Leader AE, Censits JH, et al. Decision support and shared decision making about active surveillance versus active treatment among men diagnosed with low-risk prostate cancer: a pilot study. *J Cancer Educ.* 2018;33(1):180-185.

30. Tamura-Lis W. Teach-back for quality education and patient safety. *Urol Nurs.* 2013;298:267-271.

31. DiMatteo MR. Variations in patients' adherence to medical recommendations: a quantitative review of 50 years of research. *Med Care.* 2004;42:200-209. doi:10.1097/01.mlr.0000114908.90348.f9.

32. Zolnierek KB, DiMatteo MR. Physician communication and patient adherence to treatment: a meta-analysis. *Med Care.* 2009;47(8):826-834. doi:10.1097/MLR.0b013e31819a5acc.

33. Peterson AM, Takiya L, Finley R. Meta-analysis of trials of interventions to improve medication adherence. *Am J Health Syst Pharm.* 2003;60:657-665.

34. Haynes RB, Ackloo E, Sahota N, McDonald HP, Yao X. Interventions for enhancing medication adherence. *Cochrane Database Syst Rev.* 2008;CD000011.

35. Alperstein D, Sharpe L. The efficacy of motivational interviewing in adults with chronic pain: a meta-analysis and systematic review. *J Pain.* 2016;17(4):393-403. doi:10.1016/j.jpain.2015.10.021.

36. Palacio A, Garay D, Langer B, Taylor J, Wood BA, Tamariz L. Motivational interviewing improves medication adherence: a systematic review and meta-analysis. *J Gen Intern Med.* 2016;31(8):929-940. doi:10.1007/s11606-016-3685-3.

37. Miller WR, Rollnick S. *Motivational Interviewing: Helping People Change.* 3rd ed. New York, NY: The Guilford Press; 2013.

38. Stewart EE, Fox CH. Encouraging patients to change unhealthy behaviors with motivational interviewing. *Fam Pract Manag.* 2011;18(3):21-25. http://www.aafp.org/fpm/2011/0500/p21.html. Accessed March 27, 2018.

39. Lindson-Hawley N, Thompson TP, Begh R. Motivational interviewing for smoking cessation. *Cochrane Database Syst Rev.* 2015;CD006936.

40. Bender BG, Lockey RF. Solving the problem of nonadherence to immunotherapy. *Immunol Allergy Clin North Am.* 2016; 36(1):205-213. doi:10.1016/j.iac.2015.08.014.

41. Ekong G, Kavookjian J. Motivational interviewing and outcomes in adults with type 2 diabetes: a systematic review. *Patient Educ Couns.* 2016;99(6):944-952. doi:10.1016/j.pec.2015.11.022.

42. Tuccero D, Railey K, Briggs M, Hull SK. Behavioral health in prevention and chronic illness management: motivational interviewing. *Prim Care.* 2016;43(2):191-202. doi:10.1016/j.pop.2016.01.006.

43. Barnes RD, Ivezaj V. A systematic review of motivational interviewing for weight loss among adults in primary care. *Obes Rev.* 2015;16(4):304-318. doi:10.1111/obr.12264.

44. Resnicow K, McMaster F, Bocian A, et al. Motivational interviewing and dietary counseling for obesity in primary care: an RCT. *Pediatrics.* 2015;135(4):649-657. doi:10.1542/peds.2014-1880.

45. VanBuskirk KA, Wetherell JL. Motivational interviewing with primary care populations: a systematic review and meta-analysis. *J Behav Med.* 2014;37(4):768-780. doi:10.1007/s10865-013-9527-4.

46. Hoppe MH. *Active Listening: Improve Your Ability to Listen and Lead.* Greensboro, NC: Center for Creative Leadership; 2006.

47. Fields SA, Johnson WM. Physician-patient communication: breaking bad news. *W V Med J.* 2012;108(2):32-35.

48. Marcus JD, Mott FE. Difficult conversations: from diagnosis to death. *Ochsner J.* 2014;14(4):712-717. PMCID: PMC4295750. Accessed September 20, 2016.

49. Baile WF, Buckman R, Lenzi R, Glober G, Beale EA, Kudelka AP. SPIKES—a six-step protocol for delivering bad news: application to the patient with cancer. *Oncologist.* 2000;5(4):302-311. http://theoncologist.alphamedpress.org/content/5/4/302.long. Accessed March 27, 2018.

50. Back AL, Arnold RM, Baile WF, et al. Efficacy of communication skills training for giving bad news and discussing transitions to palliative care. *Arch Intern Med.* 2007;167(5):453-460. doi:10.1001/archinte.167.5.453.

51. Schell JO, Green JA, Tulsky JA, Arnold RM. Communication skills training for dialysis decision-making and end-of-life care in nephrology. *Clin J Am Soc Nephrol.* 2013;8(4):675-680. http://cjasn.asnjournals.org/content/8/4/675.long. Accessed March 27, 2018.

52. Fujimori M, Uchitomi Y. Preferences of cancer patients regarding communication of bad news: a systematic literature review. *Jpn J Clin Oncol.* 2009;39(4):201-216. http://jjco.oxfordjournals.org/content/39/4/201.long. Accessed March 27, 2018.

53. Koenig H, King D, Carson VB. *Handbook of Religion and Health.* 2nd ed. Oxford, UK: Oxford University Press; 2012.

54. Best M, Butow P, Olver I. Doctors discussing religion and spirituality: a systematic review. *Palliat Med.* 2016; 30(4):327-337.

55. Griffiths J, Wilson C, Ewing G, Connolley M, Grande G. Improving communication with palliative care cancer patients at home—a pilot study of SAGE & THYME communication skills model. *Eur J Oncol Nurs.* 2015;19(5):465-472.

56. Henoch I, Danielson E, Strang S, Browall M, Melin-Johansson C. Training intervention for health care staff in the provision of existential support to patients with cancer: a randomized controlled study. *J Pain Sympt Manag.* 2013;46(6):785-794.

57. Coyle N, Manna R, Shen MJ, et al. Discussing death, dying, and end-of-life goals of care: a communication skills training module for oncology nurses. *Clin J Oncol Nurs.* 2015;19(6):697-702.

58. Ting-Toomey S, Kurogi A. Facework competence in intercultural conflict: an updated face-negotiation theory. *International Journal of Intercultural Relations.* 1998;22(2): 187-225. https://doi.org/10.1016/S0147-1767(98)00004-2.

59. Spector RE. *Cultural Diversity in Health and Illness.* 7th ed. Upper Saddle River, NJ: Pearson; 2009.

60. Spector RE. Heritage assessment. *Cultura de los Cuidados.* 2001;9:71-81. http://rua.ua.es/dspace/handle/10045/5076. Accessed March 27, 2018.

61. Purnell LD. *Guide to Culturally Competent Health Care.* 3rd ed. Philadelphia, PA: F. A. Davis; 2014.

62. Gudykunst WB. *Bridging Differences: Effective Intergroup Communication.* 2nd ed. Thousand Oaks, CA: Sage; 1994.

63. Gallois C, Callan V. *Communication and Culture: A Guide for Practice.* Chichester, England: Wiley; 1997.

64. Hajek C, Giles H. New directions in intercultural communication competence: the process model. In: Greene JO, Burleson BR, eds. *Handbook of Communication and Social Interaction Skills.* New York, NY: Routledge; 2003:935-957.

65. Limited English proficiency (LEP): a federal interagency website. http://www.lep.gov. Accessed July 17, 2016.

66. Ryan C. Language use in the United States: 2011. American Community Survey Reports. ACS-22. https://www.census.gov/prod/2013pubs/acs-22.pdf. Published 2013. Accessed March 27, 2018.

67. Kandula NR, Lauderdale DS, Baker DW. Differences in self-reported health among Asians, Latinos, and non-Hispanic Whites: the role of language and nativity. *Ann Epidemiol.* 2007;17(3):191-198. doi:10.1016/j.annepidem.2006.10.005.

68. DuBard CA, Gizlice Z. Language spoken and differences in health status, access to care, and receipt of preventive services among US Hispanics. *Am J Public Health.* 2008;98(11): 2021-2028. doi:10.2105/AJPH.2007.119008.

69. Fernandez A, Schillinger D, Warton EM, et al. Language barriers, physician-patient language concordance, and glycemic control among insured Latinos with diabetes: the Diabetes Study of Northern California (DISTANCE). *J Gen Intern Med.* 2011;26(2):170-176. doi:10.1007/s11606-010-1507-6.

70. National Standards for Culturally and Linguistically Appropriate Services (CLAS) in Health and Health Care. *Fed Reg.* 2013;78(185):58539-58543.

71. National Standards for Culturally and Linguistically Appropriate Services in Health and Health Care. The National CLAS Standards. U.S. Department of Health and Human Services, Office of Minority Health website. https://minorityhealth.hhs.gov/omh/browse.aspx?lvl=2&lvlid=53. Accessed April 17, 2018.

72. Karliner LS, Jacobs EA, Chen AH, Mutha S. Do professional interpreters improve clinical care for patients with limited English proficiency? A systematic review of the literature. *Health Serv Res.* 2007;42(2):727-754. https://www.ncbi.nlm.nih.gov/pmc/articles/PMC1955368/. Accessed March 27, 2018.

73. Balakrishnana V, Roper J, Cossey K, Roman C, Jeanmonod R. Misidentification of English language proficiency in triage: impact on satisfaction and door-to-room time. *J Immigr Minor Health.* 2016;18(2):369-373. doi:10.1007/s10903-015-0174-4.

74. Genoff MC, Zaballa A, Gany F, et al. Navigating language barriers: a systematic review of patient navigators' impact on cancer screening for limited English proficient patients. *J Gen Intern Med.* 2016;31(4):426-434. doi:10.1007/s11606-015-3572-3.

75. Natale-Pereira A, Enard KR, Nevarez L, Jones LA. The role of patient navigators in eliminating health disparities. *Cancer.* 2011;117(15 Suppl):3543-3552. https://www.ncbi.nlm.nih.gov/pmc/articles/PMC4121958/. Accessed March 27, 2018.

76. Primary care and public health: exploring integration to improve population health. Institute of Medicine website. http://www.nationalacademies.org/hmd/Reports/2012/Primary-Care-and-Public-Health.aspx. Published March 28, 2012. Accessed March 27, 2018.

77. Scutchfield FD, Michener JL, Thacker SB. Are we there yet? Seizing the moment to integrate medicine and public health. *Am J Prev Med.* 2012;42(6):S97-S102. doi:10.1016/j.anepre.2012.04.001.

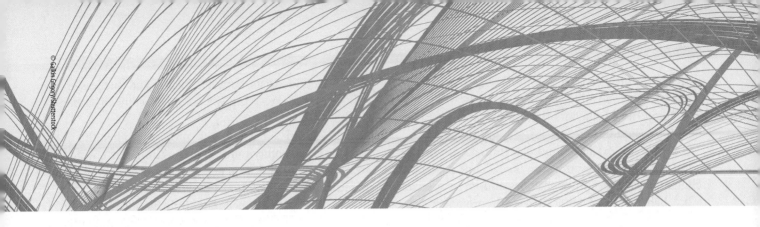

CHAPTER 10

School Health

Elisa Beth McNeill

LEARNING OBJECTIVES

By the end of this chapter, the reader will be able to:

- Explain why schools are a logical place for health promotion.
- Describe the connection between academic success and health outcomes.
- Identify the leading indicators contributing to health outcomes.
- Explain the need for skills-based health instruction.
- Describe the Whole School, Whole Community, Whole Child (WSCC) model.
- Summarize the resources available to enhance the effectiveness of health education.

▶ Introduction

This chapter describes why schools are a good place to start developing healthy behaviors and preventing the establishment of unhealthy behaviors, and how health communication can be used to affect these behaviors. Although we do not often think about what we learned about health in schools (remember learning about body parts and hygiene and why you should not use drugs?) as health communication, health education inherently includes health communication principles. To illustrate how this occurs in school settings, we present key statistics on youth risk behaviors, describe programs designed to counteract these behaviors, and provide program examples along with available resources to promote and communicate about health in schools. Having a working knowledge of how schools contribute to the landscape of health promotion and health communication will enhance opportunities and the ability of

the health communicator to contribute to promotion efforts in academic arenas.

▶ Schools Are a Logical Site for Health Communication

Accessibility to large populations of youth makes schools a logical place to provide knowledge, develop skills, and build positive attitudes related to appropriate lifetime health behaviors. Health and education impact individuals, society, and the economy. Nearly 95% of young people aged 7 through 17 in the United States are enrolled in schools, making school health programs one of the most efficient strategies for health promotion and for providing health communication.[1] Youth need to develop the competence necessary to assist them in making healthy lifestyle choices as they grow. The role of school-based health education, which inherently includes health communication using both interpersonal and group-based strategies, is to promote positive health behaviors while discouraging risky behaviors that can negatively impact health into adulthood.

A primary predictor and determinant of positive adult health outcomes in youth is academic success.[2-4] Higher rates of healthy behaviors and lower rates of risky behaviors are associated with proficient academic skills.[5-7] In fact, a negative association exists when comparing academic performance to participation in risky health behaviors. Data from the national Youth Risk Behavior Survey (discussed further later in this chapter) reveal students with higher grades are less likely to engage in selected risk behaviors compared to classmates who earn poorer grades (**FIGURE 10-1**).[8] For example, in 2015 (the most recent year this information was collected), of students making mostly *A*s, 24% reported using marijuana one or more times during their life compared to 66% of students making mostly *D*s and *F*s. Similarly, 23% of those making As were currently sexually active (having sexual intercourse with at least one person during the 3 months prior to the survey), compared to 46% of those making mostly *D*s and *F*s. Vaping, violence, and lack of physical inactivity are other health risk behaviors that are consistently linked to poor test scores, lower grades, and reduced educational attainment.[9-11] Although the data do not prove causation, they clearly suggest students who do not engage in health-risk behaviors receive higher grades. One thing is clear:

A connection exists between health and success in school that makes schools a sound place to promote health.

A second advantage of promoting health in schools is the ability to focus on building self-efficacy in practicing health-related behaviors using skill-based educational approaches. Health education programs that provide accurate information typically show improvements in health knowledge and attitudes; however, there is little correlation related to changes in risk taking and desirable behavioral outcomes.[12,13] To accomplish the difficult task of attaining and sustaining health behavior change, evidence suggests skills-based approaches are more effective than teaching knowledge alone.[14] Skills-based approaches do include health knowledge and attitude development; however, they differ from traditional methods by focusing on the aptitudes needed to make the most positive health-related choices. In a skills-based tactic, the emphasis is on the development of intra- and interpersonal skills, critical thinking, and decision-making skills that can be applied to a wide range of health behaviors.

Skills-based approaches utilize "…student centered and participatory methodologies, giving participants the opportunity to explore and acquire health promoting knowledge, attitudes and values and to practice the skills they need to avoid risky and unhealthy situations and adopt and sustain healthier life styles."[14(para 9)] For example, **role playing** in response

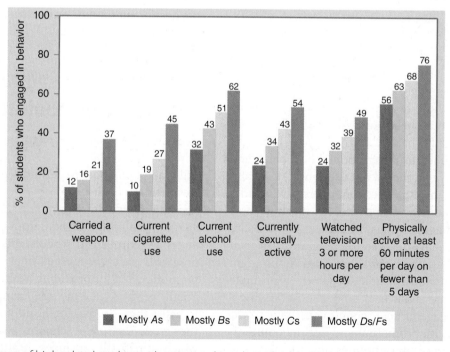

FIGURE 10-1 Percentage of high school students who engaged in selected risk behaviors, by type of grades earned—United States, Youth Risk Behavior Survey, 2009.

BOX 10-1 Social Inoculation Theory

Theorist W. J. McGuire suggested attitudes could be inoculated against persuasive attacks in much the same way that one's immune system can be inoculated against viral attacks.[a] In order to strengthen a person's adoption of healthy behaviors, one needs to strengthen the attitudes and beliefs about the importance of the behavior. Exposing individuals to "weakened" versions of a situation enables the person to activate their existing defenses by generating possible solutions to resolve the conflict. To strengthen the defense, it is critical the individual does more than just think about how they would respond; the individual needs to perform the actions. The inoculation works because it causes the individual to think carefully, deeply, and critically to determine the best course of action. Getting individuals to think for themselves is the foundation of the social inoculation approach. When people actively generate their own ideas and must vigorously defend them, they develop stronger attitudes, beliefs, and behaviors.[b]

[a] McGuire WJ. Inducing resistance to persuasion: some contemporary approaches. In: Berkowitz L, ed., *Advances in Experimental Social Psychology*. New York, NY: Academic Press; 1964:191-229.
[b] Compton J, Jackson B, Dimmock JA. Persuading others to avoid persuasion: inoculation theory and resistant health attitudes. *Frontiers Psychol.* 2016;7:122. doi:10.3389/fpsyg.2016.00122.

to a given scenario is a frequently used methodology that allows students to practice strategies for handling a potentially health-threatening experience in a safe setting. The learner must evaluate the scenario, using intrapersonal skills to critically think about the consequences of potential actions, and then apply interpersonal skills to communicate their decision. Role playing, as a method, is highly connected to the concepts of **social inoculation theory** in which, similar to receiving a vaccination, the learner is exposed to a small dose of a situation in order to explore their capacity to manage it. A good example of this is having students role play responses to being offered drugs or alcohol or to having unprotected sex. **BOX 10-1** provides an overview of social inoculation theory.

Allowing learners to practice behaviors in a nonthreatening situation gives them the opportunity to experiment or try out different solutions, thereby developing the skills needed if the actual situation should arise in the future. If the desired behavioral outcomes are going to occur, ample time must be dedicated to skill building and providing opportunities for practice. Because children in the United States spend, on average, about 6.8 hours a day in school, these settings provide the most viable arena for practice and skill development.[15]

▶ Leading Health Issues and the Youth Risk Behavior Surveillance System

When people think of health, they typically associate it with being physically active and eating healthy. These two aspects are definitely influential in their contribution to overall health; however, they represent only two of the dimensions that make up one's

health. Many factors contribute to the overall health of children and adolescents, including priority health risk behaviors that significantly contribute to leading causes of death, disability, and social problems. These behaviors are commonly referred to as the six leading risk factors for youth because they are often established during childhood and early adolescence.[16] The behaviors of greatest concern include[16]:

- Unhealthy dietary practices
- Use of tobacco
- Use of alcohol and other drugs
- Inadequate participation in physical activity (PA)
- Sexual behaviors connected to unintended pregnancy or sexually transmitted infections (including HIV)
- Actions contributing to unintentional injuries and violence

In order to develop effective and impactful prevention strategies, it is critical to identify which behaviors put youth at risk. Since 1991, the Centers for Disease Control and Prevention (CDC), as part of the **Youth Risk Behavior Surveillance System (YRBSS)**, have administered a biannual cross-sectional survey in odd-number years to monitor changes in behaviors associated with the six leading health risks.[17] During each administration of the **Youth Risk Behavior Survey (YRBS)**, data are collected from more than 3.8 million high school students in over 1700 separate surveys.[17] "YRBSS data are used widely to compare the prevalence of health behaviors among subpopulations of students; assess trends in health behaviors over time; monitor progress toward achieving 21 national health objectives for Healthy People 2020...."[17(p1)] The data are used to guide development and evaluation of school and community policies, programs, and practices designed to decrease health-risk behaviors and improve health outcomes among youth.

For example, data from the 2015 YRBS reveal that although the prevalence of cigarette smoking among high school students (11%) is being reported at the lowest levels since 1991 (28%), the use of e-cigarettes is posing new challenges, with 24% reporting e-cigarette use in the last 30 days.[18] Additionally, survey findings suggest the use of technology while driving continues to be a risk behavior of concern. Among high school students nationwide, 42% of students who had driven motor vehicles during the past 30 days had texted or emailed while driving.[18] These data suggest promotion efforts targeting e-cigarettes and the use of technology while driving are currently needed. Further analysis of the 2015 YRBS results also showed changes in obesity and sedentary-related behaviors, such as use of computers or other screens. The percentage reporting using a computer three or more hours per day for non-school-related work nearly doubled, from 22% in 2003 to 42% in 2015.[18] The increase in sedentary-related behaviors clearly suggests health promotion efforts need to concentrate on increasing opportunities for PA among youth. The YRBSS data are useful for those working in schools because they provide valid and reliable data to support the need for targeted health communication and health promotion programs and interventions.

The YRBS data also offer a snapshot of changes in the health behaviors of youth over time. The national YRBS has been collected in the spring every two years since 1991; thus, we have a reliable source documenting the changes in trends. **FIGURE 10-2** provides a sample of representative national data of both public and private 9th- through 12th-grade students in the United States describing the trends in the prevalence of alcohol use between 1991 and 2015.[19]

At first glance there appears to have been no change in the prevalence of alcohol use from 2013 to 2015 for the following indicators: ever drank alcohol, drank alcohol before age 13 years, and currently drank alcohol (at least one drink on one day during the 30 days prior to the survey). However, if you look at the overall trends from 1991 to 2015, it is evident that alcohol use by 9th through 12th graders has declined.[19] Some questions these changes in trends might cause

---

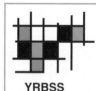

Trends in the Prevalence of Alcohol Use
National YRBS: 1991–2015

The national Youth Risk Behavior Survey (YRBS) monitors priority health risk behaviors that contribute to the leading causes of death, disability, and social problems among youth and adults in the United States. The national YRBS is conducted every 2 years during the spring semester and provides data representative of 9th through 12th grade students in public and private schools throughout the United States.

Percentages													Change from 1991–2015[1]	Change from 2013–2015[2]
1991	1993	1995	1997	1999	2001	2003	2005	2007	2009	2011	2013	2015		
Ever drank alcohol (at least one drink of alcohol on at least 1 day during their life)														
81.6	80.9	80.4	79.1	81.0	78.2	74.9	74.3	75.0	72.5	70.8	66.2	63.2	Decreased 1991–2015 Decreased 1991–2007 Decreased 2007–2015	No change
Drank alcohol before age 13 years (for the first time other than a few sips)														
32.7	32.9	32.4	31.1	32.2	29.1	27.8	25.6	23.8	21.1	20.5	18.6	17.2	Decreased 1991–2015 No change 1991–1999 Decreased 1999–2015	No change
Currently drank alcohol (at least one drink of alcohol on at least 1 day during the 30 days before the survey)														
50.8	48.0	51.6	50.8	50.0	47.1	44.9	43.3	44.7	41.8	38.7	34.9	32.8	Decreased 1991–2015 Decreased 1991–2007 Decreased 2007–2015	No change
Drank five or more drinks of alcohol in a row (within a couple of hours on at least 1 day during the 30 days before the survey)														
31.3	30.0	32.6	33.4	31.5	29.9	28.3	25.5	26.0	24.2	21.9	20.8	17.7	Decreased 1991–2015 Increased 1991–1999 Decreased 1999–2015	Decreased

[1] Based on linear and quadratic trend analyses using logistic regression models controlling for sex, race/ethnicity, and grade, p < 0.05. Significant linear trends (if present) across all available years are described first followed by linear changes in each segment of significant quadratic trends (if present).
[2] Based on t-test analysis p < 0.05.

Where can I get more information? Visit **www.cdc.gov/yrbss** or call 800-CDC-INFO (800-232-4636).

FIGURE 10-2 Trends in the prevalence of alcohol use—National YRBS: 1991–2015.

one to ask include: What factors could be contributing to the decline in the prevalence? Could the decrease be a consequence of health promotion efforts targeting adolescent alcohol use? When reviewing the data associated with binge drinking, the data indicate a decrease in the number of 9th- through 12th-grade students reporting they had drunk five or more drinks of alcohol in a row within a couple of hours on at least 1 day during the 30 days before the survey. But a closer look reveals an increasing trend in prevalence of binge drinking from 1991 to 1999. These data provided the evidence needed to support the inclusion of information on binge drinking as part of alcohol misuse prevention programs. The decrease in students reporting binge drinking from 1995 to 2015 could be related to including prevention strategies targeting binge drinking as part of alcohol misuse prevention. Similarly, national data have been used to call attention to obesity rates and the need to address sedentary behaviors in youth; thus, national survey data are a powerful tool that can be used to justify and shape the direction of health communication and health promotion.

▶ Promoting Movement and Physical Activity in All Academic Classrooms

Changing health behavior through classroom-based education works when using **skills-based health education**. One example of classroom-based education is how to incorporate PA into schools. The concern over childhood and adolescent obesity has resulted in a realization of the need to provide youth with more opportunities to be physically active. When teaching strategies in health education are being implemented from more of a skills-based approach, there is a natural ability to incorporate PA as part of instruction. Educators and scientists recognize the vital role of physical, cognitive, and brain health in education.[20] Studies show physically active children are better able to perform academically than peers who are not as physically active.[21,22] As sedentary lifestyle behaviors increase while time in physical education classes in our public schools decreases (theoretically to provide additional opportunities for academics), the need to incorporate movement in the classroom has become more prevalent.[23] There is a push to integrate occasions for PA through comprehensive approaches. This means PA is no longer isolated to recess or the physical education class. Instead, opportunities for PA are becoming the responsibility of teachers in all academic subjects.[24] Teachers who provide instruction

in core academic areas such as mathematics, science, reading, writing, and social sciences are also intentionally embedding PA into their teaching methodologies throughout the whole school day as a mechanism to increase the overall rates of PA for students.[25] Incorporation of PA into the classroom is easy to do and can occur in a variety of ways. For example, when learning to spell words, a class of students might toss a rubber ball to each other calling out the next correct letter, then finish the activity with a jumping jack when the word is spelled correctly. Station-work types of activities allow students to move around the room and give students the opportunity to stand and walk as part of content exploration. **TABLE 10-1** provides some additional examples of ways to incorporate PA as part of instruction.

Technology has also enhanced the ability to incorporate PA in the classroom. There are numerous websites and applications (apps) available for classroom use that encourage and track movement and PA. Many of these provide a variety of options for short movement breaks, often referred to as "brain breaks," that allow students to get up and move. Brain breaks are based on the premise that students need regular downtime throughout the day to refocus the brain for learning concepts and retention of factual information.[26] Using movement, or educational kinesiology, increases the oxygen in the bloodstream and leads to improved concentration, which enhances children's readiness to learn.[27] The three types of brain breaks commonly used are relaxation and breathing breaks, highly physically active, and content-related activities.[28] **TABLE 10-2** summarizes a few examples of activities for each type of brain break.

One example of a website frequently used to incorporate brain breaks in classrooms is called *Go Noodle*. This website has numerous choices for teachers to get children dancing, singing, doing yoga poses, or performing other types of movement for short intervals of time. There are also opportunities for teachers, or individual specialists working with students, to deliver content while using the Go Noodle activities; for example, students might hop and clap to the rap music in a video as they count the number of syllables in a word. As the popularity for incorporating PA as part of a class lesson increases, it is likely we will continue to see additional technology applications that are valuable resources to promote health.

Even the design of the school environment can allow PA to permeate the school culture.

In 2015, a document titled, *The Physical Activity Design Guidelines for School Architecture*, presented recommendations of core principles for designing

TABLE 10-1 Incorporating Physical Activity as Part of Instruction

Activity	Description
Measure Around the Room	Ask students to measure a variety of things in the room—chairs, desks, doors, windows—using yardsticks or rulers. Students could also use body parts to estimate lengths (e.g., the pointer finger is 2 inches long and the distance from the elbow to wrist is 10 inches). Record measurements in a log or use to create a graph.
Switch-off	Record an assignment on the board (e.g., p. 124, problems 1–20). Have students write their name on the paper and complete problem one. Then, when everyone has finished with problem one, have them stand up and move to the next desk, check their classmate's answer to problem number one, and then do problem number two. Continue until every student has completed and checked every problem.
Human Body Map	Use the human body as a "map" for learning new information in different subjects. In geography, provide students sticker labels to record the names of countries in South America. If the head is Venezuela, then where is Argentina?
Charades	Have students pantomime (act out) words, phrases, or actions without speaking. For example, students could act out states of matter, the rotation of planets, the meaning of vocabulary words, or the different rhythms of a heartbeat.
Fact-Family Relay Race	Write two parts of a fact family on the board. Break the students into groups and have one member come up to the board and complete that fact family, and then write two parts of another fact family. Have the student then toss a beanbag to the next member of the group, who will solve the next fact family.
Recycle (Nature) Walk	Students record in a journal items they see that could be reused or recycled while taking a 3-minute nature walk (inside or outside the school building).
Pattern Dancing	Students create a dance that represents a pattern in math. For example, to demonstrate an ABCB pattern, they could do a hop, a skip, a spin, and a skip.
Yoga Pose	Ask a multiple-choice question, and then have the students move their body into the pose to represent their response; for example, (a) star pose, (b) rainbow pose, (c) ragdoll pose, and (d) tree pose.

21st-century schools that serve as havens for promoting lifelong health and learning by creating a health infrastructure.[29] The suggested school design should integrate movement as part of the daily routine by designing child-centric active navigation routes; for example, schools might paint a hopscotch outline down the hallway or paint commands of actions to perform on each step of the staircase as a means to increase PA. Inclusion of exterior features like playgrounds, gardens, and nature spaces in the schoolyard, which are designed for diversity and universal access, can also increase the daily dose of PA and movement throughout the school community.[29]

A second principle suggested in the guideline is the use of dynamic furniture that is designed to encourage children's natural physical movements and is meant for growing bodies: stand-biased desks for youth, ergonomic roll-swivel chairs with seat surfaces that move in three dimensions, and a variety of postural options create an active environment tailored to the movement needs of children.[29] Standing desks allow students to alternate between sitting on a stool and standing while working. "Stand-biased classrooms can interrupt sedentary behavior patterns among students in kindergarten through grade 12 (and beyond) during the hours they spend at school, and this can be done simply, at a low cost, and without disrupting classroom instruction time."[30(p1853)]

These trends of including opportunities for PA as part of the built environment and content delivery open new prospects for the health communications

TABLE 10-2 Examples of Brain Break Activities by Type

Type	Description	Examples
Relaxation and breathing breaks	Uses breathing techniques to calm the brain Designed to change breathing patterns and facilitate oxygenation of the brain	▪ *Equal breathing:* Students inhale for a count of four and exhale for a count of four. ▪ *Abdominal breathing:* Students place one hand on the chest and another on the abdomen while taking 6–10 deep breaths through the nose, ensuring the diaphragm is moving (not the chest). ▪ *Skull shining breath:* Students take a long, slow inhale followed by a quick, powerful exhale generated from the lower belly. ▪ *Progressive relaxation:* Students work through the body, tensing and relaxing different muscle groups while maintaining slow, deep breaths. ▪ *Guided visualization:* Students imagine a peaceful place while focusing on maintaining slow, deep breaths.
Highly physical breaks	Designed to get students moving vigorously to oxygenate the brain and release muscle tension	▪ *Cardiovascular intensive:* Movements are performed (jumping jacks, squats, hop or run in place, kick boxing, or dancing).
Content-related activities	Designed to oxygenate and destress by promoting moderate-level physical activity	▪ *Sit down, stand up:* For example, students could stand to indicate an answer is true or sit to represent a false answer. ▪ *Four corners:* Students walk to the corners of the room to discuss opinions about content. ▪ *Match the meaning:* Definitions of vocabulary words are placed in locations around the room. Students walk around the room to identify the location of the correct definition to the words on their worksheet. The activity can be set up as a race or students can be given a designated amount of time to complete the task.

Reproduced from Weslake A, Christian BJ. Brain breaks: help or hindrance? *Teach Collection Christian Educ.* 2015;1(1):38-46.

specialist. The ability to move out of traditional venues for delivery of health promotion, like the health and physical education classes, facilitates a multidisciplinary approach to promoting health, which may help students recognize how their health is part of everything they do.

▶ Systems Approaches to Promoting Health in Schools

Factors contributing to the creation of effective school-based health promotion are well recognized. The *Achieving Health Promoting Schools: Guidelines for Promoting Health in Schools* document provides insights on what works and what may inhibit impactful health promotion.[31] Among other recommendations, the document highlights the important role of promoting and communicating about health from a holistic perspective; for example, schools that use a whole-school process, rather than primarily a classroom learning approach, and explore health issues within the context of students' lives and community expand efforts by minimizing the promotion of health in silos. Many factors contribute to health behavior; therefore, the need to strategically promote health from a systems perspective is essential. "A **systems approach to health** is one that applies scientific insights to understand the elements that influence health outcomes; models the relationships between those elements; and alters design, processes, or policies based on the resultant knowledge in order to produce better health at lower cost."[32(p5)] Using a systems approach, schools and communities have the ability to coordinate efforts from a variety of resources to provide more consistent and effective health promotion interventions.

Perhaps the best example of a school-based systems strategy to promote the health of schoolchildren is the **Whole School, Whole Community, Whole Child (WSCC) model** (FIGURE 10-3). Using the same concept as the ecological model, the focus of the WSCC model is directed at the whole school, with the school, in turn, drawing its resources and influences from the community and addressing the needs of the child.[33]

The WSCC model calls for a collaborative approach to learning and health, across the individual child, school, and community to meet the needs and reach the potential of each child. It makes accountable all who are part of the school and community to see themselves as responsible for both learning and health, and diagrammatically highlights the relationship between the

school and the community.[33] Systematically promoting the health and well-being of students, staff, classrooms, and schools leads to developing environments conducive to effective teaching, communicating, and learning.[33] Enhancing connectedness between the factors represented in the model creates, for students, a sense of belonging and safety while helping resource providers better understand what is best practice for students to learn. Including families and the local community in the equation allows schools to extend the safety net of support by empowering key stakeholders to take an active role in the education process.[33] Although the WSCC model originated at the national level, the model's impact on schools is strengthened because its application occurs at the local level. Schools and school districts are given the autonomy to tailor approaches for implementation of the model to best suit the needs of individual districts and their students.

Ideally, the components of the WSCC model are addressed in a multidimensional approach to maximize the effectiveness of health promotion interventions. For example, in the area of nutrition and

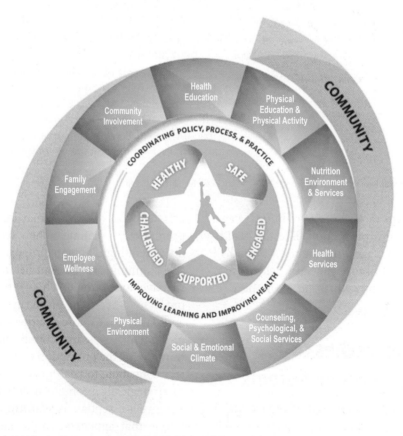

FIGURE 10-3 Whole School, Whole Community, Whole Child (WSCC) model.
Reproduced from ASCD. Whole School, Whole Community, Whole Child. http://www.ascd.org/programs/learning-and-health/wscc-model.aspx. Accessed April 13, 2018.

environmental services, a school might elect to participate in the Food Safe Schools Program (FSSP) sponsored by the National Environmental Health Association. This program has two primary goals: addressing food safety and people's behavior to encourage the use of food safety procedures, policies, and plans.[34] Using the *Action Guide* provided by the FSSP, schools can review their current food safety policies and procedures to evaluate their own culture related to food safety. "The *Action Guide* addresses food safety requirements for the National School Lunch Act…training and education, employee health and personal hygiene, produce safety, managing food allergies, food defense, responding to food recalls, and responding to a foodborne illness outbreak."[34(para 5)] To include students in thinking about health and how these guidelines may pertain to them, students in a health education class might create an advocacy campaign promoting safe food practices on posters to be displayed in the school's cafeteria. The school may also implement a policy to require all students to be trained on how to recognize symptoms of anaphylaxis due to a food allergy. In a physical education class, students might use trainer pens to learn how to administer an epinephrine auto-injector in an emergency. In the examples described, four different components of the WSCC model are working in conjunction to promote a common goal—safe food practices. The combined efforts of the many components of the WSCC model produce a common message that may strengthen the impact of the health promotion effort.

Health promotion can be enhanced or hindered depending on the established policies and procedures within a school. Criteria representative of a healthy school environment have been identified by the CDC and used to create an online self-assessment and planning tool, known as the **School Health Index (SHI)**. Schools can use this tool to improve their health and safety policies and programs.[35] The SHI is designed to promote healthier and safer behavior in the following six critical areas[35]:

- PA and physical education
- Nutrition
- Tobacco use and prevention
- Unintentional injury and violence prevention (safety)
- Asthma
- Sexual health, including HIV, other sexually transmitted diseases, and pregnancy prevention

The SHI enables teams composed of administrators, teachers, food service personnel, students, parents, and other members of the school community to examine the extent to which a school implements the policies and practices recommended by the CDC in its research-based guidelines and strategies for school health and safety programs in eight areas and then suggest a framework for improvement.[36] A list of the modules evaluated by the SHI at both the elementary and secondary level can be found in **TABLE 10-3**.

The SHI instrument is easy to use and provides clear criteria for scoring variables. For example, in Module 6: School Counseling, Psychological, and

TABLE 10-3 Modules Evaluated in the School Health Index

Module 1	School Health and Safety Policies and Environment
Module 2	Health Education
Module 3	Physical Education and Other Physical Activity Programs
Module 4	Nutrition Services
Module 5	School Health Services
Module 6	School Counseling, Psychological, and Social Services
Module 7	Health Promotion for Staff
Module 8	Family and Community Involvement

Data from School health index: a self-assessment and planning guide [middle/high school version]. Centers for Disease Control and Prevention website. https://www.cdc.gov/healthyschools/shi/pdf/middle-high-total-2014.pdf. Published 2014. Accessed March 28, 2018.

Social Services, one of the indicators on the instrument designed for middle/high school asks[37]:

Does your school have access to a full-time counselor, social worker, and psychologist for providing counseling, psychological, and social services? Is an adequate number of these staff members provided based on the following recommended ratios?

- One counselor for every 250 students
- One social worker for every 400 students
- One psychologist for every 1000 students

3 = Yes, we have a full-time counselor, social worker, and psychologist, **and** the recommended ratios are present.

2 = We have a full-time counselor, social worker, and psychologist, but **fewer** than the recommended ratios.

1 = We have a full-time counselor, social worker **or** psychologist, **but** not all three.

0 = No, we do **not** have even one full-time counselor, social work or psychologist.

The scoring criteria are useful to schools in that they outline what is considered the ideal standard, thereby providing targets for improvement if a score of three is not achieved. The SHI provides evidence of a school's commitment to the health and well-being of its students when the scores on the instrument fall into the upper ranges.

▶ National Initiatives to Support Health Promotion for Students

On the national level, initiatives exist to augment the health promotion efforts of schools. Multiple interventions have been created by the CDC to enhance healthy behaviors in youth. The Division of Adolescent and School Health has focused on a youth media campaign called *VERB: It's what you do.* The VERB campaign uses paid advertising, marketing strategies, and partnership efforts to encourage tweens (aged 9–13 years) to be physically active every day.[38] Although tweens are the primary target, parents and adult influencers such as teachers, coaches, youth leaders, pediatricians, and other health professionals are also considered secondary members of the VERB campaign's target audience.[38] These secondary members play a critical role as models, reinforcers, and enablers for tweens to be physically active every day.

Like the VERB! campaign, the Let's Move! campaign extends its promotion of health to encourage all age groups to become more physically active. Endorsed by Michelle Obama, Let's Move! Active Schools is a national initiative to ensure that 60 minutes of PA a day is the norm for youth in K–12 settings.[39] The vision for active schools includes the integration of PA before, during, and after school with involvement from staff, families, and communities as part of the Comprehensive School Physical Activity Program.[39]

BAM! Body and Mind is a second example of a CDC initiative designed to encourage youth to make healthy lifestyle choices. Students in grades 5–8 can use the website's interactive features (games and quizzes) to find information on diseases, food and nutrition, PA, safety, stress, and the body.[40] The site offers a Teacher's Corner to enable educators to download activities and related materials for health instruction. These free resources are a valuable asset for teachers and others working with youth because they provide medically accurate information in clear and concise vignettes.

Another successful example of a national initiative to promote the health of youth is the Truth campaign. The Truth campaign is an evidence-based countermarketing campaign that has demonstrated success in the prevention of smoking initiation among at-risk youth.[41] Using fast-paced, hard-edged ads that present facts about the addictiveness, number of deaths, and disease-related complications of smoking, youth aged 12–17 years are informed on the marketing practices of the tobacco industry. A goal of the Truth campaign is to challenge youth to use all of this information to make up their own minds when deciding whether or not to smoke.[41] One common aspect of all these examples is the important role of giving youth the autonomy to choose for themselves. Instead of telling youth what to do, they are taught how to critically evaluate their choices and to use decision-making skills to determine their own health behaviors. When youth are given accurate information and provided the skills and resources necessary to make their own choices, they become empowered and are more likely to make healthy ones.

A variety of school and community programs have been created to improve the health of youth. **TABLE 10-4** summarizes a few examples. The national interventions described represent just a few examples of strategies used to promote health for youth. The multidimensional nature of health behaviors explains the need for a variety of interventions and programs to meet the social, physical, emotional, intellectual, spiritual, occupational, and environmental needs of individuals.

TABLE 10-4 Sample Interventions to Promote Health

Intervention's Purpose	Designed to increase fruit and vegetable consumption	Designed to increase physical activity and promote healthy dietary habits	Designed to promote mental, emotional, and behavioral (MEB) well-being	Designed to prevent underage drinking and nonmedical use of prescription pain reliever drugs by youth
Program Titles	■ 5-a-Day Power Plus ■ Gimme 5 ■ High 5 Flyers Program ■ Nutrition to Grow On ■ Tiny Tastes ■ Teens Eating for Energy and Nutrition at School (TEENS)	■ APPLE: **A**lberta **P**roject **P**romoting active **L**iving and healthy **E**ating ■ Bienestar ■ CARDIAC Kinder ■ Coordinated Approach to Child Health (CATCH) ■ Eat Well and Keep Moving ■ New Moves ■ Planet Health ■ The Physical Activity and Teenage Health (PATH) Program	■ Good Behavior Game ■ Parent Corps ■ THRIVE Media Campaign to Prevent Suicide and Bullying Among American Indian/Alaska Native Youth	■ Life Skills Training ■ Too Good for Drugs ■ Project Towards No Drug Abuse ■ Project Success (Schools Using Coordinated Community Efforts to Strengthen Students)

▶ Resources for School-Based Health Promotion

A plethora of resources are available to assist in the promotion of health in school settings. As mentioned earlier, the WSCC model provides a framework to direct the enrichment of the health and well-being of students. Within the Health Education component of the WSCC model, guiding documents have been generated to create a more systematic and effective approach to teaching and communicating about health. In 1995 the **National Health Education Standards (NHES)** were created to establish, promote, and support health-enhancing behaviors for students in pre-kindergarten through 12th grade.[42] The second edition of the NHES, released in 2007, provides a framework for student instruction and assessment in health. The NHES articulate what students should know and be able to do by grades 2, 5, 8, and 12.[42] In a standards-based educational approach, targets for learning are established that allow teachers to track student performance and focus instruction to meet the specific needs. The NHES outline age-appropriate and developmentally appropriate student learning expectations considered to be essential to the development of health-enhancing behaviors. The standards addressed target a comprehensive assortment of health topics, including alcohol and other drugs, healthy eating, mental and emotional health, personal health and wellness, PA, safety, sexual health, tobacco, violence prevention, and comprehensive health education curricula. The NHES highlight the importance of implementing a skills-based approach to health education. Of the eight standards, only Standard 1 focuses on the development of knowledge for students. The remaining standards are dedicated to practicing the development of skills. Standards 2 through 8 focus on students analyzing influences, accessing valid information, advocating for health, using interpersonal communication, and developing skills for decision making and goal setting.[42] The development of health standards was an important contribution toward moving away from an information only–based approach to a skill development strategy for teaching and communicating about health. The standards created a systematic guide for the planning, implementation, and assessment process of student learning in health.

The positive impact the NHES had on enriching the classroom has led to the development of other content-specific standards. The **National Sexuality Education Standards (NSES)** provide clear and consistent guidance on the essential core standards for sexuality education. The development of the NSES has resulted in a more comprehensive approach to sexuality education focused on knowledge and skill development to facilitate the ability of youth to make choices that promote healthy sexual behaviors. Additionally, standards have been developed to ensure that educators teaching sexuality have been properly trained to provide instruction. The **National Teacher Preparation Standards for Sexuality Education** were designed for use by institutes of higher education to improve the preparation of teacher candidates for instruction in sexuality education.[43] All of these standards have the common goal of improving the quality of health education by thoroughly organizing instruction and better preparing health educators' capacity for promoting healthy behaviors.

A second resource available to enrich the delivery of health instruction in the classroom is the **Health Education Curriculum Analysis Tool (HECAT)**. Whereas standards indicate what should be taught and when, the HECAT can be used by schools to select or develop appropriate and effective curricula to teach the content established in the standards.[44] "The HECAT contains process guidance, appraisal tools, and resources…to help schools revise and improve locally-developed curricula, strengthen the delivery of health education, and improve the ability of school health educators to influence healthy behaviors and healthy outcomes among school age youth."[44(p1)] Analysis tools like the HECAT, and its counterpart for

physical education, the Physical Education Curriculum Analysis Tool, enable schools to choose or develop the curriculum for the best possible health-promoting educational outcomes.

The HECAT originated out of a body of research that identified what is considered to be the **characteristics of effective health education curriculum**. According to the CDC, today's state-of-the-art health education curriculum teaches functional health information and shapes group norms along with personal values and beliefs to support healthy behaviors, while developing the essential health skills needed to adopt, practice, and maintain health-enhancing behaviors.[45] Reviews of evidence-based curricula were conducted to identify common attributes they shared, which may have contributed to their effectiveness in promoting healthy behaviors. For example, a common trait of curricula showing statistical significance in the modification of health behavior was the inclusion of opportunities to make positive connections with influential others.[45] When teachers link students with positive adult role models, mentors, community health educators, counselors, or health specialists, these influential people can function to affirm and reinforce health-promoting norms, attitudes, values, beliefs, and behaviors.[45] For some youth, positive role models are nonexistent; therefore, when curricula include opportunities to connect students with trusted people of influence, the health messaging is strengthened through reinforcement from outside resources. Fifteen characteristics, summarized in **BOX 10-2**, have been identified as essential features to include when designing health education curricula.

BOX 10-2 Characteristics of an Effective Health Education Curriculum

- Focuses on clear health goals and behavioral outcomes.
- Is theory driven and research-based.
- Addresses the values, attitudes, and beliefs of the individual.
- Addresses individual and group norms that support health-enhancing behavior.
- Focuses on reinforcing protective factors and increasing perceptions of risk when engaging in unhealthy practices and behaviors.
- Examines social pressures of influence.
- Builds personal competence, social competence, and self-efficacy through skill development.
- Provides accurate and basic functional health knowledge to promote making decisions for healthy behaviors.
- Students are engaged and the information is personalized.
- Learning strategies, materials, and teaching methods are age and developmentally appropriate.
- Teaching and learning strategies are culturally inclusive.
- Adequate time for instruction and learning is provided.
- Chances are provided to reinforce skills and positive health behaviors.
- Opportunities are given to make positive connections with influential others.
- Professional development and teacher information and training are included to enhance effectiveness of instruction.

Collectively, these 15 characteristics challenge students to assess their vulnerability for health problems, the actual risk of engaging in harmful health behaviors, and their personal exposure to unhealthy situations. Challenging students to analyze their own susceptibility to behaviors that may compromise or can maximize their health enables students to validate positive health-promoting beliefs and intentions.[43] Educators, including specialists who support the work of classroom teachers, need to recognize and use strategies that account for the important role autonomy has in the solidifying of health behaviors.

▶ Health Communication Specialists in Schools

Health communication specialists (HCSs) who design behavior change and communication campaign strategies can play an important role in the promotion of health within the school environment. The primary role of HCSs is to relay accurate and reliable health messages to their target populations. School settings provide a variety of outlets for employment that can capitalize on their training in advertising, public relations, epidemiology, and technical writing.[46] For example, an HCS might find him- or herself working in a school district's administration office with the task of communicating school news to the public and fielding questions from the media. In the role of health policy expert, the HCS might also be charged with representing the interests of a school district at the state or national political level. HCSs may also use their expertise to influence policymakers on how best to handle the health compromises experienced within schools. Additionally, HCSs may work with curriculum development experts to evaluate, critique, and promote health campaigns being implemented in the schools. As experts in communicating with individuals and communities about health matters or relaying information to the public at large about health concerns, HCSs have the capacity to enhance the promotion of health in academic settings.

▶ Conclusion

In this chapter, schools were described as ideal places to prevent the development of unhealthy behaviors and to promote healthy choices. Although only a few of the key health initiatives were discussed, it is evident that a significant number of programs designed to counteract negative health outcomes for youth exist. These programs offer opportunities for the HCS to make a positive contribution in promoting health messages.

Key Terms

Characteristics of effective health education curriculum
Health communication specialist (HCS)
Health Education Curriculum Analysis Tool (HECAT)
National Health Education Standards (NHES)

National Sexuality Education Standards (NSES)
National Teacher Preparation Standards for Sexuality Education
Role playing
School Health Index (SHI)
Skills-based health education
Social inoculation theory

Systems approach to health
Whole School, Whole Community, Whole Child (WSCC) model
Youth Risk Behavior Surveillance System (YRBSS)
Youth Risk Behavior Survey (YRBS)

Chapter Questions

1. What are three reasons why schools are considered logical places for health promotion?
2. List three of the leading indicators that determine health outcomes, and describe how they impact academic success for students.
3. Content standards for health have been developed to articulate what a health-literate person should know and be able to do. Seven out of the eight NHES are dedicated to building skills for applying or using health information. Why is there greater focus on skill building and application than the dissemination of health facts?
4. Describe an activity that might be used to incorporate the three types of brain breaks discussed in the chapter. For each example, discuss a possible positive and negative outcome of incorporating the activity in a classroom. (Go to https://www.gonoodle.com for ideas.)
5. Box 10-2 lists the Characteristics of an Effective Health Education Curriculum. Select one of these characteristics and, in your own words, explain why you believe it would have a positive impact on the health behaviors of youth.

6. Select a school and evaluate its health policies and procedures associated with Module 8: Family and Community Involvement of the School Health Index (SHI), which can be found at the following link: https://www.cdc.gov/healthyschools/shi/pdf/middle -high-total-2014.pdf. After using the discussion questions to complete the scorecard on your chosen school, describe a recommendation you might make to the school to improve its health policy or procedure. (Note: Refer to pages 3–10 of the module.)

References

1. Digest of educational statistics: 2016. National Center for Educational Statistics website. http://nces.ed.gov/programs/digest/2016menu_tables.asp. Accessed March 28, 2018.

2. Srabstein J, Piazza T. Public health, safety and educational risks associated with bullying behaviors in American adolescents. *Int J Adolesc Med Health*. 2008;20(2):223-233.

3. Policy statement on school health, 2004. Council of Chief State School Officers. https://files.eric.ed.gov/fulltext/ED486226.pdf. Accessed April 13, 2018.

4. Beliefs and policies of the National School Boards Association. National School Boards Association website. https://www.nsba.org/beliefs-and-policies-national-school-boards-association. Updated April 8, 2016. Accessed March 28, 2018.

5. National survey on drug use and health, 2007. U.S. Department of Health and Human Services, Substance Abuse and Mental Health Services Administration, Office of Applied Studies website. http://www.icpsr.umich.edu/icpsrweb/NAHDAP/studies/23782. Accessed March 28, 2018.

6. Adolescent and School Health. National Center for Chronic Disease Prevention and Health Promotion website. https://www.cdc.gov/HealthyYouth/health_and_academics/index.htm#2. Accessed January 15, 2017.

7. Wong MD, Shapiro MF, Boscardin W, Ettner SL. Contribution of major diseases to disparities in mortality. *N Engl J Med*. 2002;347(20):1585-1592.

8. Health-risk behaviors and academic achievement. Centers for Disease Control and Prevention website. https://www.cdc.gov/healthyyouth/health_and_academics/pdf/DASHfactsheetHealthRisk.pdf. Accessed April 13, 2018.

9. Carlson SA, Fulton JE, Lee SM, et al. Physical education and academic achievement in elementary school: data from the Early Childhood Longitudinal Study. *Am J Public Health*. 2008;98(4):721-727.

10. MacLellan D, Taylor J, Wood K. Food intake and academic performance among adolescents. *Can J Diet Pract Res*. 2008;69(3):141-144.

11. Spriggs AL, Halpern CT. Timing of sexual debut and initiation of postsecondary education by early adulthood. *Perspect Sex Reprod Health*. 2008;40(3):152-161.

12. Gatawa BG. *Zimbabwe: AIDS Education for Schools. Case Study*. Harare, Zimbabwe: UNICEF; 1995.

13. Grunseit A, Kippax S. Impact of HIV and sexual health education on the sexual behaviour of young people: a review update. http://www.popline.org/node/279539. Accessed January 15, 2017.

14. Skills based health education. Schools & Health website. http://www.schoolsandhealth.org/skills-based-health-education. Published 1997. Accessed March 28, 2018.

15. A day in the life. U.S. Department of Health and Human Services, Office of Adolescent Health website. https://www.hhs.gov/ash/oah/adolescent-health-topics/americas-adolescents/day.html#. Accessed January 14, 2017.

16. Youth Risk Behavior Surveillance System (YRBSS) overview. Centers for Disease Control and Prevention website. https://www.cdc.gov/healthyyouth/data/yrbs/overview.htm. Accessed January 14, 2017.

17. Kann L, Kinchen S, Shanklin SL, et al. Youth Risk Behavior Surveillance—United States, 2013. *MMWR Suppl*. 2014;63(4):1-168.

18. CDC releases Youth Risk Behaviors Survey results. Centers for Disease Control and Prevention website. https://www.cdc.gov/features/yrbs/. Updated June 9, 2016. Accessed March 28, 2018.

19. Trends in the prevalence of alcohol use—national YRBS: 1991-2015. Centers for Disease Control and Prevention website. https://www.cdc.gov/healthyyouth/data/yrbs/pdf/trends/2015_us_alcohol_trend_yrbs.pdf. Accessed March 28, 2018.

20. Basch CE. Physical activity and the achievement gap among urban minority youth [Special issue]. *J Sch Health*. 2011;81(10):626-634. doi:10.1111/j.1746-1561.2011.00637.x.

21. Ahamed Y, Macdonald H, Reed K, Naylor PJ, Liu-Ambrose T, McKay H. School-based physical activity does not compromise children's academic performance. *Med Sci Sports Exerc*. 2007;39(2):371-376.

22. Carlson SA, Fulton JE, Lee SM, et al. Physical education and academic achievement in elementary school: data from the early childhood longitudinal study. *Am J Public Health*. 20008;98(4):721-727.

23. Castelli DM, Hillman CH, Buck SM, Erwin HE. Physical fitness and academic achievement in third- and fifth-grade students. *J Sport Exerc Psychol*. 2007;29(2):239-252.

24. Trudeau F, Shephard RJ. Physical education, school physical activity, school sports and academic performance. *Int J Behav Nutr Phys Act*. 2008;5:10.

25. McMurrer, J. Choices, changes, and challenges: curriculum and instruction in the NCLB era. http://www.cep-dc.org/displayDocument.cfm?DocumentID=312. Published July 24, 2007. Accessed March 28, 2018.

26. Dinkel D, Schaffer C, Snyder K, Lee JM. They just need to move: teachers' perception of classroom physical activity breaks. *Teach Teach Educ*. 2017;63;186-195.

27. Jensen E. *Brain-Based Learning: The New Paradigm of Teaching*. Thousand Oaks, CA: Corwin Press; 2008.

28. Weslake A, Christian BJ. Brain breaks: help or hindrance? *Teach Collection Christian Educ*. 2015;1(1):38-46.

29. Brittin J, Sorensen J, Towbridge M, et al. Physical activity design guidelines for school architecture. *PLoS One*. 2015;10(7):e0132597. doi:10.1371/journal.pone.0132597.

30. Wendel M, Benden M, Hongwei Z, Jeffrey C. Stand-biased versus seated classrooms and childhood obesity: a randomized experiment in Texas. *Am J Public Health*. 2016;106(10):1849-1854.

31. *Achieving Health Promoting Schools: Guidelines for Promoting Health in Schools.* International Union for Health Promotion and Education website. http://hivhealthclearinghouse.unesco .org/library/documents/achieving-health-promoting -schools-guidelines-promoting-health-schools. Published 2009. Accessed March 28, 2018.

32. Kaplan G, Bo-Linn G, Carayon P, et al. Bringing a systems approach to health [discussion paper]. Washington, DC: Institute of Medicine and National Academy of Engineering. https://www.nae.edu/File.aspx?id=86344. Accessed April 13, 2018.

33. Whole school, whole community, whole child: a collaborative approach to learning and health. ASCD website. https:// www.cdc.gov/healthyschools/wscc/wsccmodel_update _508tagged.pdf. Accessed March 28, 2018.

34. Food safe schools program. National Environmental Health Association website. https://www.neha.org/eh-topics/food -safety-0/food-safe-schools-program. Accessed March 28, 2018.

35. School health index. Centers for Disease Control and Prevention website. https://www.cdc.gov/healthyschools/shi /index.htm. Accessed January 28, 2017.

36. School health index: a self-assessment and planning guide [elementary school version]. Centers for Disease Control and Prevention website. https://www.cdc.gov/healthyschools /shi/pdf/elementary-total-2014.pdf. Published 2014. Accessed March 28, 2018.

37. School health index: a self-assessment and planning guide [middle/high school version]. Centers for Disease Control and Prevention website. https://www.cdc.gov/healthyschools/shi /pdf/middle-high-total-2014.pdf. Published 2014. Accessed March 28, 2018.

38. Youth media campaign. VERB: it's what you do. Centers for Disease Control and Prevention website. https://www.cdc .gov/youthcampaign/. Updated March 18, 2010. Accessed March 28, 2018.

39. Let's Move! active schools. https://letsmove.obamawhitehouse .archives.gov/active-schools. Accessed January 22, 2017.

40. BAM! Body and mind. Centers for Disease Control and Prevention website. https://www.cdc.gov/bam/. Accessed January 21, 2017.

41. Allen A, Vallone D, Vargyas E, Healton CG. The Truth* campaign: using countermarketing to reduce youth smoking. In: Healthey B, Zimmerman R, eds. *The New World of Health Promotion, New Program Development, Implementation and Evaluation.* Sudbury, MA: Jones and Bartlett; 2009: 195-215.

42. National Health Education Standards. Centers for Disease Control and Prevention website. https://www.cdc.gov /healthyschools/sher/standards/index.htm. Updated August 18, 2016. Accessed March 28, 2018.

43. National teacher preparation standards for sexuality education. Future of Sex Education website. http:// futureofsexed.org/teacherstandards.html. Accessed January 28, 2017.

44. Health Education Curriculum Analysis Tool (HECAT). Centers for Disease Control and Prevention website. https:// www.cdc.gov/healthyyouth/hecat/. Accessed March 28, 2018.

45. Characteristics of an effective health education curriculum. Centers for Disease Control and Prevention website. https:// www.cdc.gov/healthyschools/sher/characteristics/. Updated June 17, 2015. Accessed March 28, 2018.

46. Health communication. Study.com website. http://study.com /directory/category/Communications_and_Journalism /Public_Relations_and_Advertising/Health _Communication.html. Accessed March 28, 2018.

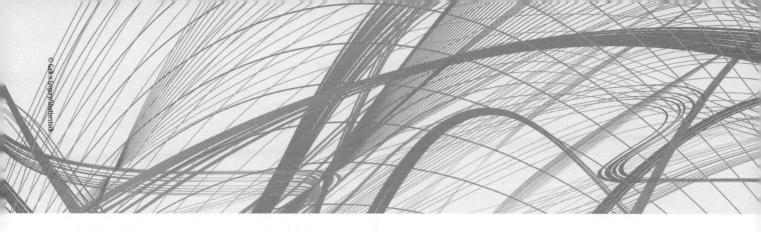

CHAPTER 11

Workplace Health

Jeannine L. Stuart and Alesha G. Hruska

LEARNING OBJECTIVES

By the end of this chapter, the reader will be able to:

- Provide a definition of and a rationale for workplace health.
- Explain how the ecological model and dimensions of wellness are relevant to workplace health.
- Explain how workplace health programs may impact employee health and productivity and impact corporate profits.
- Understand how health insurance benefits, health promotion, and occupational health and safety are interrelated.
- Explain why stress management and financial literacy should be part of a workplace health program.
- Describe what workplace practices make a company a psychologically healthy workplace and contribute to a culture of health.
- Identify communication skills needed to build a culture of health that supports workplace health goals and objectives.
- Explain why leadership involvement and support are key to a successful workplace health program and building a culture of health.

▶ Introduction

The workplace is a unique setting in and of itself. In order to function as an effective health communicator in a business setting (or with corporate stakeholders), there are a myriad of contextual and environmental factors to be understood, applied, and evaluated beyond the usual scope of the health communication profession. For example, the health communicators' triad of engage, inform, and persuade to benefit the social good is complicated by the nature of the employer–employee relationship. Additionally, unlike other settings applicable to health communicators, the primary objective of the workplace is not health, but to perform a job and earn income.[1] Indeed, a workplace can be thought of as its own ecosystem with its own organizational structure, built environment, policies, culture, norms, and values.[2,3] The corporate environment has its own jargon, external rules, regulations, and laws for applying health in the workplace. Applying a strategic health communication plan to a workplace health initiative is imperative for preventing strained employer–employee relationships and for establishing a common ground, clear communication, transparent goals, mutual trust, and clearly defined expectations.

While reading the subsequent text, health communicators will need to bear in mind perspectives from three potential audiences:

1. The *business case* from the perspective of corporate business leaders (often called the "C-suite")
2. Health and well-being from the employee perspective
3. The planners, implementers, and evaluators of workplace health programs

Health communicators have an opportunity to utilize their unique skill set in workplace health in a variety of ways. Skills and concepts such as factors that influence how nonscientific audiences process and understand scientific information and clear health communication are invaluable in communicating with various stakeholders in workplace health. In light of the significant disparity between quality research and practice, the authors of this text conclude by proposing three novel strategies from science communication and clinical outreach education that health communicators can use to market the most current research and evidence-based practices to business leaders and workplace health practitioners.

▶ Why Workplace Health?

Employed Americans spend an average of 7.6 hours per day at work,[4] thus providing an opportune site for promoting health, preventing and reducing risk factors, and managing chronic disease. The physical setting and social network of the workplace provide health professionals with the opportunity to reach individuals who may, or may not, seek health information outside of the occupational setting.[1]

The Robert Wood Johnson Foundation (RWJF) and Harvard University produced *The Workplace and Health* report, which identified and described stark differences in response to a nationally representative survey across segments of the working-age population. Forty-four percent of working adults recognize the impact work has on their overall health, with 16% to 26% reporting that their current job affects their family and social life, stress level, sleeping and dietary habits, and weight.[5] This includes more than one in five working adults with disabilities (35%), in dangerous jobs (27%), in low-paying jobs (26%), who have ever cared for sick family members (23%), with chronic illnesses (24%), working 50+ hours per week (25%), and working in retail outlets (26%), construction or outdoor work (23%), or factory or manufacturing jobs (21%).[5]

Not only does poor health contribute to increased morbidity, mortality, and reduced quality of life, but increasing healthcare costs also are placing a financial burden on the United States' workforce and businesses. Employees who miss work due to illness, or **absenteeism**, cost employers $1685 per employee each year, or $225.8 billion.[6]

Companies are continually searching for effective ways to save their bottom line and cut costs without reducing quality and care. To achieve this, a popular option is to introduce workplace health or workplace wellness programs and activities. According to the Henry J. Kaiser Family Foundation, in 2016, 83% of large companies (those with more than 200 employees) that offered health insurance benefits reported providing at least one health and wellness program activity such as weight management, smoking cessation, or health coaching.[7]

The benefits of effective workplace health programs have been well documented. According to the Centers for Disease Control and Prevention (CDC),[8] impacts include:

- Workplace health programs can lead to change at both the individual (i.e., employee) and the organization levels.
- For individuals, workplace health programs have the potential to impact an employee's health, such as their health behaviors, their health risks for disease, and their current health status.
- For organizations, workplace health programs have the potential to impact areas such as healthcare costs, absenteeism, productivity, recruitment/retention, culture, and employee morale.
- Employers, workers, their families, and communities all benefit from the prevention of disease and injury and from sustained health.

▶ A Word About Terminology

There is not one standard definition of *workplace health*. In fact, multiple terms—including corporate wellness, health and productivity management, health promotion, and employee well-being—are often used synonymously and change over time based on current trends (also depending on which side of the table you are sitting on—business owner, researcher, insurance carrier, or employee and participant). Previously referred to as *employee wellness* by the corporate world, the business industry currently uses the term *well-being*. Worker **well-being** is defined as an integrated concept that characterizes quality of life with respect to an individual's health and work-related environmental, organizational, and psychosocial factors. It is the experience of positive perceptions and the presence of constructive conditions at work and beyond that enable workers to thrive and achieve their full potential.[9]

This shift in terminology reflects the movement by corporate health and wellness decision makers working to encompass the person as a whole. This includes changing norms in business and blurring the once stringent lines between work life, home life, and recreation. In this chapter, the authors will be following the lead of the CDC and use the terminology delineated in its Workplace Health Glossary.[10]

Workplace health program (WHP) is an umbrella term that encompasses initiatives, programs, strategies, and activities intended to promote, increase, and sustain the health and well-being of employees (and occasionally their families). The CDC defines a WHP as "a coordinated and comprehensive set of strategies which include programs, policies, benefits, environmental supports, and links to the surrounding community designed to meet the health and safety needs of all employees."[10] We will unpack and describe elements of this definition later in the chapter.

Although distinct from government-mandated occupational health and safety rules and regulations and employer-sponsored health insurance, WHPs are often integrated with these components to form a comprehensive approach to workplace health. In order to promote, increase, and sustain employee health and well-being, employers may hire or designate in-house staff such as health educators, human resources managers, health insurance brokers, or third-party wellness vendors (e.g., AREUFIT Health Services, Inc. discussed later in the chapter) to implement programs with one or more of the following objectives:

- Provide resources and access to health awareness and education materials.
- Encourage healthy lifestyles intended to increase health-promoting behaviors (e.g., healthy eating, physical activity) and decrease health-risk behaviors (e.g., tobacco cessation programs and support).
- Initiate preventive health screenings, biometrics, and health risk appraisals (HRAs) to identify risk factors specific to the employee population.
- Offer chronic disease management programs targeting hypertension, diabetes, and obesity, in order to prevent worsening of health-related outcomes, improve treatment, and increase quality of life.
- Offer employee assistance programs to provide workers with *confidential* access to stress management, psychological, and substance abuse counseling and treatment.
- Provide adjunct initiatives to improve well-being (e.g., provide tools to improve financial literacy and thus reduce financial stress (discussed later in this chapter), promote mindfulness, and encourage participation of dependents and spouses).

Along with these six individual-level employee health–related objectives, a successful and sustainable WHP involves leadership support and buy-in, organizational-level policies, and an environment conducive to nurturing a culture of health (CoH), such as smoke-free campuses, access to stairwells and walking paths, and healthy vending machine options.

Workplace health programming may encompass a portion of each of these objectives as a stand-alone when entering into the realm of workplace health, with further progression into a more systematic and coordinated approach with all other program objectives for a more well-rounded and substantial WHP. Workplace health programming can be thought of as a continuum—on one end is grassroots (i.e., low budget) initiatives, and at the opposite end is a fully funded and comprehensive WHP.

▶ Evolution of Workplace Health Programs

Before continuing, health communicators involved with workplace health will need to understand the background and history of "wellness" in the workplace in the context of a changing healthcare landscape. From a perk of corporate leaders, to a piecemeal "random acts of wellness" approach, to evaluating medical and pharmacy claims data, to risk assessments, and currently to an emerging evidence base of best practices and culture of wellness, the typical vision of workplace health has evolved a great deal over the past 60 years.

Where Workplace Health Has Been

Although the concept of "wellness" is not new, its recognition and status as a vital business strategy is. The conceptualization of wellness as promoting a "holistic" notion of health (and not just the absence of disease) began to take shape in the 1950s after the introduction of the World Health Organization's definition of health in its 1948 constitution. The wellness movement of the 1970s gained traction with help from the creation of the National Institute for Occupational Safety and Health (NIOSH) in 1970, a shift in healthcare cost burden from government to employer, and the **Lalonde report**, the first government document recognizing the role of individual behavior in health.[11,12] The role of health "programs" in the workplace began as a focus on health through fitness for a select group of employees in the form of corporate fitness centers. Some fitness centers included cardiorespiratory testing as a prerequisite for entering into the program; others considered access to the fitness center as a benefit only for those who had a position of power or held an office within the executive C-suite (i.e., chief executive officer, chief financial officer, chief operating officer, chief information officer, etc.).

In 1976, Dr. Bill Hettler developed the six dimensions of wellness (DoW) in the context of academic health.[11] The six most common DoW are physical, emotional, social, intellectual, occupational, and spiritual (see **FIGURE 11-1** and **TABLE 11-1**).

Then workplace wellness progressed into executive physicals with further expansion into Lunch and Learn lectures, nutrition education, smoking cessation, 5K races, and various weight loss programs (e.g., Weight Watchers).

Wellness as a concept began to evolve with the DoW as the recognition that WHPs should include more than just the physical dimension. Faced with increased health insurance costs and scarcity of resources, WHPs shifted from their roots as a holistic wellness concept to a reflection of the biomedical model. Anything other than what could be physically

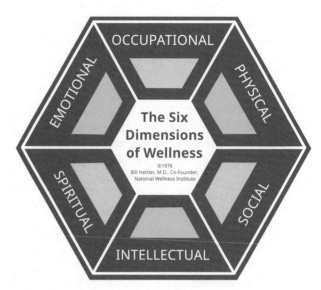

FIGURE 11-1 Dimensions of wellness.

Reproduced from Hetler B. *The Six Dimensions of Wellness Model.* ©1976. Reprinted with permission from the National Wellness Institute, Inc., NationalWellness.org.

measured through biometrics was considered "fluff." Although data were collected, most programs had conflicting and unreliable information on how to apply and evaluate these data.

Until recently, WHPs were built almost entirely around the *physical* aspects of health. Basic biometric testing, which consists of finger stick or venipuncture

TABLE 11-1 Description of the Six Dimensions of Wellness

Dimension of Wellness	Description
Physical	Encourages learning about diet, nutrition, tobacco cessation, moderate alcohol consumption, and the value of physical activity.
Emotional	Recognizes the awareness and acceptance of our own feelings. It includes the capacity to manage one's feelings and behaviors including a realistic assessment of one's limitations, ability to be autonomous, and ability to cope with stress. It also includes the ability to establish and maintain close personal relationships.
Social	Encourages contributing to one's environment and community through actively improving the world through healthier living and preserving the beauty and balance of nature.
Intellectual	Recognizes one's creative side while expanding their knowledge through learning, curiosity, problem solving, and exploration.
Occupational	Recognizes personal satisfaction and enrichment in one's work life. Occupational development is related to one's attitude about work; it involves contributing unique gifts, skills, and talents at work that are both personally meaningful and rewarding.
Spiritual	Recognizes our search for our meaning and purpose. It includes the development and appreciation for the depth and expanse of life, nature, and the universe.

Reproduced from Hetler B. *The Six Dimensions of Wellness Model.* ©1976. Reprinted with permission from the National Wellness Institute, Inc., NationalWellness.org.

blood cholesterol and glucose, blood pressure, and body mass index, along with HRAs quickly became the gold standard for many WHPs. HRAs include questions about a person's medical history, current health status, and lifestyle. These health screenings were frequently offered simultaneously with health insurance selection meetings known as open enrollment. The annual open enrollment period is the time where an employee has the opportunity to review and select a health insurance plan that is appropriate for their individual and/or family's needs and budget. Many programs to this day still consider basic biometrics along with an HRA as the foundation of their wellness program. The rationale is that "If you do not measure it, you cannot manage it." This is particularly true with current WHPs that require completion of these components in order to receive wellness credits or to remain compliant with the design of their health insurance plan or self-insured health plan. (We will revisit this concept in the section "Common Workplace Health Program Elements: Where We Are with Workplace Health.") Although still important tools, the workplace health field is beginning to see a resurgence in the DoW.

In a 2013 Aon Hewitt Health Care Survey,[13] 72% of employers were focusing their healthcare strategies on programs that would improve employees' health risks and reduce medical costs. However, within 3 to 5 years of the survey, close to half of the employer groups that had participated in the survey were intending to shift their focus toward programs that would improve workplace productivity and reduce absenteeism. Costs associated with lost productivity due to **presenteeism** are often greater than those lost to medical claims. Cost estimates from a large medical/absence database were combined to determine the prevalence and associated absenteeism and presenteeism losses. The overall economic burden was highest for hypertension, heart disease, depression and other mental illnesses, and arthritis. Presenteeism costs were higher than medical costs in most cases and represented 18% to 60% of all costs.[14]

Aon Hewitt is a leading provider of human capital and consulting services. Through a series of comprehensive industry whitepapers, the company provides expert insights based on annual survey results from health and benefit executives from companies of all sizes and industries. The 2015 Aon Hewitt Healthcare Survey reported that a top priority for employers for the following year was to increase employee awareness and effective decision making on healthcare issues by providing the employees with tools, resources, support, and advocacy.[15] For example, the Leapfrog Group aims to provide businesses and their employees with information on hospital safety, quality, and the affordability of U.S. health care. This thought process shifts away from the mindset of simply offering health insurance options to their employees toward helping them become informed healthcare consumers.

Becoming an informed healthcare consumer empowers employees to take ownership of their own health and well-being. This alters the employers' once-a-year discussion about health care during the annual health insurance open enrollment period to enrolling employees into wellness activities where consistent, small healthy lifestyle changes can have a significant impact on an employee's overall health—not to mention the companies' bottom line.

▶ Setting the Stage: The Relationship Between Health Insurance and Workplace Health Programs

Having a working knowledge of the historical context and progression of health in the workplace would not be complete without discussing it within the context of health insurance benefits. The human resources department is responsible for determining health insurance coverage and buying benefits for employee health through a variety of plans, including medical, pharmacy, dental, disability, and workers' compensation. This is important because slightly more than half (55.8%) of the working population (aged 19–64) receives health insurance benefits primarily through their employer.[7,16] As the chronic disease rates of the population rise, the cost to insure also rises. Employers are constantly challenged in finding ways to offset healthcare costs and manage the health of their employees. In most cases, healthcare costs, employee health and wellness, and occupational safety are under the direction of three distinct silos: health insurance benefits, workplace health, and occupational health and safety.[17]

Workplace health is responsible for implementing well-being initiatives primarily aimed at preventing illness and disease by sponsoring activities such as fitness programs, **biometric screenings**, and healthy food options at work. In contrast, **occupational health and safety** is responsible for preventing worker injury and illness though safe practices and policies, including Occupational Safety and Health Administration trainings, cardiopulmonary resuscitation training, and ergonomic design.[17]

Although health insurance benefits, health promotion, and occupational health and safety have three distinct corporate functions—and are frequently established as three separate business departments—integration of their goals is becoming more common as part of the company's approach to improving employee health.[17] We will revisit this concept later in the chapter.

In an effort to offset the rising cost to insure their workers, employers generally respond in one or more of the following ways: shift the cost of health care to their employees, improve the overall health of their employees through WHPs, and/or decrease/restrict health insurance benefits. Cost shifting includes increases in employee contributions toward healthcare premiums, higher out-of-pocket expenses, and an increase in the number of companies opting for **high-deductible health insurance plans (HDHPs)**. An HDHP is a health insurance plan with lower monthly premiums and higher employee out-of-pocket deductibles compared to a traditional health insurance plan.

Typically, employees contribute a portion of their monthly salary toward their employer-sponsored health insurance plan. The average worker's health insurance premium contribution for 2016 was $1129/year for single coverage and $5277/year for family coverage.[7] Between 2006 and 2016, the average premium for family coverage increased 58%, while the share of employee contribution for family coverage increased by 78%.[7] To offset the financial burden of increasing healthcare costs to the company, employers are passing on such increases to the employee. In 2016, the average premiums paid by the employer were $6435 for individual coverage and $18,142 for family coverage.[7] Projections for upcoming years do not see healthcare costs declining, but rather continuing to rise. In an attempt to contain skyrocketing healthcare costs, more companies have introduced wellness initiatives as part of their business model and long-term strategic plan.

A sample of U.S. workers were surveyed to examine their perceptions of problems, experiences, issues, and challenges related to their health in the workplace.[5] Of those surveyed, 56% of full-time workers reported that their employer offered a formal well-being or health improvement program to help keep them healthy. Among those who participated in their employer-sponsored WHP, 88% reported that these programs were important to their health, whereas only 9% said that they were not very important or not important at all to their health.[5]

Some workplaces (mostly very large corporations) have shifted from the traditional health insurance plan to a **self-insured** health insurance plan. Of workers who receive health insurance through their job, a majority (61%) are covered by a plan that's either partially or fully funded by their employer.[18] Of those workers who are insured at the workplace, 13% work at small firms (3–199 employees), and 82% are employed at large companies (200 or more employees).[18]

A self-insured health plan is where the employer takes on the cost of healthcare claims at a higher level than the traditional health insurance plan. In other words, the employer uses its own money to fund health benefits for its employees. The reason for doing so is that it allows the employer to have a better insight into the "actual" healthcare costs as opposed to those "trending" when part of the larger pooled health insurance premium plan. Workplaces that are self-insured also have the flexibility to design a health plan based on what their employees need and do not have to second guess what is best, based on a "one-size-fits-all" health plan. This type of environment helps foster a healthier workforce that embraces preventive and healthy lifestyle behaviors. These companies also typically have a greater buy-in when it comes to offering a comprehensive WHP.

Employer-sponsored health insurance coverage has become a normative business practice, so the passage of the Affordable Care Act (ACA) in 2010 marked an unprecedented change in health insurance coverage and care—and with it came an important emphasis on preventive health. This law has three important functions related to the purpose of this chapter. First, the ACA encourages employers to adopt and implement health and risk reduction programs. This includes utilizing WHPs as an opportunity for an organization to promote preventive health care at no cost to the employee as mandated by the ACA.[6] Such preventive care includes an annual physical or "well visit," eye exams, mammograms, vaccinations, and so forth. See the healthcare.gov webpage (https://www.healthcare.gov/preventive-care-adults/) for a complete list of recommended preventive screenings for adults.

Second, the ACA provides more federal funding opportunities for workplace health and well-being, including small business grants for *comprehensive* WHPs. This is especially important for small to mid-sized businesses where cost is a barrier.[6] (At the time of printing, the political landscape regarding healthcare reform may alter programs currently in place.)

Finally, over the past decade, in an attempt to drive participation, there has been an increasing emphasis by employers on offering incentives tied to participation and linking healthcare premiums (and cost sharing) to individual behaviors and disease. One of the most important workplace health provisions in the ACA and other health-related policies is that it ensures protection of workers from discrimination based on health status and genetics.

Common Workplace Health Program Elements: Where We Are with Workplace Health

Chronic diseases are responsible for 86% of our nation's healthcare costs, and therefore their identification and management are top priorities of WHPs.[19] **Health risk appraisals (HRAs)** are one of the most utilized components of WHPs, and their implementation is steadily rising.[20] Biometrics were offered in 53% of large companies, and HRAs were offered in 59% of them.[7] Conducting basic biometrics and HRAs at the workplace is a useful tool to help identify and educate employees on risk factors that can contribute to cardiovascular disease (CVD) and other chronic conditions. Additionally, preventive health screenings can be used to identify those employees who might benefit from participation in a disease management program.[21]

As HRAs target multiple health behaviors and conditions, categorizing outcomes reflects the aggregate effects of change. This provides valuable data to help evaluate the overall effectiveness of WHPs. A systematic review conducted by Soler et al. identified strong evidence of the effectiveness of HRAs when used with health education lasting 1 hour or repeating multiple times during 1 year, and that may include an array of health promotion activities.[20]

According to the CDC, CVD, stroke, cancer, type 2 diabetes, obesity, and arthritis are the most common, costly, and preventable health conditions.[19] A major contributor to heart disease and stroke, hypertension is one of the most expensive health conditions for U.S. employers.[22] Medical costs for those with diabetes are twice as high compared to their nondiabetic counterparts. In 2010, direct medical costs due to CVD were approximately $273 billion; in 2030, these same costs are expected to be as high as $818 billion.[21,23]

Evidence shows that there is a direct and strong relationship linking health and productivity in the workforce. Employees who are overweight or obese and have a comorbidity miss 450 million more days from work compared to their healthy counterparts.[24] Indirect costs associated with CVD secondary to lost productivity are projected to increase from $172 billion to $276 billion in the next 20 years.[21,23] Responsible for approximately one in five deaths in the United States each year, the economic burden of tobacco-related diseases includes roughly $170 billion annually in direct medical care and $150 billion in lost productivity.[25]

To estimate the economic burden of chronic diseases, the CDC has developed the chronic disease cost calculator, which is a downloadable tool that provides state-level estimates of medical expenditures and absenteeism costs for arthritis, asthma, cancer, CVD, depression, and diabetes (https://www.cdc.gov/chronicdisease/calculator/). Program planners can use these data to help establish program priorities, set goals, and decide which WHP components to implement.

To help offset the economic burden of risk factors and chronic disease, and promote healthy behaviors, there is an emphasis by employers to increase employee participation and engagement. To drive participation, employers use a variety of incentives and penalties, or "carrots and sticks." A common way this is done is by linking healthcare premiums to employee health-risk behaviors, or offering financial incentives tied to WHP participation. Examples include a reduction in employee health insurance premiums, cash, gift cards, additional paid time off, t-shirts, mugs, gym bags, or recognizing employees in a company newsletter as a reward for participation in the WHP. Many employers will use incentives to "nudge" behavior change.

In the 2016 RWJF and Harvard University *Workplace and Health Report*, one in four workers employed in large companies reported that the WHP offered financial incentives to participate ($n = 876$).[5] Five percent of those workers who reported working in a large company with a WHP answered that their employer imposed financial penalties for not participating.[5] In addition, one in five workers reported that their employer included wellness or health improvement programs for members of their immediate family.[5]

As tobacco-related diseases are a significant factor in escalating healthcare costs and decreased profits among employers, a growing number of companies execute a penalty on tobacco users. In 2016, 15% of large companies (200 employees or more) that offer health insurance coverage require tobacco-using workers to contribute a higher dollar amount to their monthly premium.[7] The average cost to employ a smoker is approximately $6000 more per year compared to a nonsmoking employee.[26]

Most employers who penalize tobacco-using employees simultaneously provide resources and programs to assist in their cessation efforts. For example, participation in a smoking cessation program can offset the additional fee added to the employee's health insurance premium. The insurance companies themselves are now charging a higher premium to those subscribers who use tobacco.

To support individual-level cessation efforts of the employee (and protect the health of non-tobacco users), many businesses adopt smoke-free policies in the workplace. There is strong evidence that indicate that smoke-free policies can reduce healthcare costs and are effective in reducing tobacco-related morbidity and mortality.[27] What is even more compelling for the business case is that implementing smoke-free policies in the workplace does not have an adverse economic impact on businesses.[27]

Employer-provided evidence-based tobacco cessation programs can increase productivity, morale, and retention, and decrease absenteeism, the amount of disability leave, and overall healthcare costs. **Business Pulse** is a resource from the CDC Foundation aimed at providing businesses and their employees with tools and resources to protect them from chronic disease and safety threats.[28] In 2017 Business Pulse recommended that employers, doctors, and health insurance carriers support smoking employees through a variety of interventions. These interventions include expanded access to **tobacco cessation treatments**, including individual, group, and telephone counseling and Food and Drug Administration-approved medications, and making it easier to obtain treatments by removing high copays or preauthorization for insurance to pay for treatments.[29]

Building a successful WHP can be challenging. According to the 2015–2016 Willis Towers Watson Staying@Work Survey, a number of factors are keeping WHPs from being as successful as they could be. Such barriers include inadequate resources (staff and budgets), lack of measurable return on investment (ROI), low employee engagement, lack of data to support targeted outreach, and lack of leadership support.[30]

In an effort to mitigate some of the aforementioned challenges, many governmental agencies and professional organizations are providing free assessment, planning, implementation, and evaluation resources and tools to assist employers with their WHP efforts. For instance, the CDC, the National Business Coalition on Health, the American Psychological Association (APA), Exercise Is Medicine, and the Workplace Health Research Network provide valuable resources and tools.

To help select the most clinically and cost-effective preventive health services, interventions, and policies, The Community Preventive Services Task Force provides nonbiased, evidence-based recommendations. Called *The Community Guide*, this online resource provides a summary of findings, rationale, and quality of evidence on a variety of topics such as nutrition, physical activity, obesity, and workplace health (http://www.thecommunityguide.org).

Let us revisit the six DoW to see how they might be integrated today into a well-rounded WHP (**TABLE 11-2**).

Diabetes, Tobacco, and Physical Activity

Chronic diseases, such as type 2 diabetes, and risk factors such as obesity can lead to a decline in the overall health of employees in the workplace, contribute to an increase in health-related expenses for employers and employees, and lead to lower productivity and/or days of work missed.[31] **BOX 11-1** provides examples, tools, and resources of some common workplace health initiatives geared toward preventing and managing diabetes, eliminating tobacco use, and increasing physical activity.

Stress in the Workplace

According to the 2016 RWJF and Harvard University *Workplace and Health Report*, 59% of working adults say their current job has a significant impact on their stress.[5] Although most respondents viewed their workplace as a healthy environment that supports steps to improve their health, almost half rated their workplace fair or poor in stress reduction efforts. Forty-three percent of those surveyed ($n = 1601$) said their job had a negative impact on their stress level, whereas 16% reported that their job was good for their stress level. Women were more likely to report a negative impact compared to men (46% vs. 40%, respectively). Restaurant workers, those in the medical field, followed by those in academia were the top three groups who reported their job was bad for their stress level (54%, 52%, and 47%, respectively). Additionally, workers in low-paying jobs were more concerned with stress, more likely to report that their workplace was unsupportive, and report dangerous working conditions.

In a 2014 analysis of more than 92,000 employees over an average of 2.95 years following the completion of an HRA, employees with depression were 48% more expensive in regards to their medical care costs compared to those not depressed; those reporting "high stress" levels were 8.6% more expensive.[32]

In 2016, 82% of the 1501 employees surveyed reported being in good psychological health. However, 1 in 6 employees reported that depression, anxiety, or other mental health issues made work more challenging and difficult; this was the highest

TABLE 11-2 Common Elements of Workplace Health Programs Categorized by the Dimensions of Wellness

Dimension of Wellness	Examples of Workplace Health Program Integration
Physical	Instead of sit-down meetings, have walking meetings. Minimize long-term sitting to reduce sedentary behaviors. Provide opportunities for employees to get up and move frequently throughout the day. Utilize resources from http://www.exerciseismedicine.org.
Emotional	Provide stress management classes, daily mindfulness activities, and yoga Work–life balance and flexibility Assistance for "sandwiched" employees—those responsible for both child and elder care Resources from company **employee assistance programs (EAPs)** and the American Psychological Association (http://www.apaexcellence.org)
Social	Team-building activities Retreats and boot camps Potluck lunches Cooking demonstrations Team competitions
Intellectual	Continuing education Financial literacy programs Tuition reimbursement
Occupational	Finding work that is satisfying and enriching Providing opportunities for advancement Job satisfaction Enhanced job skill training
Spiritual	Celebration of various religious holidays Diversity programming Sensitivity training

BOX 11-1 Workplace Tools and Resources for Diabetes, Tobacco, and Physical Activity

Diabetes

As of 2012, 29 million people in the United States (9.3% of the U.S. population) were diagnosed with diabetes; 27.8% of those people were considered undiagnosed diabetics.[a] In July 2016, the CDC reported that 86 million Americans had prediabetes—that is one out of three adults! Of those 86 million, 9 out of 10 of them were undiagnosed and unaware that they were prediabetic. Unlike diabetes, in which blood glucose levels are elevated, prediabetes occurs when a person's blood glucose is higher than normal but not high enough to be diagnosed as having diabetes. Without intervention, 15% to 30% of people with prediabetes will develop type 2 diabetes within 5 years. If left untreated, diabetes can lead to a variety of complications and comorbidities such as amputation, hypertension, dyslipidemia, stroke, and blindness.[b]

The CDC has developed an evidence-based lifestyle change program specifically to reduce the number of prediabetics progressing into type 2 diabetes. This program, called the National Diabetes Prevention Program (NDPP), can be implemented in the community or a workplace setting. Led by a trained lifestyle coach, this year-long program focuses on teaching healthy eating, the importance of physical activity, stress reduction techniques, and other healthy lifestyle habits to offset type 2 diabetes.

To help mitigate the high costs and health toll of diabetes, businesses can offer increased screening to identify those with prediabetes as well as expanded access to the NDPP to help workers make lifestyle changes to prevent or delay type 2 diabetes.[c,d]

(continues)

BOX 11-1 Workplace Tools and Resources for Diabetes, Tobacco, and Physical Activity *(continued)*

Tobacco

Tobacco use exists in many forms including cigarettes, cigars, pipes, hookahs (or water pipes), e-cigarettes, chewing tobacco, and snuff. It has been well documented that tobacco use increases the risk for cancer, heart disease, and stroke, and that it undoubtedly increases healthcare costs.

Cigarette smoking is the single-largest cause of preventable disease and death in the United States, killing more than 480,000 Americans each year. Smoking costs the United States more than $300 billion a year, including nearly $170 billion in direct medical care and more than $156 billion in lost productivity. Employers can reduce tobacco use and improve employee health by providing support and access to tobacco cessation programs.[e]

There are two common objectives for a workplace to develop and implement a tobacco-free policy: (1) to encourage employees to quit, and (2) to reduce nonsmoking employees' exposure to second-hand smoke.

A variety of resources are available to assist workplaces with designing and implementing a tobacco-free workplace. A full description of these resources can be found at the CDC's Workplace Health Resources webpage.[f]

Physical Activity

According to the National Health Interview Survey, which is conducted through the National Center for Health Statistics (http://www.cdc.gov/nchs/), nearly half of Americans do not meet the recommended physical activity guidelines of 150 minutes of moderate intensity aerobic exercise per week or 75 minutes of vigorous aerobic activity weekly, or a combination of the two.[g,h]

Physical activity has been shown to reduce the risk for diabetes, obesity, heart disease, and stroke, as well as depression. A new mindset has come to view exercise as medicine (http://exerciseismedicine.org) and is being embraced by physicians and healthcare professionals as an additional vital sign when assessing a patient's health (i.e., weight, blood pressure, cholesterol, glucose, and physical activity status).

Barriers to physical activity can be addressed at the workplace by providing employees with options to move more throughout their workday. Examples include onsite fitness centers, walking paths, signage at the elevators to encourage taking the stairs, and the installation of standing desks.

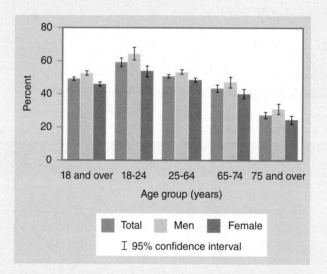

Percentage of adults who met the 2008 federal physical activity guidlines for leisure-time aerobic activity, by age group and sex: United States, 2015

Reproduced from National Health Interview Survey, 2015, Sample Adult Core component. https://www.cdc.gov/nchs/data/factsheets/nhis_2016.pdf.

[a] About Prediabetes & Type 2 Diabetes. https://www.cdc.gov/diabetes/prevention/prediabetes-type2/index.html. Accessed May 4, 2018.

[b] About Diabetes. https://www.cdc.gov/diabetes/basics/diabetes.html. Accessed May 4, 2018.

[c] CDC helps business tackle the burden of rising healthcare costs. CDC Foundation website. http://www.cdcfoundation.org/pr/2016/cdc-helps-business-tackle-burden-rising-healthcare-costs. Published June 22, 2016. Accessed March 31, 2018.

[d] What is the national DPP? Centers for Disease Control and Prevention website. https://www.cdc.gov/diabetes/prevention/about/index.html. Accessed March 31, 2018.

[e] Tobacco Use: A threat to workplace health and productivity. CDC Foundation website. https://www.cdcfoundation.org/businesspulse/tobacco-use. Accessed May 4, 2018.

[f] Workplace health resources. Centers for Disease Control and Prevention website. https://www.cdc.gov/workplacehealthpromotion/tools-resources/workplace-health/tobacco-use-cessation.html. Accessed March 31, 2018.

[g] Exercise or Physical Activity. https://www.cdc.gov/nchs/fastats/exercise.htm. Accessed May 4, 2018.

[h] ACSM Issues New Recommendations on Quantity and Quality of Exercise. http://www.acsm.org/about-acsm/media-room/news-releases/2011/08/01/acsm-issues-new-recommendations-on-quantity-and-quality-of-exercise. Accessed May 4, 2018.

percentage reported since the APA first asked this question in 2013 (16% in 2016; 11% in 2015; 14% in 2014, and 15% in 2013).[33] The top five stress factors reported by employees were low salaries, lack of growth or opportunity for advancement, heavy workloads, unrealistic job expectations, and long hours.[33] Personal and work-related stress are

a widespread concern for employers.[34] To many employers, a happy worker equals a healthy and productive worker.[34] Upon this realization, many companies are incorporating a new dimension of wellness into their workplace health initiatives— financial well-being. **BOX 11-2** illustrates the impact that financial stress can have on employee health

---

BOX 11-2 Financial Stress and Employee Health and Well-Being

Jeannine L. Stuart, PhD

More than one-third of U.S. workers experience chronic work stress, with low salaries, lack of opportunity for advancement, and heavy workloads topping the list of contributing stress factors.[a] Financial stress can be one of the biggest stressors for an employee because it impacts their lives both at home and at work. According to the American Psychological Association, money worries are one of the top stressors for Americans. Nearly three-quarters (72%) of adults report feeling stressed about money at least some of the time, and nearly one-quarter say that they experience extreme stress about money. (On a 10-point scale, 22% rate their stress about money during the past month as an 8, 9, or 10.) In some cases, people are even putting their healthcare needs on hold because of financial concerns.[a]

For adults living in low-income households (less than $50,000/year) and thus who hold lower-paying jobs, financial insecurity and stress are greater compared to higher-income households (those who make more than $50,000/year). Those living in lower-income households are twice as likely to report finances as a barrier to healthy lifestyles. Forty-four percent of lower-income Americans say paying for out-of-pocket healthcare costs is a very or somewhat significant source of stress (compared with 34% of higher-income Americans). For those lower-income Americans who have out-of-pocket healthcare costs, 31% say they have difficulty paying for these costs (compared with 14% of higher-income Americans with out-of-pocket healthcare costs).

Women who say their stress about money is high (8, 9, or 10 on a 10-point scale) are more likely than women who say they have low stress about money (1, 2, or 3 on a 10-point scale) to say they engage in sedentary or unhealthy behaviors to manage their stress. These unhealthy behaviors include watching television/movies for more than 2 hours per day (55% vs. 38%), surfing the Internet (57% vs. 34%), napping/sleeping (41% vs. 23%), eating (40% vs. 19%), drinking alcohol (21% vs. 9%), or smoking (19% vs. 7%). All of these unhealthy coping mechanisms lead to poorer health, increased presenteeism, decreased performance at work, and potentially increased healthcare costs.

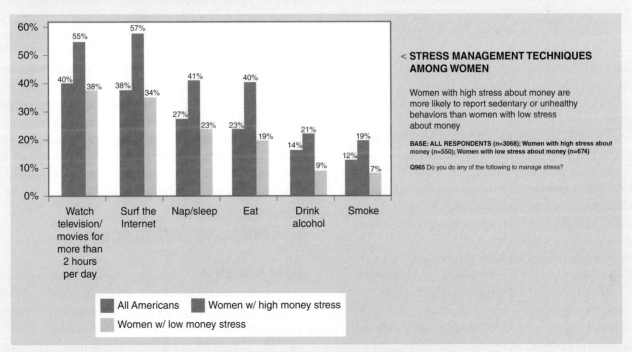

STRESS MANAGEMENT TECHNIQUES AMONG WOMEN

Women with high stress about money are more likely to report sedentary or unhealthy behaviors than women with low stress about money

BASE: ALL RESPONDENTS (n=3068); Women with high stress about money (n=550); Women with low stress about money (n=674)

Q965 Do you do any of the following to manage stress?

Legend: All Americans | Women w/ high money stress | Women w/ low money stress

(continues)

BOX 11-2   Financial Stress and Employee Health and Well-Being   *(continued)*

In addition to unhealthy behaviors, distractions associated with financial stress can potentially lead to more accidents and more mistakes. Like physical health, financial health can have a significant impact on corporate performance.

To help employees deal with financial stress, many companies are offering financial literacy programs as part of a financial wellness piece. Financial literacy programs are designed to provide knowledge and skills to manage financial resources for a lifetime of financial well-being. Such programs are much more than learning how to balance a checkbook or how to comparison shop; rather, these programs include financial and retirement literature, courses in debt management, assistance with home buying, and saving for their children's college. Financial well-being is more about financial security than monetary compensation. Low financial well-being has been shown to increase anxiety and depression, impact quality of sleep, and manifest itself in a variety of physical symptoms (i.e., headache, back pain, etc.).

Financial wellness programs can be used to recruit and retain employees. Financial wellness is not unlike any other components of the WHP in that, if delivered correctly, financial wellness can increase productivity by decreasing the distractions associated with financial stress and burdens, attracting new talent, and promoting employee loyalty.

[a] American Psychological Association. *Paying with Our Health: Stress in America.* https://www.apa.org/news/press/releases/stress/2014/stress-report.pdf. Published February 4, 2015. Accessed March 31, 2018.

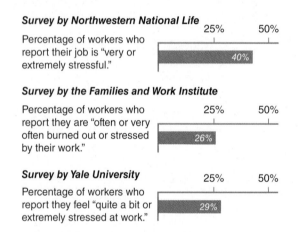

FIGURE 11-2   What workers say about stress on the job.

Reproduced from National Institute for Occupational Safety and Health. *Stress...at Work.* Publication Number 99-101. Concinatti, OH: U.S. Department of Health and Human Services; 1999. https://www.cdc.gov/niosh/docs/99-101/.

and well-being and highlights financial literacy as a method of stress management support.

According to the APA's 2016 *Work and Well-Being Survey*, only 41% of employees say that their employer helps them develop and maintain a healthy lifestyle or assists them with meeting their mental health needs.[33] Job stress is estimated to cost U.S. industry more than $300 billion a year in absenteeism; turnover; diminished productivity; and medical, legal, and insurance costs.[35] Healthcare costs are generally 50% greater for those employees who report high levels of stress compared to their less-stressed counterparts.[36] **FIGURE 11-2** shows what workers say about stress in their jobs.

The APA's 2013 Psychologically Healthy Workplace Award winners reported an average employee turnover rate of 6% compared to 38% nationally.[37] In surveys completed by the winning organizations, on average, fewer than one in five employees (19%) reported experiencing chronic work stress, compared to 35% nationally, and 84% of employees said they were satisfied with their jobs, versus 67% across the U.S. workforce.[37] Only 11% of employees at these organizations said they intended to seek employment elsewhere within the next year, compared to almost three times as many (31%) nationwide.[37] **BOX 11-3** illustrates the criteria for a psychologically healthy workplace and an example of one.

▶ Health Coaching

Health coaching, also referred to as wellness coaching, is a self-paced process in which a health professional helps facilitate healthy lifestyle behavioral change by challenging a client through self-inventories, motivational interviewing, and goal setting. A health coach's primary concern is to provide a safe, nonjudgmental environment that will help facilitate long-lasting behavioral change. There are many formats in which health coaches are utilized: in person, face-to-face meetings, telephonic coaching, and coaching via online wellness portals. Health coaching, discussed in **BOX 11-4**, is an emerging field in the wellness industry with a variety of certifications available.

▶ Tools and Technology

Data Analytics

Data are universally used to track and evaluate progress. This concept is no different when it comes to evaluating WHPs. As discussed earlier in this chapter, corporate executives and human resources professionals want to see the impact that their wellness initiatives have on cost savings and reduced

BOX 11-3 AREUFIT Health Services, Inc.: An Example of a Psychologically Healthy Workplace

Jeannine L. Stuart, PhD

Since 2006, the American Psychological Association (APA) Center for Organizational Excellence has been recognizing companies both large and small with the annual Psychologically Healthy Workplace awards. After completing a rigorous competitive evaluation and selection process, awards are initially presented at the state level with award winners having the option to be nominated for the national award.

Companies vary as much as their individual employees, so organizational categories for recognition include the following:

- Large for-profit (> 1000 employees)
- Medium for-profit (250–999 employees)
- Small for-profit (< 250 employees)
- Not-for-profit
- Government/military/educational institutions

Candidates are evaluated on workplace policies and programs in the following areas:

- *Employee involvement:* Employee involvement can increase employee job satisfaction, reduce employee turnover, increase productivity, and enhance the quality of services delivered.
- *Health and safety:* Health and safety programs focus on improving and maintaining the physical health of employees through screening, assessment, prevention, and treatment of health risks. It also can encompass mental health by assisting employees in managing their stress. In addition to improved productivity and reduced absenteeism, companies may see a reduction in work-related injuries through participation in health and safety programs.
- *Employee growth and development:* Growth and development opportunities can include learning new skills, pursuing further academic training, and providing opportunities to implement this new knowledge. Such programs will keep employees motivated and help them work to their fullest potential.
- *Work–life balance:* Work–life balance programs help employees with work- and non-work-related demands. Such programs may include, but are certainly not limited to, flexible work schedules, the ability to work from home, and employee assistance programs (EAPs). Such programs can promote good mental health, reduce absenteeism, improve productivity, and reduce employee turnover.
- *Employee recognition:* These programs honor and recognize employees for a job well done. Acknowledgement of an employee's efforts makes them feel valued to the company, enhances job satisfaction, and promotes a sense of well-being.

Other factors taken into consideration during the selection process include employee attitudes and opinions, communication within the organization, and the organization's WHP program and organizational performance.[a]

An Example of a Psychologically Healthy Workplace

AREUFIT Health Services, the winner of the Pennsylvania Psychologically Healthy Workplace Award for 2012 and 2016, is a small for-profit business that has established a series of policies and resources aimed at enhancing the quality of working life and well-being of its employees. These organizational policies are designed to promote a culture of health for full- and part-time employees, student interns, and volunteers. AREUFIT is constantly striving to improve the working environment, which includes the physical, psychosocial, occupational, organizational, and economic wellness of the organization. Examples include walk-and-talk meetings with management, eating lunch as a "family," flexible work schedules that help employees manage personal demands outside of the office, being a dog-friendly organization, allowing babies/children in the office when child care options are limited, and offering its full-time staff a 1-hour massage per month. Other initiatives include participating in a local community sustained agriculture (CSA) farm share program for its employees and families, providing a gym membership reimbursement program, supporting local charities, and closing the office twice a year and engaging in an all-employee volunteer activity (volunteering at a local food bank and farm). Team-building activities include volunteering, bowling, and interactive challenges.

The owners at AREUFIT promote an open door policy for employees to feel comfortable in communicating with executive leadership. Having an open door policy gives the employees the opportunity to share ideas or concerns, offer opinions, or simply catch up on the workday's events. AREUFIT's focus is on the whole employee. Work impacts life, and life impacts work.

[a] APA's Psychologically Healthy Workplace awards. American Psychological Association Center for Excellence website. http://www.apaexcellence.org/awards/national/. Accessed March 31, 2018.

healthcare costs. There are many web-based data analytic platforms available to integrate health and pharmacy claims, HRAs and biometric screenings, employee participation in wellness initiatives, and human capital (i.e., payroll, employee turnover, employee skill sets, etc.). Such analytics help corporate decision makers in determining where to implement targeted wellness initiatives, policies, and programs to lower healthcare spending and quantify savings in regards to the wellness ROI. Tracking data

BOX 11-4 Health Coaching

Jeannine L. Stuart, PhD

Health coaching has been used to improve lifestyle behaviors known to prevent or manage chronic conditions. Methods in which health coaching (also known as wellness coaching or lifestyle coaching) can be delivered include face-to-face meetings, telephonic coaching, secure email communications, Skype or Facetime, or a secure web-based platform.

Health coaching is very different than seeking direct medical advice. Effective health coaches are facilitators of change. They help the client establish realistic goals and create a plan to meet those goals.

Health coaching using nonphysician healthcare providers has been successful in assisting prediabetics and diabetics to manage their chronic condition. The CDC's National Diabetes Prevention Program (NDPP) utilizes the knowledge of lifestyle coaches who have been specially trained to facilitate the program to help participants learn new skills, set goals, and encourage success in meeting goals as well as to help motivate them. This program is delivered in a variety of methods: in-person individual and group meetings, online programs, or a combination of these.[a]

Prediabetics who take part in a structured lifestyle change program can reduce their risk of developing type 2 diabetes by 58% (71% for people over 60 years old). This finding was the result of a program that helped people lose 5% to 7% of their body weight through healthier eating and 150 minutes of physical activity a week. It does not take a drastic weight loss to make a significant impact.[b] Although the health coach is not qualified to make a diagnosis or advise on medical treatments, they can provide guidance based on their knowledge and training.

The field of health coaching has become very popular in recent years. Health coaching certifications and websites have popped up all over the internet. So how does a consumer know if a health coach is properly trained? The International Consortium of Health and Wellness Coaches (ICHWC; http://www.ichwc.org) has created national standards for certification—in partnership with the National Board of Medical Examiners—to launch the National Board for Health and Wellness Coaches.

These standards identify the core competencies, knowledge base, and skill sets necessary to become a national board-certified health and wellness coaching professional. The skills and tasks established by the ICHWC and listed in the 2017 Health and Wellness Coach Certifying Examination booklet include: (1) activities that take place in the initial stages of the coaching process, (2) developing and maintaining the health and wellness coaching relationship, (3) activities that address the client's evaluation and integration of progress, and (4) professional behavior of coaches.[c]

[a] National Diabetes Prevention Program. Centers for Disease Control and Prevention website. https://www.cdc.gov/diabetes/prevention/index.html. Accessed April 1, 2018.

[b] Research-based prevention program. Centers for Disease Control and Prevention website. https://www.cdc.gov/diabetes/prevention/prediabetes-type2/preventing.html. Accessed April 1, 2018.

[c] Health and wellness coach certifying examination. National Board of Medical Examiners website. http://www.nbme.org/pdf/hwc/HWCCE_boi.pdf. Published 2017. Accessed May 4, 2018.

over time allows thoughtful decisions to be made regarding enhancements, changes, or discontinuing components of the WHP. For more information on how to use, compile, analyze, and interpret health claims data, see the CDC's workplace health promotion assessment website (http://www.cdc.gov/niosh/docs/99-101/).

Technology

Technology has changed the way we do business, how we view the world, and how we communicate. Access to smartphones, tablets, and wearable technology devices, or "wearables" (i.e., Fitbits, Garmin, and Apple Watch) are commonplace. Incorporating such devices into wellness programming seems like a natural progression in health communications. Popular digital health tools include fitness, nutrition, and weight loss apps. Social media can be used to track participation and engagement, provide encouragement, and disseminate a variety of health-related material. Some web-based wellness program portals include apps to

keep employees engaged and up to date on the company's WHP activities.

Telemedicine is a form of digital health that has gained traction over recent years. It involves connecting employees with a health professional using audiovisual capabilities through a secure internet and health portal connection. Such portals can be accessed via smartphones, tablets, and computers (i.e., mHealth). A plus to having telemedicine available to employees is that it allows them to have immediate access to a healthcare professional regardless of location, time of day, or day of the week.

According to the National Alliance of Healthcare Purchaser Coalitions (formerly the National Business Coalition on Health), employers will make telemedicine available to employees in states where it is allowed, and it expects the number of employers doing so to rise significantly by the year 2020.[38] Supporters of telemedicine tout that the cost savings are too great to ignore. Whereas the average emergency department visit costs $700, an urgent care visit costs approximately $150, and a physician's office visit costs

$100, the average telemedicine session is approximately $40 per visit. Employers see this as an opportunity to deliver additional healthcare options despite the increasing costs of medical care.[39]

▶ Emerging Trends: Where Workplace Health Is Going

Health and well-being efforts may be most effective at improving productivity when they are part of a broader approach that entails a full understanding of how the workplace climate influences health. Employers should pay special attention to helping employees manage the demands of their jobs and cope with work-related stress in efforts to maximize employee performance.

A 2009/2010 Towers Watson report found that companies with the most effective health and productivity programs achieved 11% more revenue per employee, delivered 28% higher shareholder returns, and had lower medical trends and fewer absences per employee.[40(p2)]

The Workplace Health Model

According to the CDC's **Workplace Health Model**, building a workplace health program should involve a coordinated, systematic, and comprehensive approach.

A **coordinated approach** to workplace health promotion results in a planned, organized, and comprehensive set of programs, policies, benefits, and environmental supports designed to meet the health and safety needs of all employees. A **comprehensive approach** looks to put interventions in place that address multiple risk factors and health conditions concurrently and recognizes that the interventions and strategies chosen influence multiple levels of the organization including the individual employee and the organization as a whole. A WHP should be created using these two approaches in a series of strategically planned steps, or a **systematic process**.

The CDC recommends the following four steps (also shown in **FIGURE 11-3**) for building a workplace health promotion program: (1) workplace health assessment, (2) planning the program, (3) implementing the program, and (4) determining impact through evaluation.[8]

Comprehensive and cutting-edge WHPs see the value of integrating the three business departments discussed earlier—health insurance benefits, health promotion, and occupational health and safety—in a collaborative effort to ultimately improve health and corporate performance. Just as the DoW illustrate each component as part of the whole, the same holds

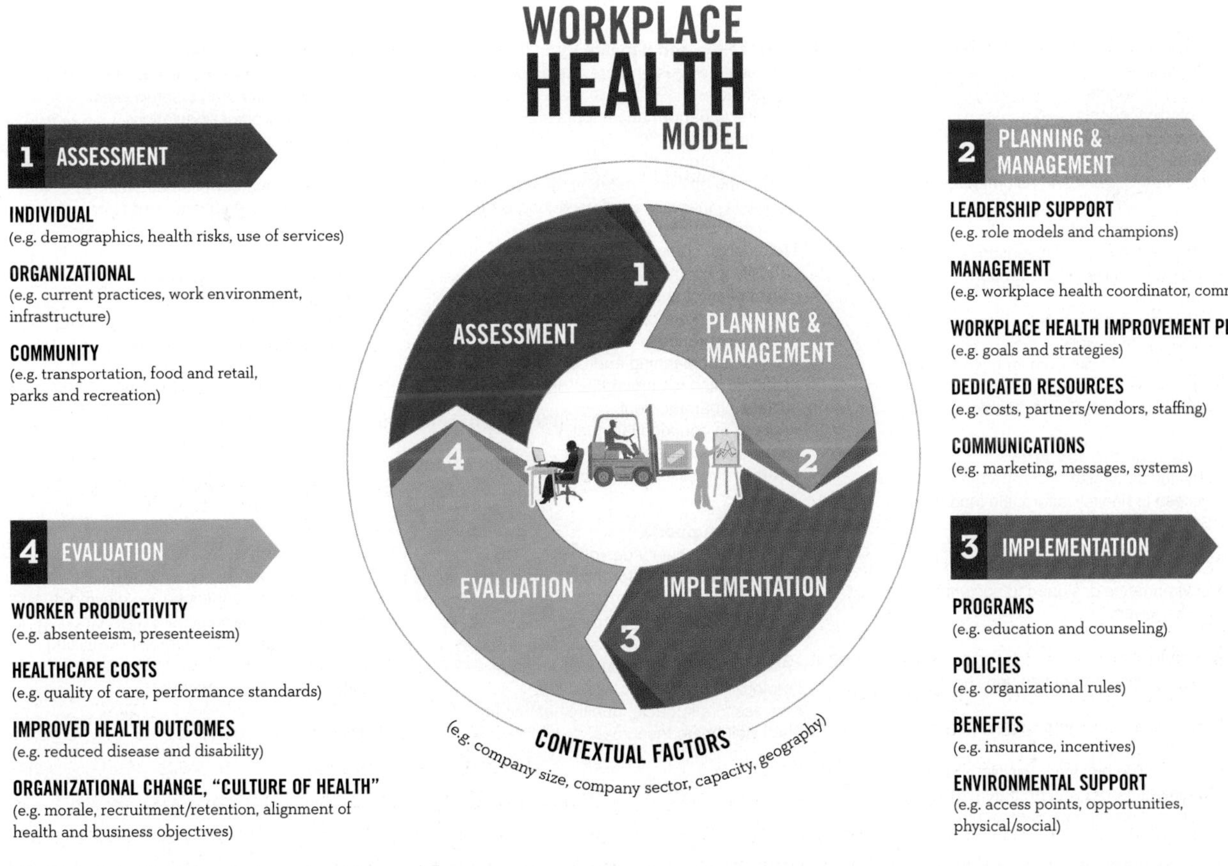

WORKPLACE HEALTH MODEL

1 ASSESSMENT

INDIVIDUAL
(e.g. demographics, health risks, use of services)

ORGANIZATIONAL
(e.g. current practices, work environment, infrastructure)

COMMUNITY
(e.g. transportation, food and retail, parks and recreation)

2 PLANNING & MANAGEMENT

LEADERSHIP SUPPORT
(e.g. role models and champions)

MANAGEMENT
(e.g. workplace health coordinator, committee)

WORKPLACE HEALTH IMPROVEMENT PLAN
(e.g. goals and strategies)

DEDICATED RESOURCES
(e.g. costs, partners/vendors, staffing)

COMMUNICATIONS
(e.g. marketing, messages, systems)

4 EVALUATION

WORKER PRODUCTIVITY
(e.g. absenteeism, presenteeism)

HEALTHCARE COSTS
(e.g. quality of care, performance standards)

IMPROVED HEALTH OUTCOMES
(e.g. reduced disease and disability)

ORGANIZATIONAL CHANGE, "CULTURE OF HEALTH"
(e.g. morale, recruitment/retention, alignment of health and business objectives)

3 IMPLEMENTATION

PROGRAMS
(e.g. education and counseling)

POLICIES
(e.g. organizational rules)

BENEFITS
(e.g. insurance, incentives)

ENVIRONMENTAL SUPPORT
(e.g. access points, opportunities, physical/social)

(e.g. company size, company sector, capacity, geography) **CONTEXTUAL FACTORS**

FIGURE 11-3 CDC workplace health model.

true for the employee, corporate production, and overall profits.

Workplace health promotion programs are more likely to be successful if occupational safety and health is considered in their design, execution, and evaluation. A growing body of evidence indicates that workplace-based interventions that take coordinated, planned, or integrated approaches to reducing health threats to workers both in and out of work are more effective than traditional isolated programs. Integrating or coordinating occupational safety and health with health promotion may increase program participation and effectiveness and may also benefit the broader context of work organization and environment.[8]

Total Worker Health (TWH) is a program advocated through the CDC's NIOSH that involves "policies, programs, and practices that integrate protection from work-related safety and health hazards with promotion of injury and illness prevention efforts to advance worker well-being."[9] The design of this program advocates for a holistic approach in understanding the factors that contribute to worker health and well-being. As previously discussed, risk factors once considered unrelated to work do, in fact, influence the employees' health and, thus, their work performance. Again, in order to consider an employee's overall well-being, we must consider the whole person and all of the DoW with program planning and design.

FIGURE 11-4 illustrates a wide-ranging list of issues that are relevant to advancing worker well-being through a TWH approach. The list of issues relevant to TWH was revised, retitled, and published in November 2015 with input from stakeholders. This updated list reflects an expanded focus for TWH that recognizes that new technologies, new working conditions, and new emerging forms of employment present new risks to worker safety, health, and well-being. Understanding and reducing those risks are important elements of TWH. Additionally, this expanded focus recognizes that there are linkages between health conditions that may not arise from work but that can be adversely affected by work. A TWH approach advocates for the integration of all organizational policies, programs, and practices that contribute to worker safety, health, and well-being, including those relevant to the control of hazards and exposures, the organization of work, compensation and benefits, built environment supports, leadership, changing workforce **demographics**, policy issues, and community supports.[41]

Control of hazards and exposures
- Chemicals
- Physical agents
- Biological agents
- Psychosocial factors
- Human factors
- Risk assessment and risk management

Organization of work
- Fatigue and stress prevention
- Work intensification prevention
- Safe staffing
- Overtime management
- Healthier shift work
- Reduction of risks from long work hours
- Flexible work arrangements
- Adequate meal and rest breaks

Built environment supports
- Healthy air quality
- Access to healthy, affordable food options
- Safe and clean restroom facilities
- Safe, clean and equipped eating facilities
- Safe access to the workplace
- Environments designed to accommodate worker diversity

Leadership
- Shared commitment to safety, health, and well-being
- Supportive managers, supervisors, and executives
- Responsible business decision-making
- Meaningful work and engagement
- Worker recognition and respect

Compensation and benefits
- Adequate wages and prevention of wage theft
- Equitable performance appraisals and promotion
- Work-life programs
- Paid time off (sick, vacation, caregiving)
- Disability insurance (short- & long-term)
- Workers' compensation benefits
- Affordable, comprehensive healthcare and life insurance
- Prevention of cost shifting between payers (workers' compensation, health insurance)
- Retirement planning and benefits
- Chronic disease prevention and disease management
- Access to confidential, quality healthcare services
- Career and skills development

Community supports
- Healthy community design
- Safe, healthy and affordable housing options
- Safe and clean environment (air and water quality, noise levels, tobacco-free policies)
- Access to safe green spaces and non-motorized pathways
- Access to affordable, quality healthcare and well-being resources

Changing workforce demographics
- Multigenerational and diverse workforce
- Aging workforce and older workers
- Vulnerable worker populations
- Workers with disabilities
- Occupational health disparities
- Increasing number of small employers
- Global and multinational workforce

Policy issues
- Health information privacy
- Reasonable accommodations
- Return-to-work
- Equal employment opportunity
- Family and medical leave
- Elimination of bullying, violence, harassment, and discrimination
- Prevention of stressful job monitoring practices
- Worker-centered organizational policies
- Promoting productive aging

New employment patterns
- Contracting and subcontracting
- Precarious and contingent employment
- Multi-employer worksites
- Organizational restructuring, downsizing and mergers
- Financial and job security

FIGURE 11-4 Issues relevant to advancing worker well-being through Total Worker Health®.

Reproduced from Total Worker Health® is a registered trademark of the U.S. Department of Health and Human Services. Total Worker Health®. Centers for Disease Control and Prevention website. http://www.cdc.gov/niosh/twh/totalhealth.html.

An important key factor to understand is that TWH is *not* a wellness program; rather, it recommends that employers and workers collaborate to design safe and healthy workplaces that support all workers, regardless of individual or legal differences (e.g., employees vs. contractors, temporary workers or contingent workers) in both their professional and personal health goals.[41] For example, one TWH initiative, **productive aging**, is dedicated to supporting employees across the life span, including the aging workforce. **APPENDIX 11A** contains an interview that highlights the importance of designing workplaces that are "age-friendly."

Where many WHPs fall short is in focusing on changing only *individual* health behaviors (such as tobacco cessation, weight management, and biometric screenings); in contrast, the TWH design focused on how the employees' environment influences their well-being. Remember, the primary goal of a WHP is the reduction of risk factors in order to reduce the company's healthcare costs. Often such programs place the burden of change on the individual without addressing the overall influences that the physical workspace and the psychological impact that work itself has on the employee's health; for example, van Berkel and colleagues found that shift work, sleep deprivation, perceived stress, noise levels, ergonomically correct workstations, access to healthy food, and time spent commuting can significantly influence health.[1]

With more employees working from home or working remotely, traveling as a large part of their job, and using enhanced technology, the traditional "workplace" is no longer an office cubical in a corporate office building. As the workplace environment itself changes, program design, implementation, and the offering of incentives present their own unique challenges, supporting the notion that one size does not fit all.

The TWH program takes into account that the workplace is any space where work is performed; for instance, the workplace may now include not only an office building, but also a motor vehicle, an outdoor space, and any other physical space where work is performed. Each of these physical environments presents a unique situation that may impact the employee's health and well-being. **BOX 11-5** shows an example of TWH in use at L.L.Bean.

BOX 11-5 Promising Practices for Total Worker Health: A Safety Redesign Jump-Starts Health and Well-Being for L.L.Bean's Aging Workforce

Chia-Chia Chang and Deborah Roy

At L.L.Bean, Maine's quintessential outdoor clothing and equipment company, the workforce is growing older. Although advancing age improves problem-solving and teamwork skills, it also adds risk, especially for older workers with physically demanding tasks. Acknowledging this truth helped L.L.Bean look beyond its established safety and health infrastructure, says Deborah Roy, MPH, RN, COHN-S, CSP, Corporate Director for Health, Safety, and Wellness. The company began taking decisive steps to optimize work processes and prevent injury and illness for all their workers, not only their older ones.

Unique Workforce Considerations

When people come to work at L.L.Bean, many become lifelong staff members because they know the company values its workers and embraces active living. However, low turnover means that employees who were hired in their 20s still have physically demanding jobs 25 or 30 years later. With an average employee age of 50, L.L.Bean's team shares many of the age-related challenges common in workplaces nationwide. Reduced flexibility of the neck and spine, lower grip and lifting strength, and limits to range of motion all become more likely as workers age. Older workers are also more likely to have one or more chronic diseases such as arthritis, diabetes, and obesity. These issues make a focus on injury and illness prevention an absolute necessity.

Integration of Prevention

Ms. Roy's team approached the challenge by focusing on one of the highest-risk areas: materials handling in the warehouse. L.L.Bean already had some critical preventive strategies in place: most workers usually were assigned materials-handling activities only twice a week and were rotated to other tasks every couple of hours. Workers were also given three sets of paid 5-minute rest and stretch breaks a day. Even still, Deborah felt more should be done.

L.L.Bean next turned to a variety of technologies to further reduce the safety and health risks to workers. Solutions for work processes included a mix of robotics, vacuum-driven lift-assist devices, and adjustable pallet lifts. This approach aligned well with the space, capital, and sustainability needs of the business. Now, for much of the year, a single robot and an operator are sufficient for handling products, but at peak volume the robot along with three workers using

(continues)

BOX 11-5 Promising Practices for Total Worker Health: A Safety Redesign Jump-Starts Health and Well-Being for L.L.Bean's Aging Workforce *(continued)*

vacuum lift-assist devices and pallet lifts can safely do the work. This mix has helped the company to reduce risk while working with existing floor space and meeting changing demands. The vacuum lifts reduce weights to less than 10 pounds, and the pallet positioners allow loads to be at optimal height. Since the system was installed in the summer of 2014, no back injuries have been reported while using this technology. Feedback from workers has been very positive, particularly from those using the vacuum lift-assist devices, which make the work safer but still provide a sense of individual-level control.

Jump-Starting Cardiovascular Fitness

L.L.Bean piloted Jump Start, a voluntary conditioning program to benefit workers on and off the job. It aims to increase cardiovascular fitness and endurance, build muscle mass, and improve flexibility with a 12-week supervised aerobic activity and strength-training program. Sessions are offered three times a week, and workers can participate for 45 minutes of paid company time during their work shift. Besides providing a qualified fitness instructor, L.L.Bean also consults with physical therapy professionals to add customized program components to meet the physical demands of specific jobs.

Early Results: Reduced Injuries, Improved Health and Well-Being

The program's launch results exceeded expectations. In a 2013 analysis, L.L.Bean found that at the end of the 12-week program, participants showed improvements in muscle strength, endurance, and flexibility, as well as in resting heart rate and cardiovascular endurance. Although weight reduction was not a goal of the program, 29% of the participants lost weight. In addition, 62% of workers reported having more energy and 29% reported less stress. The other focus of the program was to "jump start" employees into their own exercise program or get them interested in existing classes. L.L.Bean found that workers' compensation cases were reduced from 10 to 2 cases in the same group of workers, with reductions in both compensation costs and medical costs. Adding these cost reductions to the estimated savings from avoided obesity, physical inactivity, and high blood pressure, the company estimates that there was a cost avoidance of $3.15 for every dollar spent (based on the company's initial cost estimates in 2012).

Leadership Commitment to Program Success

L.L.Bean continues to offer Jump Start, tailoring it to other departments. It constantly improves the program according to results and feedback from participants. Ms. Roy emphasizes that leadership support is critical to the program's success. "Employees need to feel truly supported by their supervisors when they are going to class every week. Providing paid company time for participation in the program and letting managers and workers plan the session schedule demonstrate the company's commitment to worker safety and health," she adds. L.L.Bean is committed to ongoing organizational interventions to keep workers safe, healthy, and just as vibrant as life itself in the scenic state of Maine.

Reproduced from National Institute of Occupational Safety. Promising practices for total worker health: a safety redesign jump-starts health and well-being for L.L.Bean's aging workforce. *Total Worker Health in Action!* August 2016;5(3). https://www.cdc.gov/niosh/twh/newsletter/twhnewsv5n3.html. Accessed April 2, 2018.

▶ Creating a Culture of Health Within the Workplace

"The whole is greater than the sum of its parts."

—Aristotle

Our current healthcare system is reactive. We place far more value on identifying and managing individual risk factors and curing specific diseases than on prevention. This individualistic, biomedical healthcare culture is similarly reflected in workplace health. Akin to a patient within our fragmented healthcare system, it is difficult to impossible for employees to improve and sustain health and thrive within an unsupportive work atmosphere averse to change and limited to understanding health within the context of a singular focus on individual risk factors, behavior, and responsibility.

This reductionist approach is not only ineffective, limiting employee health and workplace strategies to focusing primarily on individual determinants of health and lifestyle, but also often leads to a "blaming the victim" mentality and fails to grasp the employee perspective.[1] Both employers and employees agree that individual behavior is an important cause of illness[42]; however, failure to recognize the reciprocal nature of policy, community, organizational, and interpersonal determinants in the ecological model and factors outside the individual's control (i.e., environmental influence on disease risk) can negatively affect the employee's self-efficacy, confidence, autonomy, and feelings of solidarity within the organization, and lead to stigma and negative psychological effects.[1,34,42,43] Before embarking on a workplace well-being endeavor, we should remember the words of social epidemiologist S. L. Syme:

> …most important, even if everyone succeeded in lowering their risk profiles [serum cholesterol, blood pressure, cigarette smoking, obesity, physical inactivity, poor diet], new people would continue to enter the at-risk population forever because we rarely target those social forces in society that cause the problem in the first place.[44(p vii)]

A large majority of the population (62%) recognizes the influence their family and friends have on their health.[42] As the evidence base on social and environmental determinants of health has begun to progress within the last 20 years, we have begun to see their impact on the health of individuals. Creating a **culture of health (CoH)** or human-centered culture is a proactive approach to integrating organizational-level initiatives and policies that support traditional, individually based strategies. Another important aspect that has a significantly broader research base than culture (albeit less popular in contemporary business writing) is organizational *climate*.[45] The **climate of a workplace** refers to workers' "shared perceptions of and meaning attached to the policies, practices, and procedures employees experience and their associated behaviors."[45(p362)] This includes what is valued, expected, and rewarded by those within the organization.[45] Although the distinction between these two terms is important, this chapter will use CoH as a concept that includes both.

A very simplistic example of supporting a CoH would be implementing a corporate policy in which healthy snacks and drinks are provided at corporate meetings instead of sugary drinks and unhealthy foods. Another example might include charging a higher price for unhealthy foods in the vending machine and a lower price for healthier snack options.

Organizational Culture and Leadership

"Culture is caught, not taught!"[46]

The physical workspace has received increased attention within the last few years, sparking a new concept in workplace health called **active design**. Active design "tackles the issue at the level of environmental design, organizational culture and policy; it addresses those features of the built environment that have been proven to support daily physical activity and healthy eating."[47] Architect Brian E. Mann describes using active design principles in creating healthy workplaces in **APPENDIX 11B**. Engelen and colleagues reported that a change in workplace design decreased sitting time and employee lower back pain, and increased standing time.[47] Additionally, improvements in design elements such as high-tech ventilation, natural light from windows, and an open floor plan led to increased motivation for employees to come to work, improved indoor air quality and temperature, and better connectivity with coworkers.[47]

When seeking to improve health, people are more likely to engage in healthy behaviors that are attached to values related to quality of life, such as being more productive and independent, and that are communicated as health-related actions and how they make us feel, look, and function.[48]

Similarly, when engaging employers and other stakeholders in a discussion on implementing WHPs, communications should be centered around what will benefit the underlying company values and priorities (e.g., reducing medical claims, improvements in productivity such as absenteeism and presenteeism, etc.).[48] These concepts are part of an important shift in the way corporate leaders are starting to understand health in the workplace and beginning to integrate WHPs into their strategic business plan.

There is substantial evidence that social networks (family, friends, and relatives whom an individual interacts with day-to-day), including coworkers, can have proactive or adverse effects on individual health, depending on the values, norms, and culture of the network.[49] Additionally, individual differences in self-esteem, socioeconomic status, self-direction at work, control over one's environment, and sense of social support can all impact health outcomes.[49] Incorporating an employee's spouse, especially if they are part of the corporate health insurance plan, is a strategy that many companies are taking in an attempt to manage healthcare costs and employee health outcomes.

Perceived employer support is essential to creating a CoH. Although 54% of workers report their employer supports their efforts to improve personal health, this feeling differs with pay, type of job, and race/ethnicity. Twenty percent of low-paid workers report unsupportive work environments compared to 7% of workers earning average to high pay, 23% of disabled workers, as opposed to 8% of workers without disabilities, and 15% of workers in dangerous jobs.[5] Additionally, black (85%) and Hispanic

(83%) workers are less likely than white workers (91%) to say their workplace is supportive of their taking steps to improve personal health and that their employers provide a smoke-free environment (26% Hispanics, 20% blacks, 9% whites).[5]

Participatory Approach: Employee and Community Involvement

In their seminal text, Green and Kreuter stated that, "Total [community] participation in developing good policies or plans should be neither expected nor targeted….Nevertheless, broad participation through a representation process should be sought in the diagnosis of needs, [because] some of the people least 'skilled' at planning…will bring other valuable assets to the planning table."[48(pp46-47)]

UMass Lowell, a NIOSH center of excellence, offers a free online Healthy Workplace Participatory Program toolkit to assist employers in implementing the TWH approach by engaging employees in the design and implementation of workplace health and safety programs (http://www.uml.edu/research/cph-new/healthy-work-participatory-program). A variety of tools to assist employee engagement in health program planning are available including surveys, sample meeting agendas and activities, informational guides, instruction manuals, and program flyers.

Many companies have a long-standing tradition of being involved with and connecting with their local communities. Terms frequently used are *corporate citizenship*, *corporate social responsibility*, and *corporate philanthropy*. Examples of corporate involvement with the community include volunteering, sponsorship of local events (e.g., 5K runs), senior leadership serving on community boards, and mentoring youth. Through community involvement, employees improve relationships with not only the community, but also senior management and coworkers. This comradery leads to a sense of belonging and employee well-being and promotes a CoH.

Demonstrate Leadership and Engage Mid-level Management

Forty-four percent of employees believe their employer is extremely or very supportive in getting and keeping them healthy, and more than 37% feel the same about their direct manager or department head. Yet a key missing ingredient for a successful wellness program is top-level leadership support.[30]

In addition, leadership influence is often more effective if leaders are accessible, visible to others, and viewed as participating in the WHPs themselves. Visible leadership participation in WHPs sets an example for employees and also conveys the message that both the WHP and the company's employees are valued.[30]

Referring back to the 2016 APA Well-Being Survey, 73% of employees with senior management who show support through involvement and commitment to well-being initiatives said their organization helps employees develop a healthy lifestyle, compared with just 11% who work in an organization without leadership support.[33] The survey found widespread links between support from senior leaders and a variety of employee and organizational outcomes, including belief that the employer believes in the value of health and safety programs, likelihood to recommend their workplace as a good place to work, a good relationship with leadership and fellow coworkers, and job satisfaction.

Corporate leaders must focus on sustainability. For a WHP to be effective, leaders and WHP coordinators must motivate their employees over time by providing clear and concise communications to employees at all levels of personnel. Such communications should reinforce the importance and value of the workplace health campaign. Other actions to promote a sustainable WHP include hiring full-time staff dedicated solely to the WHP, allocating funds to support the WHP, strategic communications, incentivizing participation, and the inclusion of employees of all ages, job duties, and social and economic backgrounds. Some corporations will even include dependents in the WHP.

Strategic Communication Plan

The application of the strategic health communication plan crafted specifically for a workplace setting can accomplish a number of important functions (APPENDIX 11C), including building trust, ensuring confidentiality, educating participants, instilling motivation, and marketing program offerings.

Additionally, from a recent literature review, interviews with subject matter experts, and site visits of successful workplace health programs, Kent and colleagues detailed five key principles of strategic communication in workplace health. These include well-defined objectives, materials and messages that are tailored and targeted, multichanneled messages, optimum timing, frequency and placement of messages, and ongoing bidirectional communications between employees and employers to gather input and feedback.[46]

Build Trust and Ensure Confidentiality

When it comes to health equity and quality of life, the workplace is a setting where ethics and social justice are rarely considered, yet their importance cannot be overstated. There is a continuing push and pull between the motivation and goals of the employer and other stakeholders compared to those of the employee. There are many reasons companies are engaging in employee health, including improvements in employees' health, well-being, and quality of life; however, workplace health is rarely exclusively altruistic. Consequently, the health communicator's triad of engage, inform, and persuade in benefit of the social good is more nuanced and complicated. First and foremost, employee input, participation, and engagement are critical to the success of a health-related program. In order for this to happen, trust between the employer and employee is essential. Employers must present clear and transparent goals while ensuring that employee personal health information is protected.

According to Green and Kreuter, people are more likely to support policies, initiatives, "even regulations if they can see clearly how such efforts address their social and economic concerns or contribute to their quality of life in addition to their health."[48(p32)] It is recommended that managers at all levels actively communicate health and wellness values by setting examples, creating norms, and sharing information.[46] Such information should include how biometric screening, HRAs, and health insurance claims data are being used and that at no time are an employee's individual health data available to managers, coworkers, or their employer. After deidentifying any individual employee characteristics, data are analyzed and then reported back to the employer in aggregate format only. The trust of supervisors and coworkers has been shown to be directly related to quality of information, and workers feel less vulnerable when information is accurate, relevant, and timely.[50] Trust in top management is related to adequacy of information, indicating that communication needs to be focused on overall program strategy, goals, and expectations.

Educate and Motivate

As businesses are starting to realize, initiating a successful WHP is not as simple as it appears to be. More often than not, employers still have a "build it and they will come" attitude.[3] Just as education alone is not enough to nudge behavior change, an employee health program alone cannot move the needle on health costs or outcomes. Using self-determination theory as a lens to study employee motivation, van Scheppingen and colleagues found the value of "healthy living" can, in fact, be caught through "transference of autonomous

regulation"; this means that if an individual is working toward being healthy in one behavior, it can serve as a catalyst to engage in other healthy behaviors and also contribute to a healthy work style that can readily adapt to work demands.[51] The catch is that this is associated with individuals who are internally motivated, as opposed to those who are externally motivated by incentives. For those employees who have not yet developed the self-motivation to adopt new healthy behaviors, financial incentives can provide the encouragement for them to do so.[52]

Tailoring health information and resources to specific subpopulations within the workplace is an important aspect of strategic workplace health communication. Quantitative data, such as a comprehensive needs assessment, and qualitative data that identify and investigate employee knowledge, attitudes, beliefs, and values tied to health and its role in the workplace are essential to tailoring intervention programs, content, and communication to the specific needs of a workplace. A systematic review and meta-analysis of the presenteeism literature found that programs that included organizational leadership, a supportive work culture, health risk screening, and programs tailored to the needs of employees were more successful at increasing productivity at work.[53] In fact, tailoring content and messages through multiple media channels with respect to cultural competence, values, and beliefs, and considering factors that influence comprehension such as low health literacy and stress, can ameliorate potential challenges such as low participation that contribute to lowered effectiveness.[4,6,54]

Participation and engagement are not created equal among all employees, even within the same organization. For example, employees who work for companies with more focus on individual responsibility, better known as a "pay or play strategy"[55] or "forced accountability,"[46] can result in concern and worry over cost incentives and privacy, as well as lowered trust, and can negatively influence program satisfaction and participation.

Although worthwhile, creating a CoH is challenging and can be an overwhelming prospect for employers. Motivating employees over an extended period of time may present a challenge to WHP coordinators. In addition to maintaining employee participation and continued engagement, financial restrictions, limited ROI, inability to measure program effectiveness, and dwindling leadership support can all present their own set of barriers to creating a CoH. Utilizing free and low-cost resources and tools provided by academic, nonprofit, and governmental organizations is invaluable to help in overcoming these challenges.

Health Communication and Public–Private–Academic Partnerships

It could be argued there has never been a greater disparity between research, evidence, and practice in any other field than workplace health. We are at a point where academia, government, nonprofits, and grassroots community groups are partnering with the business community to work together for the health of employees and the greater community. And business leaders are acknowledging the need for evidence-based practice to push the needle on their bottom line. Employers have expressed a desire for more credible information and guidance with which to make decisions regarding WHPs. To this effect, as employers seek to leverage their bottom line through promoting health and safety programs in their business, they are struggling with sources of information.[56]

Researchers and academics can look to science communication and clinical outreach education for novel strategies to disseminate the most current evidence to workplace health practitioners and business leaders. One example, as suggested by Kuehne and Olden,[57] is to provide lay summaries of research articles. For example, an initiative by the Health Research Enhancement Organization (HERO; http://hero-health.org/hero-reviews-of-industry-research/), HERO Reviews of Industry Research publishes article reviews with plain language summaries and information regarding their applicability to practice for health and well-being programs. Another approach to synthesize scientific jargon to a business audience is through academic detailing. Originally used as a tactic for the pharmaceutical industry to increase product sales, Dr. Jerry Avorn developed academic detailing as a strategy for impartial academics to "market" best clinical practices and evidence to practicing physicians. Academic marketing utilizes experienced practitioners with excellent interpersonal skills to evaluate available evidence, condense and translate it so that it is immediately applicable to improve real-life decisions, and package the information into a format with engaging graphics, headlines, and illustrations, and tailored to the clinician's behavior and current understanding.[58] Academic detailing has proved effective in numerous healthcare settings; therefore, the authors have proposed that health communicators apply it in the workplace health setting. To the authors' knowledge, to date there has been only one intervention utilizing academic detailing in the workplace.[59]

▶ Return on Investment

The success and perceived value of a WHP is often tied directly to corporate financial savings. The most common method businesses use to justify WHPs and quantify their value is through measuring their **return on investment (ROI)**. There have been conflicting reports regarding the ROI for health and well-being programming.[60] Many of these conflicting data have been because wellness programming, measurement, and outcomes vary a great deal from one organization to the next. Remember, when it comes to WHPs, one size does not fit all. Fortunately, through systematic reviews and analysis of recent data, it is evident that cost savings can occur with health risk reduction and improved health outcomes. The most often cited reasons for a company to offer a WHP include improved employee health, control of healthcare costs, increased productivity, and decreased absenteeism.[61] Each of these reasons is quantifiable and able to be analyzed, thus making it possible to calculate the ROI of a WHP. As an example, a study published in the *Journal of Occupational and Environmental Medicine* found that employees who participated in a workplace weight loss program experienced lower healthcare costs and reported a better quality of life.[62]

An analysis of approximately 21,000 employees across six large employer groups examined the association of changes in health risk status and the change in healthcare costs. The average age of the employees was 44 years with an even distribution of men and women. This study analyzed the data from both medical and pharmacy claims combined with HRA and biometric data. The study results showed that the fastest and largest ROI in the smallest number of employees was with those who had chronic disease. By engaging these employees in WHP programming with the goal of not incurring any additional health risks, it was possible to lower healthcare costs. Employers who engaged both healthy employees and chronically ill employees maximized their ROI because their strategies were focused on both prevention and risk reduction as well as the avoidance of incurring additional health risk for those already ill, thus reducing the increase in healthcare costs. In this analysis, it is evident that savings were a result of both disease management and lifestyle management programming.[63]

The value of a successful WHP may also include nonfinancial factors such as job satisfaction, social cohesion, a sense of belonging to a work team, employee engagement, and involvement. For example, according to the Community Preventive Services Task Force, obesity prevention programs at workplaces may enhance employee self-confidence, improve the relationship between management and labor, and boost profits by increasing employee productivity and reducing medical care and disability costs.

But limitations exist in both research and practical application. Realizing the limitations of ROI methodologies in WHP, researchers are identifying more sophisticated economic summary measures. In the pharmaceutical literature, spending up to $50,000 is deemed cost-effective if these dollars save at least 1 quality-adjusted year of life. By contrast, investments in WHPs are held to significantly higher standards. Erfurt, Foote, and Heirich used a cost-effectiveness ratio (CER) of cost per 1% additional reduction or prevention in CVD risks as an indicator of economic efficiency. Compared to the control group, CERs were found to be between $14 and $73 per 1% risk reduction over a three-year period for high-risk participants, and between $11 and $73 for participants of moderate risk.[64] As businesses are demanding more data-driven evidence in order to continually support WHPs, those working in worksite health should stay abreast of research on the most effective methods to measure economic and health-related outcomes.

▶ Conclusion: The Work–Health Connection

It is unrealistic when planning, implementing, and evaluating a WHP to not acknowledge the connection between a person's work and their overall health and well-being. For most of us, work is how we spend the majority of our waking hours. Thus, work can have a powerful impact on our risk for injury, mental and physical stress, management of chronic disease, fostering of healthy lifestyles, and ability to balance both our professional and personal lives. Work determines our wages and can influence our access to health and

dental care. So when developing an effective WHP, a workplace health professional needs to review *all* factors that can and will ultimately influence a worker's health, safety, and overall well-being. An engaged workforce driven by leadership support will create a CoH in the workplace, promote acceptance, and give value to the WHP.

Although approximately 83% of companies offer some type of WHP or activity, only 7% of employers implement the program components required to make these programs successful and financially viable.[65] Creating a CoH means providing a variety of activities for all employees to participate in. The traditional workplace consists of a diverse group of people who gather in one place for a common goal. Health and well-being initiatives should embrace such diversity and recognize where each individual employee is in obtaining their personal health-related goals. A positive diversity climate—workplaces that support racial/ethnic diversity—can have a significant impact on organizational performance.[45,66] Given the right tools and the opportunity to be autonomous, employees can develop the intrinsic motivation to sustain healthy behaviors.[51]

Healthy workplace strategies should be evidence-based, include each section of the DoW within an ecological approach, and work to integrate the pieces of the TWH model into every aspect of the company's business practices and policies. Additionally, employers need to provide a work environment that nurtures and helps facilitate and support healthy behaviors. Employees cannot succeed in health and/or productivity if their work environment is hostile or toxic; their employer places unrealistic expectations upon them; they do not have opportunities for personal or professional growth and autonomy; and they do not have leadership support. A successful WHP works only when the employer sees value in its employees' ability to succeed, their health, and their well-being. Such an organization would offer a collaborative work environment—one of trust and open communication.

Key Terms

Active design
Absenteeism
Biometric screenings
Business Pulse
Climate of a workplace
Comprehensive approach
Coordinated approach
Culture of health (CoH)
Demographics
Employee assistance programs (EAPs)
Health risk appraisals (HRAs)
High-deductible health insurance plans (HDHP)
Lalonde report
Occupational health and safety
Presenteeism
Productive aging
Return on investment (ROI)
Self-insured
Systematic process
Tobacco cessation treatments
Total Worker Health (TWH)
Well-being
Workplace health
Workplace Health Model
Workplace health program (WHP)

Chapter Questions

1. Discuss the relationship between the DoW and how they can be integrated into a WHP's CoH.
2. Provide two examples of how the ACA has influenced employer-sponsored health insurance plans and WHPs.
3. Identify four of the most expensive medical conditions for employers.
4. How is TWH different from a traditional WHP?
5. List three job stressors and how they might impact employee health and employer health costs.

References

1. van Berkel J, Meershoek A, Janssens RM, Boot CR, Proper KI, van der Beek AJ. Ethical considerations of worksite health promotion: an exploration of stakeholders' views. *BMC Public Health*. 2014;14(1):458. doi:10.1186/1471-2458-14-458.
2. Lynch WD, Sherman BW. Missing variables: how exclusion of human resources policy information confounds research connecting health and business outcomes. *J Occup Environ Med*. 2014;56(1):28-34. doi:10.1097/JOM.0000000000000068.
3. Environmental scan: role of corporate America in community health and wellness. Health Enhancement Research Organization (HERO) website.http://hero-health.org/wp-content/uploads/2014/12/HERO-EnvScanFinaltoIOM.pdf. Published 2014. Accessed April 2, 2018.
4. American time use survey summary. U.S. Department of Labor, Bureau of Labor Statistics website. https://www.bls.gov/news.release/atus.nr0.htm. Published June 27, 2017.
5. National Public Radio, Robert Wood Johnson Foundation, Harvard University, T.H. Chan School of Public Health. *The Workplace and Health*. July 2016. https://www.rwjf.org/content/dam/farm/reports/surveys_and_polls/2016/rwjf430330. Accessed May 6, 2018.
6. Workplace health promotion. Using the workplace to improve the nation's health: at a glance 2016. Centers for Disease Control and Prevention website. https://www.cdc.gov/chronicdisease/resources/publications/aag/workplace-health.htm. Accessed April 2, 2018.
7. The Kaiser Family Foundation, Health Research & Educational Trust. *Employer Health Benefits 2016 Annual Survey*. http://files.kff.org/attachment/Report-Employer-Health-Benefits-2016-Annual-Survey. Published 2016. Accessed April 2, 2018.
8. Workplace health model. Centers for Disease Control and Prevention website. https://www.cdc.gov/workplacehealthpromotion/model/index.html. Accessed April 2, 2018.
9. Lee MP, Hudson H, Richards R, Chang CC, Chosewood LC, Schill AL, on behalf of the NIOSH Office for Total Worker Health. *Fundamentals of Total Worker Health Approaches: Essential Elements for Advancing Worker Safety, Health, and Well-Being*. https://www.cdc.gov/niosh/docs/2017-112/. Published December 2016. Accessed April 2, 2018.
10. Workplace health glossary. Centers for Disease Control and Prevention website. https://www.cdc.gov/workplacehealthpromotion/tools-resources/glossary/glossary.html#W. Updated December 8, 2015. Accessed April 2, 2018.
11. Miller JW. Wellness: the history and development of a concept. *Spektrum Freiz*. 2005;27:84-106. http://duepublico.uni-duisburg-essen.de/servlets/DerivateServlet/Derivate-35061/11_miller_1_05.pdf. Accessed April 2, 2018.
12. Lalonde M. *A New Perspective on the Health of Canadians: A Working Document*. Ottawa, Canada: Government of Canada; 1974.
13. *Aon Hewitt 2013 Health Care Survey*. Aon Hewitt website. http://www.aon.com/attachments/human-capital-consulting/2013_Health_Care_Survey.pdf. Published 2013. Accessed April 8, 2018.
14. Goetzel RZ, Long SR, Ozminkowski RJ, Hawkins K, Wang S, Lynch W. Health, absence, disability, and presenteeism cost estimates of certain physical and mental health conditions affecting U.S. employers. *J Occup Environ Med*. 2004;46(4). http://journals.lww.com/joem/Fulltext/2004/04000/Health,_Absence,_Disability,_and_Presenteeism_Cost.13.aspx. Accessed April 2, 2018.
15. 2015 health care survey. Aon Hewitt website. http://www.aon.com/human-capital-consulting/thought-leadership/health/2015-health-care-survey.jsp. Accessed April 2, 2018.
16. Garfield R, Majerol M, Damico A, Foutz J. *The Uninsured: A Primer. Key Facts about Health Insurance and the Uninsured in America in the Era of Health Reform*. Supplemental Tables. Menlo Park, CA: The Kaiser Commission of Medicaid and the Uninsured; 2016:i-21.
17. Jinnett K. *Get the Watch Working: Integration Across Benefits Purchasing, Health Promotion and Health Protection*. San Francisco, CA: Integrated Benefits Institute; 2016. https://www.ibiweb.org/wp-content/uploads/2018/01/Full-_IBI_Get_the_Watch_Working-_Integration_Across_Benefits_Purchasing-Health_Promotion_and_Health_Protection.pdf. Accessed May 6, 2018.
18. 2016 employer health benefits survey. Henry J. Kaiser Family Foundation website. http://kff.org/report-section/ehbs-2016-summary-of-findings/. Published September 14, 2016. Accessed April 2, 2018.
19. Chronic disease prevention and health promotion. Centers for Disease Control and Prevention website. https://www.cdc.gov/chronicdisease/. Published November 14, 2016. Accessed April 24, 2017.
20. Soler RE, Leeks KD, Razi S, et al. A systematic review of selected interventions for worksite health promotion. *Am J Prev Med*. 2010;38(2):S237-S262. doi:10.1016/j.amepre.2009.10.030.
21. Arena R, Arnett DK, Terry PE, et al. The role of worksite health screening: a policy statement from the American Heart Association. *Circulation*. 2014;130(8):719-734. doi:10.1161/CIR.0000000000000079.
22. Business pulse: lowering healthcare costs, improving productivity. CDC Foundation website. https://www.cdcfoundation.org/businesspulse/health-costs. Accessed April 24, 2017.
23. Heart disease and stroke cost America nearly $1 billion a day in medical costs, lost productivity. CDC Foundation website. https://www.cdcfoundation.org/pr/2015/heart-disease-and-stroke-cost-america-nearly-1-billion-day-medical-costs-lost-productivity. Published April 29, 2015. Accessed April 2, 2018.
24. CDC healthy workforce infographic. CDC Foundation. http://www.cdcfoundation.org/businesspulse/healthy-workforce-infographic. Accessed April 2, 2018.

25. Economic trends in tobacco. http://www.cdc.gov/tobacco /data_statistics/fact_sheets/economics/econ_facts/. Published March 3, 2017. Accessed April 24, 2017.

26. Tobacco use: a threat to workplace health and productivity. CDC Foundation website. https://www.cdcfoundation.org /businesspulse/tobacco-use. Published 2017. Accessed April 24, 2017.

27. Reducing tobacco use and secondhand smoke exposure: smoke free policies. Community Preventive Services Task Force website. https://www.thecommunityguide.org /sites/default/files/assets/Tobacco-Smokefree-Policies .pdf. Published November 2012. Accessed April 2, 2018.

28. Business pulse. CDC Foundation website. http://www .cdcfoundation.org/businesspulse. Published 2017. Accessed April 24, 2017.

29. Business pulse: tobacco use: a threat to workplace health and productivity. CDC Foundation website. http:// www.cdcfoundation.org/businesspulse/tobacco-use -infographic#productivity2. Accessed April 24, 2017.

30. 2015/2016 Staying@work—United States research findings. Willis Towers Watson website. https://www .willistowerswatson.com/en/insights/2016/04/2015-2016 -staying at-work-united-states-research-findings. Published 2016. Accessed April 2, 2018.

31. Workplace safety and health. Centers for Disease Control and Prevention website. http://www.cdc.gov/features /workingwellness/. Published July 7, 2015. Accessed April 23, 2017.

32. Goetzel RZ, Pei X, Tabrizi MJ, et al. Ten modifiable health risk factors are linked to more than one-fifth of employer-employee health care spending. *Health Aff (Millwood).* 2012;31(11):2474-2484. doi:10.1377/hlthaff.2011.0819.

33. 2016 work and well-being survey. American Psychological Association Center for Organizational Excellence. http:// www.apaexcellence.org/assets/general/2016-work-and -wellbeing-survey-results.pdf?_ga=1.263105292.128624032 4.1435114200. Accessed April 2, 2018.

34. Pescud M, Teal R, Shilton T, et al. Employers' views on the promotion of workplace health and wellbeing: a qualitative study. *BMC Public Health.* 2015;15(1). doi:10.1186 /s12889-015-2029-2.

35. Rosch PJ. The quandary of job stress compensation. *Health Stress.* 2001;3:1-4.

36. National Institute for Occupational Safety and Health. *Stress... at Work.* Publication Number 99-101. Concinatti, OH: U.S. Department of Health and Human Services; 1999.

37. Psychologically healthy workplace awards and best practices honors 2013. American Psychological Association website. http://cwfl.usc.edu/worklife/docs/2013-phwa-magazine.pdf. Accessed April 2, 2018.

38. News. National Alliance of Healthcare Purchaser Coalitions website. http://www.nationalalliancehealth.org/News. Accessed April 24, 2017.

39. Shutan B. Telemedicine offerings double within past year. Employee Benefit Adviser website. https://www .employeebenefitadviser.com/news/telemedicine -offerings-double-within-past-year. Published November 16, 2016. Accessed April 2, 2018.

40. 2009/2010 North American staying@work report: the health and productivity advantage. Watson Wyatt Worldwide website. https://www.towerswatson.com/en-US/Insights /IC-Types/Survey-Research-Results/2009/12/20092010 -North-American-StayingWork-Report-The-Health -and-Productivity-Advantage. Published December 2009. Accessed April 2, 2018.

41. Total Worker Health. National Institute for Occupational Safety and Health website. https://www.cdc.gov/niosh/twh /totalhealth.html. Published November 13, 2015. Accessed April 23, 2017.

42. National Public Radio, Robert Wood Johnson Foundation, Harvard University T.H. Chan School of Public Health. *What Shapes Health.* January 2015. https://www.rwjf.org/content /dam/farm/reports/surveys_and_polls/2015/rwjf418340. Accessed May 6, 2018.

43. Resnik DB. Genetics and personal responsibility for health. *New Genet Soc.* 2014;33(2):113-125. doi:10.1080/14636778. 2014.905195.

44. Berkman LF, Kawachi I, Glymour M, eds. *Social Epidemiology.* 2nd ed. New York, NY: Oxford University Press; 2014.

45. Schneider B, Ehrhart MG, Macey WH. Organizational climate and culture. *Annu Rev Psychol.* 2013;64(1):361-388. doi:10.1146/annurev-psych-113011-143809.

46. Kent K, Goetzel RZ, Roemer EC, Prasad A, Freundlich N. Promoting healthy workplaces by building cultures of health and applying strategic communications: *J Occup Environ Med.* 2016;58(2):114-122. doi:10.1097/ JOM.0000000000000629.

47. Engelen L, Chau J, Bohn-Goldbaum E, Young S, Hespe D, Bauman A. Is active design changing the workplace? A natural pre-post experiment looking at health behaviour and workplace perceptions. *Work.* 2017;56(2):229-237. doi:10.3233/WOR-172483.

48. Green LW, Kreuter MW. *Health Program Planning: An Educational and Ecological Approach.* 4th ed. New York, NY: McGraw-Hill; 2005.

49. Cockerham WC, Hamby BW, Oates GR. The social determinants of chronic disease. *Soc Determinants Health Approach Health Disparities Res.* 2017;52(1 Suppl 1):S5-S12. doi:10.1016/j.amepre.2016.09.010.

50. Thomas GF, Zolin R, Hartman JL. The central role of communication in developing trust and its effect on employee involvement. *J Bus Commun 1973.* 2009;46(3):287-310. doi:10.1177/0021943609333522.

51. van Scheppingen AR, de Vroome EMM, ten Have KCJM, Zwetsloot GIJM, Bos EH, van Mechelen W. Motivations for health and their associations with lifestyle, work style, health, vitality, and employee productivity: *J Occup Environ Med.* 2014;56(5):540-546. doi:10.1097/JOM.0000000000000143.

52. Schmidt H. Wellness incentives, equity and the 5 groups problem. *Am J Public Health.* 2012;102(1):49-54.

53. Cancelliere C, Cassidy JD, Ammendolia C, Côté P. Are workplace health promotion programs effective at improving presenteeism in workers? A systematic review and best evidence synthesis of the literature. *BMC Public Health.* 2011;11(1):395.

54. Hampson S, Kirsten Z, Singh T. Workplace health protection and promotion communication: current perspectives: issues in occupational health—peer reviewed. *Occup Health South Afr.* 2016;22(5):17-20. https://journals.co.za/content /ohsa/22/5/EJC195967. Accessed April 2, 2018.

55. Wright BJ, Dulacki K, Rissi J, McBride L, Tran S, Royal N. Does skin in the game matter if you aren't playing? Examining participation in Oregon's public employee health engagement model. *Am J Health Promot.* June 2016. doi:10.4278/ajhp.150120-QUAN-678.

56. Loeppke R, Taitel M, Haufle V, Parry T, Kessler RC, Jinnett K. Health and productivity as a business strategy:

a multiemployer study. *J Occup Environ Med.* 2009;51(4): 411-428. doi:10.1097/JOM.0b013e3181a39180.

57. Kuehne LM, Olden JD. Opinion: lay summaries needed to enhance science communication. *Proc Natl Acad Sci.* 2015;112(12):3585-3586. doi:10.1073/pnas.1500882112.

58. Avorn J. Academic detailing: "marketing" the best evidence to clinicians. *JAMA.* 2017;317(4):361-362. doi:10.1001/jama .2016.16036.

59. Depression management at the workplace (DMW). Clinicaltrials.gov website. https://clinicaltrials.gov/ct2/show /NCT01013220. Updated December 16, 2014. Accessed April 2, 2018.

60. Mattke S, Liu H, Caloyeras JP, Huang CY, Van Busum KR, Khodyakov D, Shier V. *Workplace Wellness Programs Study: Final Report.* Santa Monica, CA: The RAND Corporation; 2013.

61. Pronk N. Best practice design principles of worksite health and wellness programs. *ACSMs Health Fit J.* 2014;18(1):42-46. http:// journals.lww.com/acsm-healthfitness/fulltext/2014/01000 /Best_Practice_Design_Principles_of_Worksite_Health.12 .aspx. Accessed April 2, 2018.

62. Michaud TL, Nyman JA, Jutkowitz E, Su D, Dowd B, Abraham JM. Effect of workplace weight management on health care expenditures and quality of life. *J Occup Environ Med.* 2016;58(11). http://journals.lww.com /joem/Fulltext/2016/11000/Effect_of_Workplace _Weight_Management_on_Health.3.aspx. Accessed April 2, 2018.

63. Nyce S, Grossmeier J, Anderson DR, Terry PE, Kelley B. Association between changes in health risk status and changes in future health care costs: a multiemployer study. *J Occup Environ Med.* 2012;54(11):1364-1373. doi:10.1097/JOM .0b013e31826b4996.

64. Erfurt JC, Foote A, Heirich M. The cost-effectiveness of worksite wellness programs for hypertension control, weight loss, smoking cessation, and exercise. *Pers Psychol.* 1992;45(1):5-27.

65. Goetzel RZ, Ozminkowski RJ. The health and cost benefits of work site health-promotion programs. *Annu Rev Public Health.* 2008;29(1):303-323. doi:10.1146/annurev .publhealth.29.020907.090930.

66. Gonzalez JA, DeNisi AS. Cross-level effects of demography and diversity climate on organizational attachment and firm effectiveness. *J Organ Behav.* 2009;30(1):21-40. doi:10.1002 /job.498.

Appendix 11A

Productive Aging in the Workplace

Anita L. Schill and L. Casey Chosewood

▶ Managers' Buzz

Addressing the health and safety needs of the aging workforce continues to be a high priority. The National Center for Productive Aging and Work (NCPAW), a NIOSH Center hosted by the Office for Total Worker Health, focuses on aging across the working life and specifically on the concept of productive aging. This issue's Total Worker Health Exclusive highlights the role that work plays in our lives as we age and the importance of designing work and workplaces that are age-friendly.

Recently the staff of *TWH in Action!* caught up with Bermang Ortiz, Public Health Advisor, National Center for Productive Aging and Work, NIOSH and Juliann Scholl, PhD, co-director of National Center for Productive Aging and Work, NIOSH to discuss the concept of productive aging in the context of work and to get an updated look at the Center's current portfolio.

Q: We've been talking about an aging workforce in the United States for more than a decade now. Is this still an issue for employers and workers?

A: Absolutely. The U.S. population continues to age significantly. Today's workforce is a reflection of that. For example, people 65 years or older accounted for about 15% of the U.S. population in 2015, but that percentage will increase to 22% by 2050.[1] In addition, workers 55 or older are increasing in number, and will account for nearly 25% of the labor force in 2024.[2] For workers entering the job market now, it will not be uncommon to be working for 6 decades or more. It's also important to note that today's economy is demanding that many of us work longer than we planned. But as folks work longer, they'll be exposed to both traditional work hazards and newly emerging ones that we have not well-characterized yet. Productive aging provides a useful perspective on how to address the challenges and opportunities presented by a lengthening of the working life span and the particular needs of an aging workforce.

Q: Your NIOSH Center focuses on the concept of "productive aging." How did this concept first arise and how do you define it?

A: In the 1980s, gerontologists advocated for a more balanced discussion about aging, focusing more on the productive abilities of older individuals—not only on the strains they might pose to society's resources. Out of this effort, the concept of productive aging emerged.[3] Since then, productive aging has been defined in different ways, but the common thread for us at NIOSH is that older individuals bring many assets to the workplace, such as greater job knowledge and safer work practices.

Drawing on this perspective, the National Center for Productive Aging and Work (NCPAW) defines productive aging as an approach that emphasizes the positive aspects of growing older. It highlights the ways that workers can make important contributions to their own lives, their communities and organizations, and to society as a whole. Productive aging also highlights the need for workplaces to provide safe and healthy work environments that make it possible for workers to function optimally and thrive at all ages. Consistent with Total Worker Health®, NCPAW's concept of productive aging takes a comprehensive, integrated approach to understanding the aging process across the life span, including the physical, mental, and social aspects of a worker's well-being.

Q: There's lots of stereotypes out there about older workers. I understand in NCPAW you are working to shatter some of these old myths.

A: We are! Productive aging helps us see past the stereotypes of older workers as being unproductive, unadaptable, or unsafe. Although aging can bring losses in physical and cognitive abilities that may affect job performance, older workers possess valuable years of work experience. They have fewer nonfatal injuries, have fewer conflicts with coworkers, and often have advanced skill levels. These positive attributes often more than compensate for declines in other areas. Because of individual variabilities in physical and cognitive losses, age alone is not a sufficient indicator of health and work capacity.

Q: What guidance can the Center offer organizations and workers?

A: The NCPAW productive aging perspective offers workers, employers, and occupational safety and health professionals a theoretical framework to follow for workers of every age. By developing and implementing programs and policies that support the changing work capacities of workers over the working life span, employers can minimize work-related safety and health hazards. As a result, they will benefit from gains in recruitment, retention, competitiveness, and productivity in the long term. Workplaces designed as "age friendly" meet multigenerational workforce needs by minimizing exposures to work-related safety and health hazards. For instance, "age friendly" workplaces are those that prioritize workplace flexibility, matching tasks to abilities, encourage teamwork, and invest in training to build worker skills. These and other practices ensure that younger workers reach later life without injury or illness and older workers maximize their changing abilities by working without injury or illness.

For more information on productive aging and work, visit NCPAW or contact ncpaw@cdc.gov.

References

1. He W, Goodkind D, Kowal P. An aging world: 2015. International Population Reports. U.S. Census; 2016.
2. Toossi M. Labor force projections to 2024: the labor force is growing, but slowly. *Monthly Labor Rev.* 2015:1-32.
3. Butler R. *Productive Aging: Enhancing Vitality in Later Life.* New York, NY: Springer; 1985.

Appendix 11B

Design Considerations for a Healthy Workplace

Brian E. Mann

It might seem fundamental to think that a healthy, comfortable worker would be a productive worker, and it follows that health and comfort would be dependent on the design of the workplace. Despite this logic, the healthy workplace is a complex concept that is difficult to quantify and involves seemingly conflicting ideals—the profit motive of management versus the cost of providing worker comforts. Nonetheless, owners and managers at many levels in businesses small to large are increasingly aware of the benefits to the bottom line that accrue from thoughtfully designed workplaces that are sensitive to workers' physical and emotional well-being.

A network of disciplines and professionals is growing around the healthy workplace movement including executives, management, shareholders, human resources professionals, healthcare providers, regulators (both in government and in the quasi-governmental code agencies), lawyers (of course), interior designers, and architects. These stakeholders have varied interests, constituencies, and perspectives and, as noted previously, sometimes conflicting ideals. We are focused here on the design of workplaces, so we will focus on the role of the architect, who is chiefly responsible for the look and feel of spaces, albeit in collaboration with and subject to the needs and wants of the other stakeholders, primarily the owner/client and regulators.

It is helpful to have an understanding of the set of tools architects use in their work as they pertain to places where people work. This partial list (in no particular order) captures some of the basic building blocks of the physical environment that have real influence on the health and well-being of workers:

- Size of space from small to large
- Scale of space as it relates to the average human form
- Proportion of space narrow to wide, tall or squat
- Light: natural and artificial
- Ventilation: natural and artificial
- Temperature: warm or cold
- Color
- Texture
- Noise
- Ergonomics

Architects mix these blocks into lobbies and offices and hallways and cafeterias; factory floors and loading docks and warehouses; waiting rooms and exam rooms and surgical suites; classrooms and auditoriums and teachers' lounges; and much more—the combinations and cross-disciplinary permutations are seemingly endless. Architects work to a set of parameters, known as the program, that collectively establish the needs of the client, the physical attributes of the land or building space, the regulatory limitations of the particular project, and more. The architectural process is then a sort of puzzle-solving effort of organizing the building blocks in the service of the program to yield a good solution among the limitless number of possibilities. The process involves prioritizing and weighing the many factors into formulations that might value workers' health anywhere along a spectrum from "don't care" to "absolutely critical."

In the United States' early-20th-century Progressive Era, worker safety and to a smaller extent health became important components of reform. As the economy transformed from agricultural to industrial, factory floors and offices emerged as the primary locus of production where, in general, workers were valued no more than raw material. Cultural and economic factors devalued individuals such that the notion that worker health and well-being were not at odds with productivity seemed antithetical to capitalist dogma. Nineteenth- and early-20th-century workplaces were brutal places and often deadly. Galvanized by the horrific tragedy at the Triangle Shirtwaist Factory fire in 1911, reformers began a long march toward improving conditions in workers' built environments. These improvements to safety, working conditions, and to a smaller extent worker well-being formed the basis for the modern building codes. These sets of guidelines regulate everything from building size and combustibility to egress patterns to number of plumbing fixtures to the amount of natural light and fresh air to handicapped accessibility and much more, and they form a framework for architects that ensures, at a minimum, a level of safety and accommodation for building occupants including both workers and the public at large. These codes regulate across every conceivable use from industrial to office to medical to retail to places of assembly like theaters and malls and also to residential uses including homes, apartment buildings, and hotels. These guidelines are revisited on an ongoing basis as the nature of work and workers has changed. Architects have often been at the forefront of these changes. In his revolutionary 1904 Larkin Company office building in Buffalo, New York (demolished in 1950), Frank Lloyd Wright made worker comfort a priority. His design emphasized natural light, employed air conditioning, and featured worker amenities like a communal cafeteria—elements that are at the core of workplace design today.

The challenge for today's architects, working in an increasingly complex world that is both more enlightened and more sensitive, is to find "one-size-fits-most solutions" by identifying and managing risks in the interest of protecting and promoting worker health and well-being. But this has to happen with the understanding that the benefits accrue to both the worker and the business. Determining how improvements in workplace design will foster improvements in worker health is complex. What are the fundamental components of worker health as the workplace environment itself changes? AS the National Institute for Occupational Safety and Health (NIOSH) states, the traditional workplace is no longer limited to an office building, factory floor, or warehouse. Although managing physical risks is relatively straightforward (keep hands away from blades), it is more difficult yet no less important to manage the impact of physical and/or psychological risks. For the architect, designing for physical well-being reflects modern medical opinion and now includes, in addition to minimizing risks for bodily harm, managing stress and promoting physical fitness.

Design considerations for health in the workplace can be divided into two main spheres, the built environment (physical characteristics of the workspace) and human factors. Together, these two spheres make up the applied science of human factors and ergonomics (HF/E). HF/E "promotes a human-centered approach to the design of work systems and technology that considers physical, cognitive, social, organizational, environmental and other relevant factors of human-systems interactions, broadly defined, in order to make them compatible with the needs, abilities and limitations of people, with the ultimate goal of optimizing human wellbeing and overall system performance."[1(p xxi)] Within these spheres are work spectrums, along which different attributes of the work environment and work activities vary. Analyzing the project program within this framework gives a picture of the specific environment and the behaviors within it. Among the work spectrums are the following:

- *Work type:* Industrial, medical, office, etc.
- *Atmosphere:* Frenzied to calm, quiet to loud
- *Culture:* Casual to formal
- *Energy:* Dynamic to sedentary
- *Demographic:* Young to old
- *Bodily risk:* Dangerous to safe

Targeting some ideal standard within the work spectrums allows the architect to both design healthier spaces and take into consideration any necessary modifications; for example, although a noisy factory floor is unavoidably stressful, locating the employee lounge far from noise exposure can ameliorate the acute effects of physiological stress. The next sections describe some ideal building blocks that contribute to healthy workspaces.

Noise

The impact of noise on well-being cannot be overstated. Beyond the obvious discomforts of loud machinery, two noise issues have large negative effects on well-being. First, the subtle buzzing, beeping, whirring, and clicking from the many machines that adorn the workspace from cellphone to copier aggregate to overwhelm the brain's noise-filtering mechanisms and can cause heightened sensitivity, distraction, and stress. Second, in many modern workplaces, open communal work areas inevitably feature a cacophony of voices that also overwhelm and distract. These problems can be amplified by hard surfaces that reflect and propagate sound. Good design recognizes this potential and manages it by isolating the little noises and controlling loud ones through sound absorption and sound masking and by providing areas of quiet retreat.

Management was quick to adopt the concentrated open office model as a nod to efficiency and modernity without recognizing the direct impact of noise on the workers within. Designers, too, are often seduced by hard materials and open well-lit spaces, and are handcuffed by low ceilings such that they contribute to a problem not easily fixed after the fact. Noise needs to be considered at every level of design. For more information on noise exposure and preventing hearing loss, see NIOSH's Preventing Hazardous Noise and Hearing Loss During Project Design and Operation.[2]

Ergonomics

The body is a mechanical machine with levers and joints and lots of supporting cables. Given the amount of time spent at work, it is surprising how little thought has gone into idealizing the operation of this machine. Chronic ailments including back and wrist pain, eye strain, and headaches plague workers, radically reduce productivity, and burden the healthcare system. It is astonishing how many bad chairs there are—and it is crucial for designers and management to select comfortable, adjustable chairs for their employees. Macro factors like providing and incentivizing exercise ranging from active breaks to walkable areas to full-on fitness are not yet sufficiently integrated into workspace culture. In addition, each individual's working space can be tailored to their needs without adding much if anything to cost. A template to analyze everything from neck angle to foot placement can easily be created and systematically deployed.

Room to Work: Size, Scale, and Proportion

Allocate sufficient space per employee to safely and comfortably perform their work. In many settings this is a minimum of 15 square feet per person. Congested or compressed (too narrow or low) spaces can trigger a physiological stress response.[3] There are architectural theories that presume ideal proportions of space as a function of the human body (see LeCorbusier's Module) or some naturally occurring mathematical arrangement (see the Golden Ratio or Fibonacci).

Room size is interdependent with light, color ventilation, and noise, because each of these variables can be positively or negatively amplified in small spaces.

Businesses must, of course, trade off space per employee with cost per unit of space (rent, maintenance, and conditioning) so a balance must be struck. Good, efficient space planning can provide for adequate employee space while tightening space in other low-impact areas. New work/life balance spaces are adding common amenity spaces, promoting exercise at work, and arranging flexible work areas that may provide smaller individual units of workspace but compensate with areas of relief.

Light

Light is a dominant factor in workspaces and influences all the other major categories of design. Owners are often unaware of the importance of good lighting, and there is a small premium to pay for the design of and the number and types of fixtures necessary to produce it. Nowhere in the design process is the argument for initial investment with long-term payoff more critical.

Different tasks demand different amounts of light, and there is a wide variation of personal comfort with respect to amount and quality of light at work. Nevertheless, light matters a lot, and there is now a great deal of evidence that poor quality light is a primary cause of stress and illness in the workplace. Studies show that the fluorescent lighting that prevailed in workplaces for decades operated at a frequency low enough to be perceived audibly as a buzz and visually as an on/off strobe effect. This caused countless headaches and led to fatigue and stress. Newer generation high-frequency fluorescent and now LED-based light generation have largely solved this problem. However, issues of light color (and resulting contrast), brightness, and glare continue to affect the workplace. Well-designed lighting is flexible and should include individually controlled task lighting as well as intelligent control that adjusts for changes in natural lighting in the space. The light should be naturally warm and minimize shadows and glare, particularly on computer monitors.

Ventilation

Fresh air, either natural or introduced into the mechanical system, is critical to minimizing illness. Code mandates the introduction of fresh air into the makeup of the air distributed into a building. Opening windows is no longer an alternative in many places, either because there are not windows or because opening them short circuits the heating/cooling system. Mechanically provided ventilation can be noisy, poorly balanced, or drafty. In larger or older buildings, the mechanical system is a complex system of airflow that must be well designed and should include levels of localized control. Designers are now returning to an old technology, ceiling fans, to provide a softer, more natural airflow in spaces.

Heating and cooling are primary cost contributors and thus are primary business considerations. But owners need to think beyond efficiency to the effect of good air on employee well-being and productivity. For more information on indoor environmental quality, see NIOSH's indoor environmental quality webpage.[4]

Temperature

Few conditions are more personal than temperature, and providing for individual temperature comfort is one of the most challenging areas of design. Solutions range from managing sunlight to desk fans, and although there are ideal ranges of temperature in a space, providing individualized temperature control within those ranges is difficult.

Management is often primarily concerned with cost, and it is easy to dismiss the concerns of the employee who is too hot or too cold, but few factors affect performance more than this simple comfort.

Color

Few factors are more psychologically complex than color, but ever since color theorists began their study and painters began their active color experimenting in the 19th century, there has been at least a tacit understanding that color can evoke emotions and that there is a correlation between color and mood. This is not purely objective science; it bears an individualized component and is broadly sensitive to many of the other core design factors. This is further complicated by the importance of color in corporate branding and messaging. There is a strong argument for the use of muted earth tones suggesting nature. Good design deploys color to identify and differentiate spaces, reducing monotony in the work environment. Workers frequently adorn their spaces with both personal items and artwork, and these mechanisms are broadly calming and actively color based. Color is often dismissed, making workspaces uninspiring and bland. Therefore, it is important to think more critically about color and its effect on employees.

References

1. Karwowski W. Neuroergonomics: a complex systems perspective. In: Johnson A, Proctor RW, eds. *Neuroergonomics: A Cognitive Neuroscience Approach to Human Factors and Ergonomics*. New York, NY: Palgrave Macmillan; 2013: xxi-xxiv.

2. Preventing hazardous noise and hearing loss during project design and operation. National Institute for Occupational Safety and Health website. https://www.cdc.gov/niosh/docs/2016-101/pdfs/2016-101.pdf. Published 2015. Accessed April 2, 2018.

3. Wells NM, Evans GW, Cheek KA. Environmental psychology. In: Frumkin H, ed. *Environmental Health: From Global to Local*. 3rd ed. San Francisco, CA: John Wiley & Sons; 2016:203-230.

4. Indoor environmental quality. National Institute for Occupational Safety and Health website. https://www.cdc.gov/niosh/topics/indoorenv/default.html. Accessed April 2, 2018.

Appendix 11C

Developing a Workplace Health Communication Plan

Successful implementation of the workplace health program depends, in large part, on how the employees react to the changes. Even the slightest misunderstanding can result in major disruptions. Thus, regular and consistent communication is a vital component of the overall program and fosters an organizational commitment to employee health. Employees are key stakeholders and should be informed of the program's purpose; the actions taken; the reasons for and results of those actions. Consistency comes from repetition and uniform presentation from all levels of the organization and over time will create a culture of health.

▶ Develop a Communications Plan

The development of a communications plan can accomplish several things for the program including[1]:

- Increased awareness and recognition of the program
- Increased awareness of workplace health and safety risks
- Increased awareness of workplace health promotion opportunities for employees
- Increased trust between management and employees
- Increased program participation
- Improved health-related behaviors
- Ultimately, improved employee health

Well-designed communications can:

- Increase employees' knowledge and awareness of a health issue, problem, or solution
- Influence or reinforce perceptions, beliefs, and attitudes
- Refute myths and misconceptions
- Prompt action
- Demonstrate or illustrate health-promoting skills
- Show the benefits of behavior change

- Educate employees on the organization's position on a health issue or policy
- Increase demand or support for health promotion programs and services
- Strengthen organizational relationships
- Realign the social rules or standards for workplace behavior

However, communication usually must be combined with other strategies such as implementing a health-related program, policy, or benefit to:

- Overcome systemic barriers, such as insufficient access to health promotion programs and services
- Cause sustained behavior, culture, and environmental change—from employees adopting and maintaining new health behaviors, to the organization adopting and maintaining new policies
- Change the physical or psychological aspects of the work environment

▶ Clearly Communicate the Workplace Health Program Goals and Objectives

Materials and messages should be culturally competent, that is, understood by and applicable to individuals from different cultures, race or ethnicities, or languages; relevant, and at a sufficient level of health literacy.

Health Literacy is the degree to which individuals have the capacity to obtain, process, and understand basic health information and services needed to make appropriate health decisions, as defined by the National Library of Medicine and as used in Healthy People 2010. According to the 2003 National Assessment of Adult Literacy, more than 77 million adults in the United States demonstrate basic or below basic health literacy skills.

▶ Effectively Market Program Offerings to Employees

Messages should include both the program's marketing strategy, as well as the reasons behind the program's strategic direction. If employees are unaware of the health promotion opportunities available to them, they are unlikely to participate, and without sufficient participation, program success cannot be achieved. Employees also need to be aware of what the program is trying to achieve for both individual employee health and the employer's bottom line.

Brand the Health Strategy, Including a Logo

■ The workplace health program should be branded, including a logo, and used in all communication materials.

Define the Target Audience(s)

■ Identify the employee group(s) who will be the subject of the communication efforts.
■ Consider identifying subgroups for tailored messages, in view of such demographic factors as job category, education level, or age.
■ Engage employees to learn as much as possible about their demographics; their knowledge, attitudes, and beliefs related to health promotion; their needs and interests; and opportunities and barriers for employees to access health information.
■ Conduct a situation analysis to determine overall strengths, weaknesses, opportunities, and threats related to the current employee communication strategy. For example, opportunities could include the addition of "outward-facing" components such as health and social responsibility activities that support good causes in the community or activities that promote a good work environment.

Use a Variety of Message Channels Such as Email, Newsletters, Intranet, Etc.

■ Multiple communication channels should be used to ensure that employees receive the information they need to make informed decisions; these channels may include email, bulletin boards, newsletters, the intranet, presentations, and direct communication from management, a representative of the wellness council, and coworkers.
■ Consider the optimum timing and frequency of message delivery to reach the intended employee audience(s).
■ Consider pretesting and revising of messages with representatives of the target audience.

Recognize and Celebrate Success

■ Employee success stories should be highlighted, shared, and celebrated to help motivate others to make lifestyle changes.
■ Employees can also be recognized and supported using incentives as rewards for meeting individual health behavior goals.
■ Recognition can also be achieved for the overall efforts of the workplace health program. The CDC Healthier Workplace Initiative has compiled a listing of multiple award opportunities in workplace health promotion.

Reference

1. National Cancer Institute. *Making Health Communication Programs Work*. Rockville, MD: U.S. Department of Health and Human Services; 1989.

Glossary

A

Absenteeism The time an employee spends away from work. Absences can be scheduled (e.g., vacation time) or unscheduled (e.g., due to illness or injury).

Active design An evidence-based approach to identifying architecture solutions to supporting healthy communities or workplaces by using design strategies to encourage physical activity.

Advertising Council A nonprofit organization devoted to the development and placement of public service media in the United States. Its legacy includes Smokey the Bear's "Only you can prevent forest fires," the "Tearful Indian" campaign against pollution, the crash test dummies for motor safety, "A Mind Is a Terrible Thing to Waste" for the United Negro College Fund, and more recently, "Buzzed Driving Is Drunk Driving."

Affordable Care Act of 2010 (ACA) The comprehensive healthcare reform law enacted in March 2010. The law has three primary goals: (1) make affordable health insurance available to more people by providing consumers with subsidies that lower costs for households with incomes between 1000% and 400% of the federal poverty level; (2) expand the new Medicaid program to cover all adults with income below 138% of the federal poverty level; and (3) support innovative medical care delivery methods designed to lower the costs of health care generally. Sometimes known as Patient Protection and Affordable Care Act or Obamacare.

Attitudes An individual's predisposition toward an object, person, or group that influences their response to be either positive or negative, favorable or unfavorable.

Attribution theory Focuses on the causal attributions learners create to explain the results of an activity, and classifies these in terms of their locus, stability, and controllability.

Audience segmentation Division of a large group of people into smaller, more homogenous groupings based on shared characteristics for the purpose of communication.

B

Barriers Hindrances to desired change. These may be factors external or internal to audience members themselves (e.g., lack of proper healthcare facilities or the belief that fate causes illness and is inescapable).

Baseline data Information regarding a target audience or situation prior to an intervention. Generally, these are collected to provide a point of comparison for an evaluation.

BEHAVE framework A simple and widely used framework for describing an audience, a behavioral change, a motivation, and a mechanism for change developed by the Academy for Educational Development (AED).

Behavioral beliefs The subjective probability that an object has a certain attribute; for example, a person may believe that physical exercise (the object) reduces the risk of heart disease (the attribute).

Beneficiary The person or group of people who would benefit most directly by an intervention. Sometimes the audience and the beneficiary are the same. Sometimes others are asked to act on behalf of a third-party beneficiary, as when mothers are asked to adopt behaviors that benefit their children.

Biometric screenings The measurements of physical characteristics such as height, weight, body mass index, blood pressure, blood cholesterol, blood glucose, and aerobic fitness tests that can be taken at the worksite and used as part of workplace health assessments to benchmark and evaluate changes in employee health status over time.

Business Pulse A resource from the Centers for Disease Control and Prevention Foundation aimed at providing businesses and their employees with tools and resources to protect them from chronic disease and safety threats.

C

Channel The conduit or route of information delivery (e.g., interpersonal, small group, organizational, community, mass media).

Characteristics of effective health education curriculum The Centers for Disease Control and Prevention's guidelines describing today's state-of-the-art health education curriculum.

Clear Communication Index (CCI) A research-based tool to help develop and assess public communication materials.

Click through The ratio of the number of clicks on a specific link to the number of viewers of an online page.

Climate of a workplace Workers' shared perceptions of and meaning attached to the policies, practices, and procedures at the workplace.

Closed-ended questions Questions that encourage short or single-word answers.

Cognitive dissonance A psychological discomfort caused by simultaneously holding two or more contradictory conditions. Individuals are motivated to reduce this discomfort by changing their original preferences.

Comprehensive approach A tactic to put interventions in place that address multiple risk factors and health conditions concurrently and recognizes that the interventions and strategies chosen influence multiple levels of the organization, including the individual employee and the organization as a whole.

Confirmation bias When we interpret messages such that they confirm what we already believe (e.g., "He only hears what he wants to hear").

Confirmational messages Approvals or statements of agreement; reassurances delivered in response to expressed concerns or fears.

Continuation (or expansion) plan A strategy to ensure a broader reach, diffuse expenses, and provide continuity of leadership and ownership.

Control belief An individual's belief that they have some control over their life and especially their health issues; a positive factor in improving health behavior.

Coordinated approach An approach that results in a planned, organized, and comprehensive set of programs, policies, benefits, and environmental supports designed to meet the health and safety needs of all employees.

Cost-effectiveness The degree to which something is effective or productive in relation to its cost.

Creative brief A document that includes information that will be needed by a creative team in order to develop concepts and messages. It contains information about the primary target audience as well as settings, channels, and activities for reaching them. Promising message variables and thoughts on what materials will be needed are included. Secondary audiences are also profiled.

Cultural competence The ability to understand and relate to behavioral patterns that are determined in part by membership in racial, ethnic, and social groups. This term is used to emphasize the major role of social factors (age, income, education, living circumstance, etc.) in successful patient–provider communication. (In common usage it is often limited to gender, ethnic, and nationality issues.)

CulturalCare A practice that acknowledges and respects patients' underlying beliefs about health and illness as well as the meanings patients assign to specific conditions and their preferred methods of treating disease and illness.

Culturally and Linguistically Appropriate Services (CLAS) Developed to provide a common understanding and consistent definition of culturally and linguistically appropriate healthcare services. They were proposed as one means to correct inequities in the provision of health services and to make healthcare systems more responsive to the needs of all clients.

Culture of health (CoH) A proactive approach to integrating organizational-level initiatives and policies that support traditionally individually based strategies.

Customer journey An individual's experience that begins with becoming aware of an offering and continues through actions taken.

D

Demographics Statistical characteristics of human populations such as age, sex, race, ethnicity, and country of origin. Used to study trends in population growth and change.

Deontological principles Ethical or moral principles that can be used to guide behavior (e.g., the golden rule, do the right thing, do the least harm, respect the individual, etc.).

Diffusion of innovations (DI) A theory by E. Rogers that addresses change in a group rather than an individual. This could be a classroom, an organization, or a community. The theory describes how new ideas, or innovations, are spread within the group. According to this theory, innovations are spread via different communication channels within social systems over a specific period of time.

Direct costs The part of a budget that contributes directly to a program's outputs. They are made up of personnel costs (salary and benefits) as well as "out-of-pocket" costs associated with products and services not obtained through a salaried employee.

Document literacy The knowledge and skills needed to perform document tasks (i.e., to search, comprehend, and use noncontinuous texts in various formats); part of the NAAL's scoring of adult literacy.

E

Ecological model Public health definition that assumes health and well-being are affected by *interaction* among multiple determinants including biology, behavior, and the environment. Interaction unfolds over the life course of individuals, families, and communities. An ecological approach to health is one in which multiple strategies are developed to impact determinants of health relevant to the desired health outcomes.

Edutainment Entertainment, especially video games, with an educational aspect.

Elaboration likelihood model (ELM) Postulates an elaboration likelihood continuum whereby messages with personal importance are scrutinized, processed, and elaborated with care, and others may be processed with less effort using heuristics or issue-irrelevant message cues.

Emotional intelligence The ability to identify and manage one's own emotions and the emotions of others.

Empathy The ability to understand and share the feelings of another.

Employee Assistance Programs (EAPs) Worksite-based programs and/or resources designed to benefit both employers and employees. By helping employees identify and resolve personal concerns that affect job performance, they help businesses and organizations address productivity issues.

Engagement Encouraging interest or interaction.

Entertainment education (EE) The process of using media that primarily interests or amuses an audience to carry messages that inform or persuade for social good.

Ethnic identity When many people share cultural traits, such as language, appearance, food, religion, dress, and meaningful symbols, and have a common ancestral homeland.

Evaluation plan An integral part of planning that provides information to improve a project during development and implementation.

Expandability The ability of a product to accommodate additions to its capacity or capabilities.

Eye tracking Using a head-mounted camera and computer screens designed for this purpose, it is possible to detect and measure eye movements and gaze fixation as we look at an image (moving or still) or text. Our innate response to imminent danger or arousal causes our pupils to dilate and our blink rate to change. All can be measured photographically and can be used to measure reading ease as well as a subject's interest in an image, a video, or text.

F

Flesch-Kincaid Grade Level Readability Test Developed for the Navy and used by the Army to assess training manuals in the 1970s, the F-K formula uses a weighted combination of the number of syllables, words, and sentences in a passage to estimate reading grade level from fifth grade through college (or reading ease, with different weighting parameters).

Formative research The information-gathering activities conducted prior to developing a health communication strategy. It includes measurement of the extent to which concepts, messages, materials, activities, and channels meet researchers' expectations with the target audience.

Framing Words (or sometimes images) used to put a message or a data point into a desired context; for example, if your chances of winning the lottery are 1 in 1 million, a positive frame states that 1 person out of 1 million will be a big winner. A negative frame states that 999,999 people out of 1 million will lose. Different frames lead people to draw different conclusions even when the same data are being discussed.

Frequency The number of times a message gets to an audience of interest.

G

Gain-framed appeal Message designed to emphasize the advantages of performing a desired behavior.

Galvanic skin response (GSR) An electrical measure of reduced skin resistance indicative of perspiration triggered by sympathetic nervous system activity related to emotion.

Gatekeepers People who have a reputation, or perceived responsibility, for upholding standards in a community. They can help support a behavior change goal if they agree with it, or prevent its adoption if they disagree. Very often, popular clergy members, business leaders, or healthcare providers may be community gatekeepers, and it is wise to seek their input when planning an intervention.

Gender The state of being male or female, typically used with reference to social and cultural differences rather than biological ones. One's gender identity is their perception of having a particular gender, which may or may not correspond with their birth sex.

H

Health belief model (HBM) First developed to explain individual public health behaviors, such as participation in free tuberculosis screening programs. In this model, individual beliefs motivate or discourage health behaviors. These beliefs are perceived susceptibility, perceived severity, perceived benefits of interventions, perceived costs of intervention, cues to activate behavior change, and perceived ability to act (self-efficacy).

Health communication specialist (HCS) An individual who designs behavior change and communication campaign strategies; can be within a school or school system.

Health Education Curriculum Analysis Tool (HECAT) Can be used by schools to select or develop appropriate and effective curricula to teach the content established in the National Health Education standards and the Centers for Disease Control and Prevention's Characteristics of an Effective Health Education Curriculum.

Health literacy The ability to understand and use complex health information.

Health Literacy Tool Shed An online database of health literacy measures. The site contains information about measures, including their psychometric properties, based on a review of the peer-reviewed literature.

Health risk appraisals (HRAs) Assessment tools used to evaluate an individual's health. It could include a health survey or questionnaire, physical examination, or laboratory tests resulting in a profile of individual health risks, often with accompanying advice or strategies to reduce the risks.

Healthy People 2020 (HP2020) The key U.S. government process, and policy document, for developing goals and monitoring public health progress every decade.

Heritage Assessment Tool A set of tools developed to assist providers in understanding individual patients' backgrounds and the strength of ties to their home cultures.

Hierarchy of effects (HOE) The HOE model, created by Robert J. Lavidge and Gary Steiner, suggests that a consumer must go through six steps from viewing an advertisement to purchasing a product: Awareness, knowledge, liking, preference, conviction, and purchase. The hierarchy represents a progression of learning and decision making a consumer experiences as a result of advertising.

High-deductible health insurance plan (HDHP) A health insurance plan with lower monthly premiums and higher employee out-of-pocket deductibles compared to a traditional health insurance plan.

I

Immigrant A person who comes to a country to take up permanent residence.

Implementation (or tactical) plan Short-term action plan that breaks down bigger-picture goals and strategies into narrower, actionable tasks.

Inbound marketing A technique for bringing customers/clients/patients to products and services through content marketing, social media marketing, search engine optimization, and branding to attract attention, foster interest, and improve accessibility.

Indirect costs Expenses that it costs an agency to exist, but that are not tied directly to creating the program's outputs. Examples usually include office space, environmental management (heat, air conditioning, water, custodial services, etc.), and depreciation on equipment. These are usually calculated as a percentage of direct costs. Also called "overhead."

In-kind contributions In the nonprofit world in which public health often operates, this is organizations' time, space, use of equipment, and other in-house resources. These will be used to produce program outputs, but are not factored into the direct or indirect costs of the budget. Some donors will expect to see a match made of their investment through direct financial, in-kind resources or additional donations.

Integrative model (IM) Provides a practical structure for teaching learners to explore organized bodies of knowledge, which is content that consists of a combination of facts, concepts, generalizations, and their relationships.

L

Lalonde report The first government document recognizing the role of individual behavior in health.

Landing page A page on a website at which visitors arrive from somewhere else (e.g., an ad, a link). Within the realm of marketing and advertising, landing pages are used to generate further action by a visitor, either clicking through to another part of the website or gathering data by means of a form. (See http://unbounce.com for particularly useful definitions of internet marketing tools.)

Lay health advisors Members of a community who have been trained to talk about a health issue with their peers.

Limited English proficiency (LEP) When clients or patients do not speak English well enough to understand instructions or questions. Often (incorrectly) used to refer to people, and not their abilities.

Logic model A visual design of how a problem will be solved through an intervention—the structured flow of inputs, outputs, outcomes, and goals obtained.

Loss-framed appeals Messages designed to emphasize the negative outcome of performing a desired behavior.

M

Macro plan A preliminary plan that includes the analysis of the problem, including its ecological setting, the affected populations, the core intervention strategy, and any additional research necessary to understand those persons affected by the problem and/or with whom you plan to communicate.

Message testing An iterative process that involves both quantitative and qualitative research to collect consumers' attitudes toward a message of interest.

mHealth Mobile-based or mobile-enhanced solutions that deliver health. The ubiquity of mobile devices in the developed and developing worlds presents the opportunity to improve health outcomes through the delivery of innovative medical and health services with information and communication technologies to the farthest reaches of the globe.

Mindful communication Type of communication based on an objective, nonjudgmental approach, in which participants maintain a heightened state of awareness throughout their interactions.

Mixed-methods approach A research design that combines quantitative and qualitative methods. These may be sequenced or done simultaneously and triangulated.

Motivational interviewing (MI) A psychotherapeutic approach that attempts to move an individual away from a state of indecision or uncertainty and toward finding motivation to make positive decisions.

N

National CLAS Standards Guidelines intended to advance health equity, improve quality, and help eliminate healthcare disparities by providing a blueprint for individuals and health and healthcare organizations to implement culturally and linguistically appropriate services.

National Health Education Standards (NHES) Guidelines created to establish, promote, and support health-enhancing behaviors for students in grades prekindergarten through 12.

National Sexuality Education Standards (NSES) Content-specific standards that provide clear and consistent guidance on the essential core standards for sexuality education.

National Teacher Preparation Standards for Sexuality Education Standards designed for use by institutes of higher education to improve the preparation of teacher candidates for instruction in sexuality education.

Normative beliefs Perceptions about what others are doing or thinking about a health behavior or issue. Part of the integrative model (IM), along with behavioral beliefs and control beliefs.

Numeracy The ability to think and express oneself quantitatively. In reference to health literacy, it encompasses the knowledge and skills required to estimate quantities from food labels, use a glucometer or thermometer correctly, measure medicine doses, or perform any other mathematical operation necessary for nonhealth professionals to manage their own or a loved one's health care or wellness.

O

Occupational health and safety A program that is responsible for preventing worker injury and illness though safe practices and policies.

Open-ended questions Questions worded to allow an individual to respond freely in their own words.

Optimism bias The mistaken belief that one's chances of experiencing a negative event are lower or of experiencing a positive event are higher than those of one's peers.

Outbound marketing The traditional form of marketing in which a company initiates the conversation and sends its message out to an audience.

P

Patient navigators People trained to help patients navigate through the healthcare system and help interpret medical advice.

Perceptual process The sequence of psychological steps that a person uses to organize and interpret information from the outside world in order to assign meaning.

Persona The aspect of someone's character that is presented to or perceived by others.

Pilot testing A trial of a marketing package or health communication intervention in its entirety in a limited location. Results are used to fix problems before a large scale launch, or to make a "no go" decision.

Practice strategy An approach or tactic for achieving a communication goal.

PRECEDE-PROCEED model Developed by Green, Kreuter, and associates in the 1970s, the model works backwards from a desired state of health and quality of life, and asks what about the environment, behavior, individual motivation, or administrative policy is necessary to create that healthy state. PRECEDE stands for Predisposing, Reinforcing, Enabling Constructs in Educational/Environmental Diagnosis and Evaluation. PROCEED stands for Policy, Regulatory, and Organizational Constructs in Educational and Environmental Development. PRECEDE-PROCEED has nine steps: (1) social assessment, (2) epidemiological assessment, (3) behavioral and environmental assessment, (4) educational and ecological assessment, (5) administrative and policy assessment, (6) implementation, (7) process evaluation, (8) impact evaluation, and (9) outcome evaluation.

Premature death Death that occurs before the average age of death in a certain population.

Presentability A product's suitability and social acceptability in appearance.

Presenteeism The measurable extent to which health symptoms, conditions, and diseases adversely affect the work productivity of individuals who choose to remain at work.

Press advisory An alert or invitation to the media, usually to attend an event, press conference, or kick-off of a program. Provides the key information—the who, what, when, where, and why.

Press release An official written or recorded statement issued to newspapers and other media outlets to announce a program, event, or something newsworthy. It is usually provided in a news format that media could use, such as a news story with quotes, photos, and so forth.

Pretest A type of formative research that involves systematically gathering target audience reactions to messages and materials before they are produced in final form.

Primary audience The group of people most affected by a problem, and whose behavior you hope to change when planning a communication intervention.

Primary data Data observed or collected directly from first-hand experience.

Process evaluation Studies the functioning of components of program implementation. It includes assessments of whether materials are being distributed to the right people and in the correct quantities, the extent to which program activities are being carried out as planned and modified if needed, and other measures of how well the program is working. Sometimes referred to as "delivery assessment."

Productive aging An initiative dedicated to supporting employees across the life span, including the aging workforce.

Prose literacy The ability to read simple, ordinary, or complex sentences to paragraphs; part of the NAAL's scoring of adult literacy.

Public service announcements (PSAs) Typically aired or published without charge by the host channel. Can be in print, audio, or video form.

Purposeful communication Intended to gain another person's attention in order to get a desired response.

Q

Quality-adjusted life expectancy A measure of the value of health outcomes. Health is a function of both length of life and quality of life; this combines the value of these attributes into a single index number.

Quantitative literacy The ability to read, understand, and use numbers and calculations in the activities of daily living; part of the NAAL's scoring of adult literacy.

R

Race A social construct that classifies humans into groups based on physical traits, ancestry, genetics, or social relations, or the relations between these groups.

Rapport A close and harmonious relationship in which the people or groups concerned understand each other's feelings or ideas and communicate well.

Reach The number of people who actually receive intended messages.

Return on investment (ROI) An analysis used to compare the investment costs to the magnitude and timing of expected gains. For workplace health programs, this usually refers to the medical savings or productivity gains associated with the employer's investment in employee health programs.

Risk perception A judgement of the adverse consequences of a particular hazard. It can be made by an individual, a group of people, or society.

Role playing The acting out of the part of a particular person or character; for example, as a technique in training or psychotherapy.

Root cause analysis A systematic process for identifying the basic or root causes of problems and an approach for responding to them.

S

School Health Index (SHI) An online self-assessment and planning tool for schools to improve their health and safety policies and programs.

Secondary audience A group or groups of individuals that can help reach or influence the intended audience segment and who are not considered part of the problem. Secondary audiences should be identified through profiles created for the primary audiences.

Secondary data Data collected by someone other than the user, such as census data.

Selective exposure Limiting media exposure to channels that offer information and opinions with which the individual agrees.

Self-efficacy One's belief in one's ability to succeed in specific situations or to accomplish a task. One's sense of self-efficacy can play a major role in how one approaches goals, tasks, and challenges.

Self-insured Policies in which the employer assumes the financial risk for providing healthcare benefits to its employees.

Setting A location or environment where the target audience can be reached with a communication effort (e.g., a grocery store is a setting where audience members can be reached with educational pamphlets).

Sex In biology, this refers to the genetic expression of the genes inherited from one's parents. In most cases individuals are either XY or XX. Those with one X and one Y chromosome in every cell of the body are biologically male. Biologically, females have two X chromosomes in every cell.

Shared decision making (SDM) A process in which clinicians and patients work together to make decisions and select tests, treatments, and care plans.

Skills-based health education Activities aiming to change health behavior through classroom-based education.

SMOG A measure of readability that estimates the years of education needed to understand a piece of writing. SMOG is an acronym for Simple Measure of Gobbledygook.

Social cognitive theory (SCT) Developed by Bandura, this hypothesizes that individual behavior is the result of constant interaction between the external environment and internal psychosocial characteristics and perceptions. This idea has been dubbed reciprocal determinism. There are numerous constructs in SCT, including self-efficacy, which has migrated into other theories, as well.

Social determinants of health (SDH) The conditions in which people are born, live, work, and age that affect their health.

Social inoculation theory Used to explain how people may resist unwanted persuasion attempts by preparing counterarguments in advance.

Social marketing According to Lefebvre and Flora (1988), "The design, implementation and control of programs aimed at increasing the acceptability of a social idea, practice, or product in one or more groups of target adopters. The process actively involves the target population who voluntarily exchange their time and attention for help in meeting their needs as they perceive them." In this text, social marketing does *not* refer to the use of social media or social causes to promote commercial products and services. Both of these uses are common, however.

Soft launch The release of a new product or service to a restricted audience or market in advance of a full launch.

SPIKES protocol A framework for delivering difficult information about diagnosis, prognosis, and treatment options.

Stages of change (SOC) The stages that an individual moves through when modifying behavior. It is used in the transtheoretical model to integrate principles involved in behavior change from other major theoretical approaches.

Stakeholders Those who are involved in or affected by a course of action.

Strategic health communication plan A detail-level description that focuses on specific change objectives, audiences, messages, and media.

Sustainability Meeting the needs of the present generation without compromising the ability of future generations to meet their own needs.

SWOTE analysis A plan developed in the 1960s for assessment of a program's internal strengths and weaknesses, and external opportunities and threats (SWOT). We have added an *E* for ethical assessment.

Systematic process A series of strategically planned steps.

Systems approach to health Applies scientific insights to understand the elements that influence health outcomes; models the relationships between those elements; and alters design, processes, or policies based on the resultant knowledge in order to produce better health at lower cost.

T

Tailoring As in sewing, this refers to custom fitting health communication material or a message to one person's needs based on information about that individual. It is often based on theoretical constructs such as readiness stage, health beliefs, and self-efficacy; demographic factors; factors specific to a health behavior or condition; as well as the person's name and other personal information deemed relevant to the intervention. With software developed by the University of Michigan, this may be done in an online environment.

Targeting Media that use demographic, cultural, or other group references in the media or channel strategy to reach specific audiences. For example, using MTV or BET is a channel strategy to reach youth and African American audiences. Church-based outreach to promote breast cancer screening among older African American women is another targeted channel strategy. Billboards and print advertising frequently feature models of recognizable ethnicities, sex, and age to appeal to target market segments. (In the past, this was also often called *tailoring*, until truly individualized communication became feasible through the internet and informatics applications.)

Teach back method A communication confirmation method used by healthcare providers to confirm whether a patient (or caretakers) understand what is being explained to them.

Tertiary audience A group that affects the behavior of an intermediate audience that, in turn, may affect the behavior of a primary audience. The "public at large" is often considered a tertiary audience in communications directed to patients (as primary audiences) and providers or caregivers (as secondary audiences).

Text messaging An electronic communication sent to and received by mobile phone.

Tobacco cessation treatments A variety of interventions aimed at helping clients quit smoking.

Total budget The sum of direct and indirect costs, including in-kind contributions and other donations.

Total Worker Health (TWH) A CDC program encompassing policies, programs, and practices that integrate protection from work-related safety and health hazards with promotion of injury and illness prevention efforts to advance worker well-being.

Touch point Any way a consumer can interact with a business, whether it be person-to-person, through a website, an app, or any form of communication.

Transactional model of communication A way in which someone invents and attributes meaning to realize their purposes. The way this meaning is generated is through a process of encoding (by the sender) and decoding (by the receiver).

Transtheoretical model (TTM) A theory that posits that individuals move through a specific process when deciding whether to change their behavior and actually changing their behavior. The stages are precontemplation, contemplation, preparation, action, and maintenance.

U

Usability testing According to the American Marketing Association, a research step in the design and launch of a website where users evaluate the ease of use of the site's navigation, layout, and other attributes.

User testing When consumers examine both the messages and the material. Often in health communication, one would ask members of the target audience to assess messages or ideas that will be used, as well as mock-up of materials, videos, or other communication to get input on accessibility and acceptability.

Utilitarianism This theory posits that decisions should be judged by their consequences. Net utility should be maximized for all parties involved in a decision.

V

Vicarious (observational) learning The learning of various attitudes, feelings, beliefs, and emotions, not through direct exposure to a stimulus but through observing how others react to it.

W

Well-being An integrated concept that characterizes quality of life with respect to an individual's health and work-related environmental, organizational, and psychosocial factors.

Whole School, Whole Community, Whole Child (WSCC) model Designed to strengthen a unified and collaborative approach to learning and health. It focuses on the child, emphasizes a school-wide approach, and acknowledges learning, health, and the school as being a part and reflection of the local community.

Workplace health A program responsible for implementing wellness initiatives primarily aimed at preventing illness and disease by sponsoring activities such as fitness programs, biometric screenings, and healthy food options at work.

Workplace Health Model A coordinated, systematic, and comprehensive approach to achieving a healthier workplace for employees.

Workplace health program (WHP) An umbrella term that encompasses initiatives, programs, strategies, and activities intended to promote, increase, and sustain the health and well-being of employees (and occasionally their families).

Y

Youth Risk Behavior Surveillance System (YRBSS) A state-based survey to monitor priority health risk behaviors that contribute markedly to the leading causes of death, disability, and social problems among youth and adults in the United States.

Youth Risk Behavior Survey (YRBS) The survey used in the Youth Risk Behavior Surveillance System (YRBSS).

Index

Note: Page numbers followed by *b, f,* or *t* indicate material in boxes, figures, or tables, respectively.